CRANIOSACRAL THERAPY FOR CHILDREN

Also by Daniel Agustoni

Harmonizing Your Craniosacral System: Self-Treatments for Improving Your Health

Craniosacral Rhythm: A Practical Guide to a Gentle Form of Bodywork Therapy

CRANIOSACRAL THERAPY FOR CHILDREN

Treatments for Expecting Mothers, Babies, and Children

DANIEL AGUSTONI

Translated from the German by Elaine Richards
and David G. Beattie

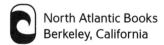

North Atlantic Books
Berkeley, California

Published by
North Atlantic Books
P.O. Box 12327   Cover photos by Tom Schneider
Berkeley, California 94712   Cover and book design by Brad Greene

Printed in the United States of America

PLEASE NOTE: The creators and publishers of this book disclaim any liabilities for loss in connection with following any of the practices, exercises, and advice contained herein. To reduce the chance of injury or any other harm, the reader should consult a professional before undertaking this health program. The instructions and advice printed in this book are not in any way intended as a substitute for medical, mental, or emotional counseling with a licensed physician or healthcare provider.

Craniosacral Therapy for Children: Treatments for Expecting Mothers, Babies, and Children is sponsored by the Society for the Study of Native Arts and Sciences, a non-profit educational corporation whose goals are to develop an educational and cross-cultural perspective linking various scientific, social, and artistic fields; to nurture a holistic view of arts, sciences, humanities, and healing; and to publish and distribute literature on the relationship of mind, body, and nature.

North Atlantic Books' publications are available through most bookstores. For further information, visit our website at www.northatlanticbooks.com or call 800-733-3000.

Library of Congress Cataloging-in-Publication Data

Agustoni, Daniel.
    Craniosacral therapy for children : treatments for expecting mothers, babies, and children / Daniel Agustoni.
        p. ; cm.
    Includes bibliographical references and index.
    Summary: "A comprehensive guide to craniosacral therapy, which releases tensions in the body in order to improve physical and emotional health, complete with hands-on techniques, methods of evaluation, case examples, and over 120 instructional photos and illustrations"—Provided by publisher.
    ISBN 978-1-58394-553-7
    I. Title.
    [DNLM: 1. Musculoskeletal Manipulations. 2. Child. 3. Infant. 4. Pregnancy. 5. Stress, Psychological—therapy. WB 535]
        615.5'42—dc23
                                                                        2012024870

1 2 3 4 5 6 7 8 9 UNITED 18 17 16 15 14 13

In gratitude to the *Breath of Life* and the *winds of change.*

ACKNOWLEDGMENTS

I would like to express my sincere thanks to the following individuals who have helped me in the preparation of this book. Their contributions have helped bring this "child" to maturity and birth:

Joachim Lichtenberg, Petra Reinmuth, and Heini Müller for reading the German manuscript and providing their comments—your assistance was as fruitful as ever.

Once again Christine Mäder looked after the Sphinx Craniosacral Institute most ably while I devoted myself to the task of writing. Petra Reinmuth worked devotedly to produce the illustrations. Tom Schneider once more assisted with the preparation of the graphics and provision of his photographs.

I sincerely thank all the parents and their children who came to the Sphinx Craniosacral Institute for the photographs.

My thanks to all the teachers of the pediatric courses I attended. Among those from whom I learned a great deal, I want to express my special thanks in particular to Joachim Lichtenberg, William M. Allen, Benjamin Shield, Peter Levine, Steve Hoskinson, Raja Selvam, Thomas Harms, Stephen W. Porges, Stanley Rosenberg, and Robert Schleip. I deeply appreciate the courage and life work of John E. Upledger (1932–2012).

I would also like to thank Elaine Richards and David Beattie for their translation and their collaboration with me in this work, and Christopher Church for his excellent, precise editing. Likewise I thank everyone involved in this project at North Atlantic Books, especially Jessica Sevey, Brad Greene, Doug Reil, and Richard Grossinger. My sincere thanks go to Benjamin Shield for his foreword and to Anthony Arnold and William M. Allen for their comments regarding this English edition.

Above all I would like to thank the participants in my pediatric craniosacral courses. Their questions stimulated my holistic perception of what is involved as well as my formulation of answers across the range of topics covered by this book.

Special thanks are due to all the parents and children I have treated over the last sixteen years at my practice and in courses. Every course of treatment has something new to teach me. Your children are wonderful teachers of love, spontaneity, vitality, and authenticity.

DANIEL AGUSTONI, SPRING 2012

CONTENTS

PART TWO

Conception, Pregnancy, Birth, and Development ... 51

PART THREE

Elements, Assessments, and Practice ... 225

PART FOUR

Treatment Examples ... 435

FOREWORD

The treatment of infants and children is one of the most important aspects of health care. Pediatric Craniosacral Therapy is foundational to this care. In this new work, Daniel Agustoni brings to the reader his vast wealth of knowledge, experience, and heart to make pediatric Craniosacral Therapy practical, accessible and understandable to his readers. For decades, the treatment of infants and children was relegated behind that of adults. In recent times pioneers such as Daniel Agustoni have proved the importance of this work and have refined its theory and technique.

Why is it so important to treat children? An osteopath recently answered this question simply: when we look at a child, we never know who or what that child can be, and when we look at an adult, we never know who or what that individual could have been. Life has its challenges, and there may be fewer greater challenges than the birth process. Every birth has its story, and even what may appear to be the simplest of births may create significant lifelong impacts on both the child and the mother. Dr. William Garner Sutherland, the founder of Cranial Osteopathy, had a favorite saying. To paraphrase, "As the twig is bent, so grows the tree." An injury, whether seemingly minor or alarmingly significant, has the potential to impact an individual for his or her entire life. Agustoni deeply understands this principle, and in this book, *Craniosacral Therapy for Children,* he gives the reader solutions to the successful treatment of many conditions that have eluded other specializations.

If we can treat someone early in life, we can prevent or resolve many conditions that would otherwise detract from who that individual will become. Early intervention with pediatric Craniosacral Therapy can positively affect developmental, structural, sensory, learning, behavioral, and personality disorders. I am often asked if every child has a clinical problem and if every child needs to be treated. I answer that not every child needs to be treated, but every child should have the benefit of evaluation. Often, Evaluation becomes Treatment. Moreover, the therapeutic techniques that Agustoni skillfully describes are not only to treat clinical problems but to enhance the lives of infants and children.

The techniques described in this book are invaluable in treating infants and children. Much of this work will only be found in Agustoni's book. And as important as it is to be able to confidently use these techniques in the treatment of children, much of this work is applicable and beneficial to adults as well. *Craniosacral Therapy for Children* goes beyond basic instruction. More than just a how-to book, it encompasses a way of being to positively influence the child, the mother, and the family.

Writing with heart and with passion for this work, Agustoni emphasizes that this work must be child-centered. He feels that establishing trust and safety are primary before we can think of doing anything clinical with our hands. Throughout this book, Agustoni conveys the importance of security and respect for the child and the family. This is crucial because very often the child has lost this sense of security, not only because of the forces of birth but often because of prior medical intervention that may have disturbed the sense of safety. By the time that the child is brought to the therapist, the child may have not only clinical conditions but apprehension due to past experiences. This wonderful book helps the practitioner to meet and resonate with the child in a way that allows the child to optimally integrate the treatment. It shows how pediatric Craniosacral Therapy not only brings out the best in the child but can bring out the very best in those treating the child as well.

Children often cannot express what is wrong with them or how they feel during treatment. This is why the skillful therapist constantly looks for cues to make certain that their touch is nurturing, not intrusive, and that the child can integrate the work and is not activated by it. Children, even newborns, give us many cues to guide us in our work. They often show us when they are deeply accepting the work and can express to the therapist how it is best to work at any given moment. The skilled therapist works not only with the infant but with the family. Simultaneously maintaining the contact and bond with the child and the family is an art that Agustoni carefully describes. It is like tai chi, navigating moment to moment everyone in the room, what is needed, the changes that occur, and the feelings of what has occurred before the treatment. It is both guiding things to be and allowing things to happen.

With this book, Daniel Agustoni has done a great service to infants and children, to their parents and families, and to practitioners of numerous fields. For therapists who want to devote their practice to the treatment of infants and children, parents who want to improve the life of their child, and women who have recently given birth or are expecting, *Craniosacral Therapy for Children* will shed positive light for all who are fortunate enough to read it.

BENJAMIN SHIELD, PHD
INTERNATIONAL INSTRUCTOR OF PEDIATRIC CRANIOSACRAL THERAPY

AUTHOR'S PREFACE
TO THE ENGLISH EDITION

Many children and parents need help at difficult times in their lives from the people around them or through professional help. The craniosacral treatment for children that I present here offers just such help. In Switzerland, Craniosacral Therapy is one of the most popular methods of complementary medicine among patients. Its ability to support healing is increasingly recognized by conventional allopathic physicians, and Swiss health insurers are prepared to contribute to the cost of treatment. Midwives, pediatricians, and parents report examples of successful craniosacral treatment in children. Could the impressive success they report be due to the fact that children's autonomic nervous systems are still so flexible and adaptable? Could it be that these "little Buddhas" still retain a profound link with core experiences such as love and joy, and with the stream and flow of life in the body? Does the cell memory of their bodies recall original primal states? Does treatment call elemental forces silently into motion? My experience tells me that all these elements contribute to self-regulation, regeneration, and healing.

The findings of recent studies in neurobiology and trauma research and the latest imaging procedures increasingly support the treatment principles and insights of complementary and alternative medicine and the phenomena encountered there. These approaches were previously dismissed with a smile or even opposed as "ineffective" or "unscientific." The concept of Craniosacral Therapy as a form of treatment in its own right and thus its practice was defined by the osteopath Dr. John E. Upledger, DO, in the 1980s. Drawing on various branches of Cranial Osteopathy, since that time Craniosacral Therapy has continued to develop in various ways. The treatment concept that I myself developed, Craniosacral_Flow®, does not employ any forced dialogue or accompaniment of the process. The principles guiding Craniosacral_Flow® follow those of salutogenesis and work in a resource-oriented way.

The willing cooperation of the child and mutual respect are important elements of the craniosacral treatment of children. The variety of options for learning and treatment available to the craniosacral practitioner make it possible to provide therapeutic support to babies and children in a playful manner tailored to the individual. When treating children, we always consider themes of bonding and attachment, appropriate boundaries, and respectful contact. It is important to build up a therapeutic relationship of trust. This helps children—and often their parents who are with them—to relax physically and emotionally, to experience their true selves, and to find lightness of being. Craniosacral treatment of children helps babies and children in different stages of development and in stressful situations. It restores the amount of vital force available to them. Minor restrictions, injuries, or handicaps can be resolved simply before they affect the individual's health and produce negative effects in later life.

My desire is to give you, the reader, the best possible impression of the strengthening and healing effect that this gentle form of body-oriented therapy has on the youngest members of our families and societies. This book presents the main foundations of the craniosacral treatment of children and a discussion of its related themes. These include an understanding of prenatal and perinatal trauma, the therapeutic value of the enactment of birth, preparatory therapy for the parents, and the special approach needed in communicating with children.

This book is particularly suitable for advanced students and practitioners of Craniosacral Therapy who already have a good basic knowledge but as yet have little experience treating children. It will provide them with insights into a resource- and solution-oriented approach as well as possible ways of designing treatment sessions. I also present concrete suggestions for treatment using effective structural techniques. This book also addresses the interests of other professionals, such as midwives, educators, psychologists, pediatricians, other bodywork practitioners, and practitioners of complementary and alternative medicine whose interests lie in body-oriented therapies.

The current developments, clear examples of treatment, and many practical tips presented here provide a deeper understanding of this subject area. Parents and family members with an interest in knowing more can also find information about the careful procedures used by pediatric craniosacral practitioners and about the levels on which this gentle method works. I do not claim to cover every single aspect of the subject in this book, nor do I claim that any one form of pediatric craniosacral treatment is "right" or "good."

The kinds of questions that craniosacral practitioners ask themselves, especially when treating children, include the following: can I, as the practitioner, attune myself spontaneously to the child, trust the therapeutic process, and accompany it interactively? How do I sense the concerns of the child and of the family members? How can I create the kind of setting that promotes trust? How do I communicate, verbally and nonverbally? What form of approach do I use to establish contact, what is that contact like, and what is the quality of the therapeutic relationship? What is the intention and quality of touch? How do I ensure that treatment is never too invasive? How do I structure the session so as to support healing changes and enable them to become established in the longer term? By constantly reflecting on such matters, we as practitioners extend our experience and expand the range of treatment options available to us.

I am deeply touched and full of gratitude to be able to accompany children and close members of their family on their journey by means of craniosacral treatment. This applies both in actual therapy in my practice and in courses. I am repeatedly struck by how interested, open, present, direct, and spontaneous young people are. All too often I see others in whom these qualities have been overwhelmed by trauma. As a craniosacral practitioner I work to try to help them reexperience and integrate these qualities in the course of the therapy.

Doing so challenges me to be in good contact with those qualities myself. I have also noticed that even quite young children are more and more frequently stressed, restless, or distracted. It makes me wonder whether, or to what extent, the contributory factors might be a stressful family situation, stress at school, too much television or sitting in front of a computer, or too little exercise.

The family members accompanying children understandably have high expectations and a great many questions. Sometimes they find it hard to comprehend just what is happening at those times in a treatment session when the practitioner spends twenty minutes or more touching a part of the body or relaxes the trunk and cranial bones while saying hardly a word. Or when children are playing unconcernedly and the practitioner accompanies their process of moving at their own speed from the treatment table to land on the prepared soft padded floor. Situations like these provide an opportunity to talk with the family member, to raise resource and solution-oriented themes, and to answer their questions.

Over the past sixteen years practicing pediatric therapy, I have experienced time and again how effective these treatments can be. Many children respond positively to craniosacral treatments, exercises in sensation and perception, and relaxation. I often find children receiving treatment able to endure the pressure of their previously existing suffering and gratefully accepting new impulses. The treatments I have had the privilege of giving to children and their parents have made me feel very humble. I have often seen what empathy, expertise, and experience can achieve when working in concert with complete trust in the enormous balancing and healing forces of humanity, nature, and the cosmos. All these experiences have moved me to write this book. I have been helped as I write by the certainty that healing processes can take place on all levels of what it is to be human—and that a great deal of suffering can be avoided or resolved in the future if this holistic method becomes better known.

Craniosacral Therapy brings children and their parents relief and joy: the craniosacral treatment of children promotes the capacity to love, bonding and attachment, and a sense of security and ease. All these can have a positive effect on the entire family system and other matters. I am confident that this can reduce the increasing hyperactivity and tendency toward violence in families and schools, among young people, and ultimately in society as a whole.

It gives me great pleasure that in addition to my two previous books, *Craniosacral Therapy for Children* is also now available in English. I hope that this book will prove helpful to many people, both professionally and privately, and so contribute to healing and bringing about changes large and small as well as what we might think of as miracles in ourselves, our children, and our world.

DANIEL AGUSTONI
BASEL, SWITZERLAND, SPRING 2012

PART ONE

Overview

HEALING AND HEALTH
FOR CHILDREN AND PARENTS

Pregnancy, birth, and the development of a child are a time of great change for both mother and father. The transition marks a turning point in life, a kind of initiation, and gives rise to hopes and fears for both parents. Changes are also important opportunities for a person's own inner healing. For the new mother and father, becoming a parent activates conscious and unconscious memories of their own prenatal period, birth, and infancy and evokes a variety of recollections from their childhood. When craniosacral practitioners treat a child, they should remember that treatment that includes more than just the structural level enables more comprehensive healing to take place. During the pregnancy and during and after the birth, both parents experience emotions such as joy, anxiety, and aggression. Usually there is some kind of link between these emotions and their own childhood experiences, since such experiences have a formative effect on personality. Instead of suppressing their feelings, mother and father can experience the healing of old wounds through conscious awareness of their own personal history. Craniosacral therapists who are familiar with primal therapy, Gestalt therapy, or family systems therapy may recognize difficulties that the parents might have and which are emerging in their bonding behavior. They can then invite the parents to seek a way forward through feeling and self-reflection. The parents might, for example, be encouraged to distinguish their own feelings better from their children's, and then to give authentic expression to what they themselves are feeling.

Pregnancy and the birth of a child change the partnership; it becomes a threesome of mother, child, and father. If this new situation is consciously recognized, and anxieties can be openly addressed without overemphasizing them, the result can be a positive one: the changed situation, and the resolution of whatever difficulty it brings, can be transformative for all concerned. When the needs, fears, and anxieties of both parents are addressed and dealt with, this brings greater trust and strengthens the partnership. When fears are resolved, it has a beneficial effect on the body and mind of the mother-to-be and on the child, because in the worst case fear can lead to tensions that cause pain. That can lead to a fear-tension-pain syndrome at the time of the birth. The resource-oriented approach aimed at resolving trauma does more than simply address the difficult issues; it also looks at what is happy and positive. This anchors the emerging pleasant bodily sensation and so prevents excessive agitation or feelings of hopelessness. It is helpful to both parents to reflect on themes from their own birth and childhood and consciously deal with them, as this can offer them both a chance to gain in maturity.

Situations during or after the birth produce a range of emotions for mother and father—not only joyful feelings but unpleasant ones too. For example, they may feel a sense of guilt, fearing that what they have done is inadequate, that they have failed; they may recall images or memories of moments of fear, or may experience a lack of sexual desire. Instead of putting the best light on such feelings or suppressing them, they may be able, perhaps with therapeutic help, to acknowledge and transform them.

Empathy and understanding of how the baby experiences the world, and insight into the world of the child as it goes through the various stages of development, give the parents greater sensitivity to their own emotional themes, assuming that the situation is a positive one. This can open up access for them to their own inner child and essential inner needs. This is a time that brings many inevitable changes. As parents face these changes, reestablishment of contact with what is essential can lay foundations for a better ordering of their own lives. Every change involving the people immediately around the child also affects him or her. The key person here will tend to be the mother. If she, and ideally the father too, receive the support of Craniosacral Therapy, it also usually brings relief to the child.

The Craniosacral Therapy treatment given to the child also indirectly provides treatment for the parents. Parents sometimes report that watching their child being treated, together with the atmosphere around the treatment, causes them too to feel relaxed. The fact that both the child and the parents are receiving professional support can also assist the healing of each individual and of the family system as a whole.

Practitioners and parents can learn an enormous amount from children. Although they are small, children are already complete beings with a great capacity for perception, with authenticity and the ability to make themselves felt, with spontaneity and the ability to feel pleasure and displeasure. All these elements indicate a strong primary personality (discussed further in section 23.2), linked by the bonds of love to the people close to them, and in touch with the ebb and flow within their bodies. There is little sense of the secondary personality, however, or of its primary basic needs, because it is the product of adaptation and conditioning. The secondary personality is something that is determined and more often directed toward consumption and recognition—and lacking in coherence and authenticity. Craniosacral treatment sessions give both the child and its parents the opportunity to recognize their own deepest basic needs and develop their primary personality.

MY FIRST CRANIOSACRAL TREATMENT OF A BABY

2

I would like to begin with an example of a treatment session, as this will illustrate what craniosacral treatment of babies can be like. It is one example of many, but gives an introductory impression of the approach. Further examples of treatment can be found in part IV.

For several years I gave craniosacral training courses that involved regularly traveling abroad. On one occasion the organizer, who is a physiotherapist, and I were invited to dinner with one of her friends, who had had a baby son—we'll call him Thomas, although that is not his real name—some six weeks earlier. Another of the guests at dinner was Thomas's grandmother. It emerged that she had also been a physiotherapist for many years and had taken a number of additional courses in her training, including one in osteopathy in her second year. There were three therapy practitioners present along with the mother and child. Later in the evening I was asked to give Craniosacral Therapy to young Thomas.

The birth process had been a long one. Following the birth it had been difficult for baby Thomas to establish contact with his mother. His sucking reflex had too often been absent or weak, leading to difficulties with his nutrition and digestion. His left shoulder was immobile, and he showed slight signs of paralysis, which looked like brachial plexus palsy.

I asked his mother what the pregnancy and birth had been like for her and the child. She replied that the pregnancy had been quite good on the whole, but that she would have liked more support from the baby's father, who had ended their relationship during the pregnancy.

The birth had been difficult: after the head had been delivered, one shoulder and arm had appeared, after which the delivery had come to a halt for a very long time. Those assisting at the birth had needed to use firm manipulation to free Thomas's other shoulder and the rest of his body. I could sense how deeply the mother felt about this. Not only was she concerned about her son's condition, she was also suffering sleepless nights. She felt overwhelmed and found it difficult to cope with her baby's endless crying and screaming. Conventional allopathic medical investigations had been done, but the treatment received so far had not achieved very much, and any improvement had been short-lived.

By that time I had fifteen years of experience as a result of the training courses I had taken as well as personal experience receiving treatments. This included primal therapy and Gestalt therapy as well as bodywork methods such as Gerda Boyesen's biodynamics, Leonard Orr's Rebirthing, and Stanislav Grof's holotropic breathwork. I had six years' experience in treating adults. I did have a fairly good capacity for empathy with the world of the newborn, and my practice had given me a familiarity with supporting such processes. I had also experienced craniosacral treatment of babies and children many times as a participant in craniosacral courses in Europe and the United States. I knew that in contrast to some of the demonstrations given in these courses, I did not want to treat any child against his or her will or even provoke a process, but that it was possible, with care, even when dealing with a highly charged nervous system, to be a companion of the process.

Although I had experience of Craniosacral Therapy in children and adolescents, I had never given treatment to a baby. I shared my concerns; nevertheless, both the practitioners present as well as the mother encouraged me to be confident and make the attempt. I knew that my touch would not harm the child but rather reduce the burden and the traumatic memory, and thus assist self-healing. I also had the agreement of his closest family caregivers, his mother and grandmother. I gave myself time before starting the treatment and trusted that when I came to offer the touch of my hands, this would happen at the right time and in the right location.

The craniosacral session was carried out in the child's own room. I began by greeting Thomas, who lay against his mother's shoulder, wriggling uncomfortably. It is understood, of course, that newborns cannot understand the actual words said to them, but they can understand the way words are expressed, the mood and subtle harmonics. I explained briefly that I would support Thomas in his spontaneous expression and his movements—and, it may well be, in his crying and screaming. I asked his mother if, when the right moment came, she would lay him down on the wide padded changing table. There was a slight air of agitation in the room, but this diminished in response to my acknowledgement and acceptance. I began by taking several conscious light breaths and grounding myself, and then said to Thomas, "In a moment I am going to touch you, if you will let me." Then, slowly, clearly, and carefully, I intuitively touched the region of his diaphragm, solar plexus, stomach, and liver with one hand. I did nothing else and waited. The baby oriented himself and looked at me with wide eyes. The expression on his face showed no sign of rejection of my touch, and nor did his breathing. I knew that the unknown journey had begun, and that this touch would encourage all kinds of actions and reactions on the physical, psychological, energetic, and instinctive level.

Thomas made various noises and took hold of the proffered finger of my other hand. We made eye contact and looked at each other for some time, and as we did so, I said to him, "That is your treatment, and I am simply supporting you in your own way, so that afterward everything will be a bit easier for you." He gave several sighs and then paused. Then the silence was broken. Thomas began to scream and cry, whether I touched him or not, and whether I was physically or emotionally close to him or farther away.

"That's what he does, that's just the way he cries. He starts in the evening and hardly stops, and it continues all night," said his mother, her voice full of concern and irritation. Then, with one hand, I touched the back of his head and neck, supporting it for some time. At the same time, with my other hand I touched and supported his pelvis and sacrum. I maintained a definite supportive touch with both hands, imposing no force. After a while I began to invite breadth, using both hands, not applying any firm, quick, or forceful pull, but more in the manner of an offer, by means of my intention. Thomas seemed to respond immediately to this invitation to space and breadth because he gave a long sigh and immediately began to make a great variety of improvised and quite smooth movements. After that he made several active, forceful movements, accompanied by screams. This time, however, the cries seemed stronger, more energetic and vital. I remained empathetic and present, from time to time checking the nearness and distance between me and the child. I felt it important for me to judge when Thomas needed nearness, and how much, and similarly when he needed space—on the physical, psychological, and energetic level.

To his mother's surprise, the periods of wild crying and screaming quite soon subsided. He would pause from time to time, interspersed with periods of sobbing and crying. Meanwhile I supported the innate impulses of Thomas's body as he made movements and as he stopped. From time to time, when he cried or screamed loudly, I touched the region of his diaphragm and solar plexus with one hand, keeping my other hand on his neck and shoulder as a supportive point of rest and calm, and following the movements Thomas made. The upper edge of my hand touched both his occiput and the occipital ridge, an invitation to more space addressed to the cranial base.

From time to time I engaged in short dialogues with the baby's mother. Thomas's recurrent periods of calm were quite new to her. During the treatment, I invited his mother to pick up her son on three occasions and consciously establish contact with him in whatever way felt right, on the physical level, visually or by sound, but above all with the heart. That was successful, but only briefly. It ended in a fresh burst of vehement crying that only stopped, gradually, when she put him back down on the changing table.

In the last third of the treatment session, the baby's left shoulder, which had been hypotonic, even lax, at the outset, began to seem more as if it belonged. Both during the periods of rest and during movement, the shoulder began to participate slightly in the movement, though still quite sluggishly. Twice during the periods of calm I sensed the craniosacral motion: it was clearly evident and quite quickly detectable in the head region, but sluggish and weak in the trunk. There were two rounds of activation, including screaming, followed by deactivation, leading through to still and apparently peaceful moments. These were followed by a third that was similar but quite short. After that I knew that the moment had come for Thomas and all the others to end the session. So again, I praised Thomas and his mother and announced that I was going to take my hands away.

The way I understood what happened was this: the stability and flexibility of my hands had given the baby the necessary security and enabled him to give expression to his difficult birth and the suffering that was weighing on him. He became able to dismantle the considerable tension present in some regions of his body. With my hands on Thomas's sacrum and occiput or on his trunk—in those places where at certain moments I sensed movement or restriction, or where I felt my hands being involuntarily drawn—I gently supported his spontaneous unwinding motions in the region of his dural tube. I did not have a specific treatment plan laid out but rather followed my intuition.

I also knew, on the basis of the courses I had attended, that the participating presence of other people can strengthen the healing potential of a treatment session, and on the other hand that inappropriate comments or questions could be a disturbing factor. In this instance, during the entire treatment there was a palpably supportive atmosphere of goodwill on the part of all the adults, which probably made it easier for Thomas and for me to deal with the strenuous highs and lows of this journey.

Following my first craniosacral treatment of six-week-old Thomas, I could not be sure how to judge its success, or whether it would achieve anything. Three days later, feedback from his mother reached me through the course organizer: the baby's feeding and digestion had improved, he was laughing more, and in particular there was more movement in his left shoulder. His periods of crying were significantly shorter, and he was easier to comfort. He was better able to go to sleep and to sleep through the night. His mother was surprised and delighted, and she sent greetings. I was pleased at the news and surprised that after such a short time Thomas was so much better. At the same time, experience of many craniosacral sessions, some with children and many with adults, had shown me that empathetic, but not sympathetic, support does break down the memories of traumatic events and bring people relief.

My experience of Craniosacral Therapy—seven years at that time —had also told me that the practitioner is not a magic healer; rather, the practitioner helps, among other things, to balance the craniosacral system. By bringing this balance, the treatment enables the Breath of Life and the potency within it to stimulate the healing forces inherent in nature. The wonderful effect of a single treatment session made a great impression on me. Not only Thomas and his mother but I too, as the provider of the therapy, felt we had received a great gift.

CRANIOSACRAL THERAPY

Craniosacral Therapy is a gentle form of treatment normally performed by a trained practitioner. It can be used as a stand-alone therapy or in combination with other methods. The origin of the term *craniosacral* is a combination of word forms for *cranium,* the head, and *sacrum,* the base of the spine. Craniosacral Therapy is carried out by applications of very gentle touch, involving such light pressure that it amounts to around 0.04 to 0.1 ounces on the head. The course of treatment can be matched to the individual—to the training, treatment approach, and experience of the practitioner and to the particular requirements of the client.

My book *Craniosacral Rhythm*[1] provides clear information on the anatomy of the craniosacral system in text, graphics, and photos that demonstrate basic techniques and give many practical tips on craniosacral treatment. It gives examples of treatment for adults and numerous answers to frequently asked questions on craniosacral treatment, and it provides a detachable poster showing a well-established basic craniosacral treatment session.

This book, therefore, does not provide detailed descriptions of the craniosacral system, its rhythm, or the basics of Craniosacral Therapy. A summary of the history of the craniosacral system, its essential principles, associated issues, and the levels on which it operates is given below, along with its areas of application.

3.1. History of Craniosacral Therapy

The origins of Craniosacral Therapy lie in Cranial Osteopathy, developed by William Garner Sutherland (1873–1954), who sensed slow movements in the body that resemble the motion of the tides; he discovered that there was a subtle "breathing" of the entire cranium and body. He called this "primary respiration" and saw it as an antecedent of pulmonary breathing and the heartbeat, and as regulating all bodily functions.[2] In his career as an osteopath, which spanned more than fifty years, he discovered various treatment options that were further developed in different ways by his students. Sutherland's later insights into the Breath of Life were passed on by his students, notably Rollin E. Becker and Ruby Day; they in turn provided personal instruction to the American osteopath James Jealous, who is today the most important representative of the biodynamics of osteopathy.

The American osteopath Randolph Stone founded Polarity Therapy, based on over sixty years of experience. Alongside osteopathic and craniosacral techniques, Polarity Therapy incorporates principles of polarity, the five elements, and ayurvedic healing methods. Teachers of Polarity, such as Franklyn Sills and later the Rolfing and craniosacral teacher Michael J. Shea, adapted the Breath of Life teachings of Sutherland, Becker, and Jealous, and fifteen or twenty years ago began to teach biodynamic Craniosacral Therapy.

Craniosacral Therapy, which originally developed from Cranial Osteopathy, became established over the last twenty-five years as a treatment in its own right; it has also seen further development, with the opening of craniosacral principles to bodywork therapists, natural health practitioners, midwives, psychologists, and educators. The craniosacral approach has also received input over the past century from psychology, psychiatry, biology, neurology, and other sciences.

The significant change from Cranial Osteopathy to Craniosacral Therapy occurred through the work of the osteopath John E. Upledger (1932–2012), who worked in a study group on the cranial sutures during the 1970s and later carried out studies of his own. In the first half of the 1980s he began to teach Upledger CranioSacral Therapy® to osteopaths and others in the United States. He incorporated the emotional state of the patient as well as dialogue—SomatoEmotional

Release®—into the treatment. There are, however, some teachers and practitioners of other craniosacral treatment approaches who are either unfamiliar with unwinding and SomatoEmotional Release® or who do not want to employ them. Today, there are many schools and practitioners offering the craniosacral method under various names and with various approaches; it has expanded, been elaborated, and been established as a form of independent treatment around the world.

Craniosacral self-treatment is used by the client for self-help between treatment sessions and following the conclusion of therapy.

3.2. Basic Principles

An overview of Craniosacral Therapy aimed at beginners is provided here; Craniosacral Therapy practitioners can skip to chapter 4.

The main parts of the body to be treated are the head (cranium), the torso, and the base of the spine (sacrum). When performing this therapy, the practitioner senses the craniosacral rhythm or the midtide by "listening" at various parts of the body, or at just one part over a longer period. The craniosacral system, or "fluid body," is treated and harmonized using specific techniques.

The **craniosacral system** consists not only of the cranium, spinal column, and sacrum but also internally of the membranes surrounding the brain and spinal cord (the meninges) and the fluid they contain, called cerebrospinal fluid (CSF). The cranium moves, and not all cranial sutures fuse with age; rather, like the continental plates on the surface of the earth, our cranial bones and sutures have a degree of mobility.

In various parts of the brain are chambers called ventricles. At certain places on the ventricle walls are extensive arterial networks where clear CSF is constantly formed from the blood. This fluid surrounds and protects the brain and spinal cord, and the substances that it contains are important for communication by our nervous and hormonal systems. The fluid is reabsorbed into the venous system,

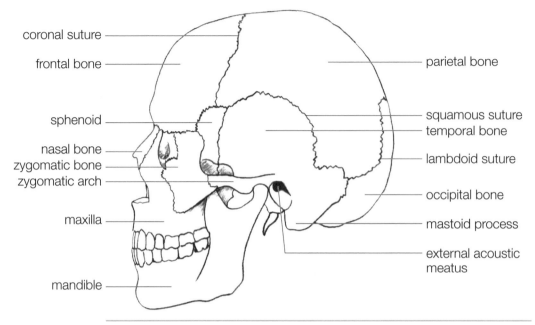

Figure 3.1. Lateral view of the cranial bones and sutures.

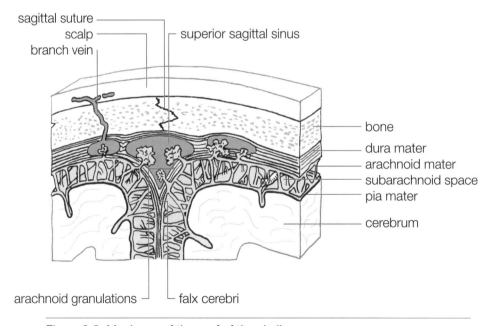

Figure 3.2. Meninges of the roof of the skull.

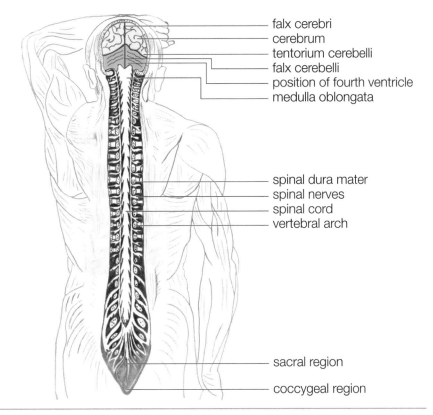

- falx cerebri
- cerebrum
- tentorium cerebelli
- falx cerebelli
- position of fourth ventricle
- medulla oblongata

- spinal dura mater
- spinal nerves
- spinal cord
- vertebral arch

- sacral region

- coccygeal region

Figure 3.3. Central nervous system with nerve exit points.

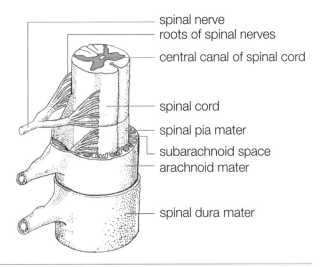

- spinal nerve
- roots of spinal nerves
- central canal of spinal cord

- spinal cord
- spinal pia mater
- subarachnoid space
- arachnoid mater

- spinal dura mater

Figure 3.4. Nerve exit points with spinal dura mater, arachnoid mater, and pia mater.

mainly in the head. Osteopaths have described it as the "highest known element" contained in the body and as "liquid light."[3] The brain and spinal cord, surrounded and buoyed by the CSF, oscillate in rhythmic harmony. The fluid protects them from such dangers as the shock of impact and injury and also provides them with nourishment and removes waste products.

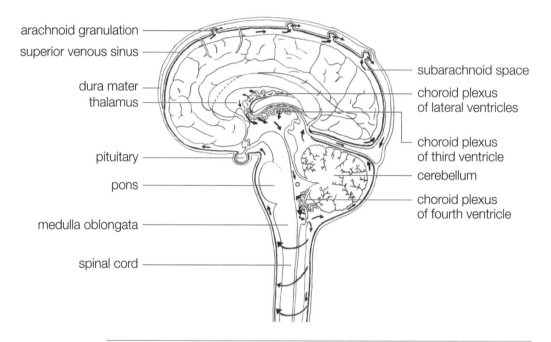

arachnoid granulation
superior venous sinus
dura mater
thalamus
pituitary
pons
medulla oblongata
spinal cord

subarachnoid space
choroid plexus
of lateral ventricles
choroid plexus
of third ventricle
cerebellum
choroid plexus
of fourth ventricle

Figure 3.5. Production, release, distribution, and absorption of CSF in the brain.

Craniosacral Therapy works on the basic assumption that the body is a whole. It sees the human person as a unity of body, mind, and soul and applies the principle that structure and function affect each other. The body has the capacity to regulate itself, heal itself, and maintain its health. However, events in our individual life histories have the effect of reducing that capacity for self-healing and maintaining health. These factors in our life histories include conception, pregnancy, birth, development, extreme events, illnesses, accidents, falls, surgical operations, and spiritual trauma. For a time, our bodies can deal with restrictions by compensating, but if the imbalance is not resolved, it has the effect of reducing the flow of life and of the body's fluids, and this can lead to disease processes.

Craniosacral treatment has the effect of widening the joint-like connections between the cranial bones, giving them better mobility. The meninges, the membranes of our central nervous system (CNS), become more elastic, and the flow of CSF is improved. This harmonizes the craniosacral system and its rhythm, in turn helping the self-regulatory capacity of all body systems, with which it is intimately connected. The cranial nerves therefore have more room, which benefits all the perceptive senses: sight, taste, smell, touch, hearing, and balance. Arterial and venous blood flow is also improved.

Another effect is to help bring the autonomic nervous system (ANS) into balance, which reduces stress and assists digestion. The relaxation of the locomotor system produces such effects as easing or resolving headaches and back pain. The state of tension of the connective tissue is one of the elements that influences whether the craniosacral rhythm can be sensed over the whole body and how even the rhythm is. Another positive effect is on lymphatic flow and freedom of respiration. Parts of the hormonal system also receive support. These control emotional reactions, sleep, hormone secretions, body temperature, and blood pressure. This multifaceted regulation strengthens our immune system.

The **craniosacral rhythm** of around six to twelve cycles per minute is an expression of what has been called "primary respiration" or the Breath of Life. Primary respiration constantly animates the perfect blueprint of existence and harmonizes the body as a whole right down to the cellular level. The practitioner evaluates the quality of motion of the craniosacral rhythm. This is evaluated in terms of strength, amplitude, symmetry, and cycles per minute. The practitioner senses each of these parameters and observes the changes in them as the treatment proceeds. This is done by "listening" with the hands to the qualities of the rhythm at various locations on the body, including the head. This enables the practitioner to find where there is freedom of the bodily structures or where they are restricted. Once specific treatment has been given, the practitioner listens again to discover whether the rhythm is now stronger or more even at a number of locations in the body, and to assess what degree of strength can be detected. The aim of treatment is more than just to improve the balance of the various qualities of the craniosacral rhythm; the effects of this improved balance are important in their own right. These include improved homeostasis, improved flow, greater exchange of all bodily fluids, and a sense of wholeness and peace. Before treatment, energy had been held in check. Now the relaxation and harmonized craniosacral rhythm make it available once more as vital energy in the service of health.

A number of different models have been proposed to explain the fascinating phenomenon of the craniosacral rhythm. The fluid pressure system is based on the assumption that the fluctuation in volume of the cerebral fluid moves the meninges and cranial bones, bringing about the craniosacral rhythm. Because the craniosacral system extends from the head via the dural tube to the sacrum and coccyx, and CSF is distributed along the spinal cord, the subtle and slow movements of the craniosacral rhythm can also be sensed at the sacrum and over the whole body, transmitted by way of free connective tissue. Another proposed explanation is the biodynamic concept, which states that the macrocosmic **Long Tide** (one cycle per one hundred seconds), arising from the dynamic stillness, generates the **mid-tide** (two to three cycles per minute) that can be sensed in and around the body, and this in turn gives rise to the craniosacral rhythm (six to twelve cycles per minute). All these rhythms act as inner healers with their own innate intelligence: self-corrections are made, manifested both in the "energy body" and in the various bodily structures and the body as a whole. Primary respiration is the same primordial force that breathes life into everything on this planet through its rhythmic ordering that contributes to the creation of form and permeates every form.

The **stillpoint** is another element of Craniosacral Therapy. From time to time, the craniosacral rhythm or the slower mid-tide will stop, and this is called the stillpoint. Some stillpoints are spontaneous, arising on their own, but they can also be induced from outside by the practitioner or in self-help. It is ultimately the wisdom of the body that decides whether a stillpoint lasts twenty seconds or three to four minutes. During the stillpoint, the entire craniosacral system and all the associated structures are able to reorganize and harmonize themselves. Essential changes relating to immaterial substances take place, and the body's ability to absorb more universal vital force is enhanced. Often a change can be observed, for example in the breathing, the tissue, or the atmosphere in the room, and the patient is felt to slip into a state of deeper relaxation. When the craniosacral rhythm resumes, the brain and spinal cord are cleansed and nourished with fresh CSF. After a stillpoint, the craniosacral rhythm or mid-tide can usually be perceived more clearly and is more even.

3.3. Application and Effect

Following the initial dialogue, the client is settled comfortably on the treatment table, lying down. The client is dressed in normal everyday clothing and remains on the treatment table for around forty-five to sixty minutes, relieved of the need to do anything. The practitioner makes a brief visual assessment, followed by a whole-body assessment. This involves palpating the texture of the tissue and joints, which provides an impression of muscle tone and the conductivity of the connective tissue. It becomes possible to recognize connections operating over the whole body, for example where strong and even motions of the craniosacral rhythm, and therefore vitality and health, are evident and where the body offers slight resistance. The practitioner encourages the balancing of the craniosacral system by sensitive listening and specific relaxation techniques, and so assists more balanced primary respiration. The treatment of structures in the pelvic region, for example, relieves strain in mothers suffering from backache and sciatic pain during pregnancy, and treatment in the shoulder and nape of the neck as well as the cranial base can help prevent problems such as tension headaches.

KEY POINT

Craniosacral treatment brings relaxation to the body inward from outside. A more even craniosacral rhythm results in improved homeostasis, maintenance of the internal environment. This harmonized rhythm begins to release restrictions working outward from inside, from the center to the periphery. Following the treatment, these vitalizing and reorganizing motions and forces also help to free restrictions in the whole body.

The touch exercised by a careful craniosacral practitioner is definite and light. This avoids causing any instinctive defensive tightening of the body. The natural unity of body, mind, and soul means that the touch and relaxation can bring about a response by different levels of what it is to be human: the level of the body, both physical and energetic; the emotional level; the mental level of mind and spirit; and the spiritual level of the soul.

The expression of primary respiration—the innate treatment plan and wisdom that is called our "inner healer," among other names—can be communicated by signals of the body. An atmosphere of stillness is felt in a room in which healing is taking place and body, mind, and soul are being experienced as a unity; instead of separation and fragmentation, we experience ourselves once more as a direct and immediate whole with all its potential.

The fact that the motions of the craniosacral rhythm, mid-tide, and Long Tide are very subtle and slow has implications for the way we detect them; this is done not by thinking and knowing, but mainly by continuously sensing. Craniosacral bodywork is training in body awareness and perception, both for the practitioner and for the client.

As well as producing harmonization and self-regulation on various body levels, it enables individuals to clearly sense emotions, important insights, and the flow of energy, for example, in their own bodies. A new sense of the body becomes possible.

Because of the great variety of ways in which this bodywork operates, it can reduce or resolve a number of different complaints over the course of a few sessions with children and parents. For example, successful treatment of backache could have the additional effect that the person no longer suffers from insomnia, or that hyperactivity is reduced. Clients often report being in a state of deep relaxation, yet at the same time conscious and wide awake. This enables them, in a protected atmosphere, to direct their attention to what their body, emotions, and spirit are saying and enables real perception of what is in the moment. In this place of stillness, we may reach a state where the various levels of perception are no longer sensed separately. Then we experience the wholeness of our humanity. Linked with the core of our being, it becomes possible to experience individually what is meaningful, vital, and healing. Religious or spiritual insights may also occur. Craniosacral bodywork has the effect of expanding consciousness, can nurture our capacity to love, and stimulates healing processes on all levels.

Practitioners should be trained in dialogue and interactive ongoing support of the healing process. They should be present and empathetic, but without identifying with the child or its parents; they must be able to establish appropriate boundaries. They need to have empathy rather than pity and to remain aware of their therapeutic responsibility.

By orienting themselves to motion and rhythms, practitioners direct their attention to health—the focus is on free motion, not on restrictions, and this strengthens what is positive and has vitality. This is fundamentally important and represents a significant part of the holistic craniosacral treatment that I teach. If the craniosacral practitioner works in a resource-oriented way, the client's sources of strength are employed to a greater extent in the treatment; this helps the client to deal better with strong emotions, pain, insights, and new body sensations. Trauma can be released from the cell memory without causing retraumatization. All cells form a living holistic matrix, as they are linked with the connective tissue and the body's fluids and are involved in an interactive process. The connective tissue and fluids are important for homeostasis and are also able to store and remember events. The connective tissue operates like a fine mesh net. It is an important connecting element among the cells and contains the pathways for nerves, blood, lymph, and CSF. The ground substance surrounds each and every cell. An attentive practitioner has a communicative link with the whole body through the connective tissue at a particular site and can sense free and inertial locations and fulcrums via the connective tissue. If the connective tissue and muscles are relaxed, it is also possible to treat individual organs and so support their function. If the client has trust both in the experienced craniosacral practitioner and in the therapeutic process, then resistant, more deeply seated trauma and restrictions can more readily begin to be released.

The practitioner can, very carefully, accompany the client verbally. This helps clients—children and adults—to sense changes with more conscious awareness. It helps to anchor new perceptions. The approach depends on the practitioner's own personal style and professional knowledge; it may be body-oriented, psychotherapeutic, systems- or spiritually oriented, or a combination of these. The practitioner accompanies the course of the treatment session directly and immediately as it progresses, adapting the approach to the situation and the needs of the child and the parents. The client, child or adult, decides whether to participate in the progress of the treatment session. They don't have to if they don't want to; it is equally legitimate for clients to go to sleep or to remain passively at rest in their center. The rest and relaxation during treatment often act as a long refreshing sleep, like bathing in an inner spring welling up within.

The person's whole body and the various regions of the brain rebalance themselves anew.

In many cases, a previous shock or traumatic event is the hidden cause behind symptoms, illnesses, and seemingly fated accidents. Usually the intensity of the trauma, high at that time, remains stored in the nervous system and tissues, down to cellular level. If clients realize and draw on their personal resources in the security of the here and now, it counters the traumatic memory and provides the basis for enduring healing of trauma. The nervous system stores the new, positive sensations. The treatment can be concluded by listening at various locations to help achieve integration and sense the change between "then" and "now." Clients are allowed to sense the body again, and this is followed by a short closing dialogue.

Reactions following a craniosacral treatment session vary considerably, depending on the individual. For some clients the feeling is one of clarity and alertness; for others it is greater relaxation and sensitivity than they have felt for a long time. Each treatment is unique. Central body systems receive important impulses toward balance, and the session continues to take effect over several hours, weeks, or months, depending on the individual. Clients may, for example, report sleeping better, a pleasant sensation of the body, and enjoyment of life. Others, after several sessions, have a greater sense of what is good or less good for them. Sometimes clients may experience a short-lived intensification of symptoms. This is completely possible and is usually a sign of a "healing crisis." In many cases stubborn physical problems are released if the client also makes changes to old habits in everyday life. This can be part of a vital reorientation and transformation.

The effect of treatment from a craniosacral practitioner can be enhanced by self-help measures; these are described in my book and audio CD *Harmonizing Your Craniosacral System*.[4]

Self-help exercises encourage perception and relaxation. Craniosacral treatment and self-treatment both operate by means of awareness through touch. This makes them more than just a successful way to combat symptoms; they provide us with the possibility of connecting with our inner selves—with the core of our being—in a protected space that offers security. At the same time we sense the link that binds us to people, nature, and the cosmos. These experiences promote our confidence in life, our composure, and our spiritual experience, and so promote our well-being and health.

3.3.1. Indications and Contraindications

With its great variety of approaches, craniosacral bodywork can be used to accompany and support the person before and during birth, over the course of physical development and in the stages of personal growth and change, and right through to the end of life. Its comprehensive effects means that Craniosacral Therapy has a wide range of application: it is helpful for regeneration and maintenance of health and also aids healing in the treatment of health problems, diseases, and syndromes.

SUCCESSFUL CRANIOSACRAL THERAPY USE WORLDWIDE

- preparing for birth
- during and after birth and during postnatal recovery
- providing the newborn with a start in life
- in speech and language therapy and special education, speech and learning difficulties, and hyperactivity
- in occupational therapy
- in dentistry
- in the treatment of chronic pain, such as back pain, headaches, and migraines
- for sleep problems, digestive complaints, and autonomic and organic disturbances

- preceding and following surgery to relax tissues or promote wound healing
- following individual cases of shock and trauma, such as falls and accidents or bad news
- following collective shock and trauma, such as natural disasters or wars, for victims and their loved ones
- in rehabilitation and care
- generally in people facing highly demanding situations privately or at work
- for well-being and spiritual growth
- for relaxation and regeneration; and in cases of burnout
- to support the dying

The craniosacral treatment of children can reduce the undesired side effects of birth and provides support to the child's respiratory pathways, cardiac function, digestion, hormonal and immune systems, and locomotor system.

See chapter 30 for a discussion of selected indications with pointers for Craniosacral Therapy. A comprehensive list of over one hundred indications for adults can be found in my textbook *Craniosacral Rhythm*.

Craniosacral treatment can also be used in mammals such as cats, dogs, and horses, as they also have a craniosacral system and craniosacral rhythms.

The most important contraindications are: acute meningitis; severe or open head injury; recent head fracture; acute intracranial bleeding, where a change in CSF pressure could prolong the bleeding; intracranial aneurysm, due to the pressure difference where a leak or rupture is already present; herniation of the medulla oblongata; heart attack or stroke in the acute phase; infection where the prognosis is unclear, for example as a result of a tick bite; and brain tumor. (See also section 6.2.)

In view of the numerous areas of application and broad spectrum of effects, it is understandable that ever more practitioners are making successful use of this method in their work, including midwives, massage therapists, naturopaths, physicians, dentists, psychologists, practitioners of complementary and alternative medicine (CAM), and other qualified health practitioners.

Craniosacral bodywork can also be learned by those without medical qualifications and family members of the chronically sick or those in need of care. For such individuals, the requirements are sound anatomical knowledge, intuition, self-reflection, and the ability to slow down and prepare for stillness. It is also necessary to have an attentive, open, clear, and centered basic attitude that allows space and adequate experience through having attended specialist courses and having received treatment sessions themselves.

Experience from craniosacral practice shows that it can alleviate many everyday complaints that have not yet reached the chronic stage, either partially or completely, in six to nine treatment sessions, before they potentially turn into serious health problems. Treatment usually leads us from the realm of the mind to a holistic sense of the body. This also has an effect on the psychological level by stimulating and encouraging healing processes. The treatment sometimes allows us to sense ourselves as light and boundless, or we may feel firmly grounded and centered. Our consciousness of sensation expands. We discover in our own experience that we are beings endowed with sensitivity; we sense that we are a unity.

THE HISTORY OF CRANIOSACRAL TREATMENT FOR CHILDREN

4

I want to begin by outlining the beginnings of osteopathy and Cranial Osteopathy, their pioneers, and their successors, and then consider developments that have taken place over the past century. Various body therapies have emerged from psychoanalysis and humanistic psychotherapy; these specifically look back to the circumstances before, during, and after birth and during the stages of development. The research carried out by Wilhelm Reich and his successors in the field of bioenergetics has extended the understanding of vital force and development in children and adolescents. Since around 1986, Craniosacral Therapy has constantly received fresh impulses from various schools of thought—psychological, bioenergetic, and spiritual—and this has expanded the approaches and treatment options for Craniosacral Therapy in infants and children.

Andrew Taylor Still (1828–1917), an American, was the founder of osteopathy. He was a man of religious faith, and it was his conviction that human beings contained within their own bodies "God's drugstore."[1] He believed that osteopathic techniques activate this resource. He recognized that health comes about when the various structures of the body are in a balanced state and there is optimum flow of all bodily fluids. Still spoke of the CSF as the "highest known element."[2]

William Garner Sutherland (1873–1954) was a pupil of Still and obtained the title of DO, doctor of osteopathy, in 1900. He was impressed by the articular surfaces of the cranium, which convinced him that they enable motion. In the first half of the twentieth century he developed Cranial Osteopathy, involving treatment approaches in the bones, connective tissue and membranes, and fluids. For a number of years he treated infants suffering from various disorders in a hospital.[3]

Still and Sutherland both offered important evidence pointing to the importance of the foramen magnum and the position of the occipital bone, with its four parts, in infants. When describing children in whom the position of the occipital bone was distorted, Sutherland used the expression "bent twig."[4] Such children are more susceptible to physical and emotional stress, and their nervous systems react more quickly to stress by exhibiting symptoms.

In the latter years of his life—after some fifty years of continuous research—Sutherland acquired some insights into what he called the Breath of Life,[5] a concept that may sound mysterious to some. He taught a selected group of pupils a form of Cranial Osteopathy that operates without the external application of any force. Rollin E. Becker refers to elements of this treatment approach in two excellent books.[6] A number of other osteopaths also dedicated themselves to Cranial Osteopathy and later taught it in Europe.

Beryl E. Arbuckle studied the intracranial membranes in stillborn infants and applied cranial osteopathic techniques to treating children, especially cases of cerebral palsy.[7] Rebecca Lippincott[8] and Anne Wales were also influential in the development of Cranial Osteopathy for the treatment of children.

Two well-known teaching colleagues spoke to me with great respect and gratitude for Viola Frymann and about her teaching. As a child she had the experience of seeing her father restored to health by osteopathic techniques, and from that time her family put their faith in osteopathy. Frymann trained in medicine and surgery, took a supplementary course in midwifery, and worked for a year of practicum in a homeopathic hospital. In 1952 she attended a course in Cranial Osteopathy in Denver. Her teacher was Sutherland, and one of his lectures, on birth trauma and nausea in newborns, awakened her interest. Frymann began to examine and treat newborns in the osteopathic hospital in San Diego and subsequently founded the Osteopathic Center for Children. She is among the pioneers of cranial osteopathic treatment of children and has carried out significant clinical research that remains important today. In 1963 she made a tracing of the cranial rhythm using an oscillograph, and in 1966 she published an impressive study that she had undertaken in which she found a dysfunction in 1,105 of the 1,250 infants with behavioral abnormalities examined in the study.[9] This dysfunction was mainly found at the spheno-occipital or sphenobasilar synchondrosis (SBS), between the sphenoid and occipital bones, the key joint of the cranial base. Another important location was the four parts of the occipital bone. Frymann compared the art of palpation—touching and listening with the hands or evaluating by means of touch—with learning to play the piano. In her treatments, she included both the structural and the spiritual level. More information on her life and work, together with interviews, personal writings, and some of her research results can be found in her *Collected Papers*.[10]

Others whose ideas have furthered the development of cranial osteopathic treatment of children include Wilhelm Reich, Otto Rank, Alexander Lowen, and Wilhelm Reich's daughter Eva Reich. Wilhelm Reich was convinced that there was a pulsatory fluctuation of expansion and contraction taking place in infants.[11] As far back as 1924, Rank believed that the trauma of birth exerts an effect on the experiences and life history of the developing person.[12] For some decades, different forms of Reichian bodywork—David Boadella's biosynthesis and Gerda Boyesen's biodynamics—have worked with vital energy, subtle pulsations, and the release of prenatal, perinatal, and biographically determined patterns. To this day, the movements of humanistic psychology, initiated by Abraham Maslow (1908–1970), transpersonal psychology, and the insights of Carl Jung have influenced teachers and practitioners of Craniosacral Therapy.

Some therapists and clients had also encountered prenatal and perinatal experiences on the basis of Fritz Perl's Gestalt therapy, Arthur

Janov's primal therapy, and breathing techniques such as Rebirthing, conscious breathing, or holotropic breathwork. This background of thought also flowed into Craniosacral Therapy. The research and writings of Ronald D. Laing and Frank Lake should be mentioned here.[13] Birth dynamics and their effects are recalled in training seminars by William Emerson and his pupils. The spiritual way of attentiveness and meditation has also enriched Craniosacral Therapy. The fundamental alert, open, and meditative attitude aids the kind of perception in which the wisdom of the body and the Breath of Life perform their work. The perinatal research carried out over decades by the early practitioners Wilhelm Reich and Rank and their successors helped to define prenatal and perinatal psychology. Reichian approaches retain a psychotherapeutic content, but other therapies work exclusively with the body.

Through the work of practitioners of these various methods who also use Craniosacral Therapy, their valuable background knowledge found its way into craniosacral treatment of children, adolescents, and adults. This brought in ideas derived from humanistic, transpersonal, prenatal, and perinatal psychology. As a result of this variety, craniosacral treatment of children can be carried out in very different ways, modified and embellished according to the school, background, and emphasis of the practitioner. For those with a neo-Reichian, prenatal and perinatal, or other emphasis, the craniosacral treatment of children offers a noninvasive body-oriented additional approach that initiates and integrates useful healing impulses. Craniosacral Therapy or Cranial Osteopathy as well as neo-Reichian therapy both regard self-regulation and pulsation as a fundamental principle of central importance.

Other pioneers who have worked for a more comprehensive understanding and have laid foundations for a gentle, more human manner of dealing with unborn and newborn babies and children are David Chamberlain in *Babies Remember Birth*,[14] Ludwig Janus, Thomas R. Verny in *The Secret Life of the Unborn Child*,[15] Frédérick Leboyer in *Birth without Violence*,[16] Maria Montessori, Emma Pikler, and more recently, Michel Odent, Aletha Solter, Raymond F. Castellino, and Thomas Harms. In recent years many craniosacral practitioners have taken courses in trauma healing, such as Peter A. Levine's Somatic Experiencing®,[17] and are making use of elements of this in their craniosacral treatments.

BASIC ELEMENTS AND HEALING IMPULSES IN THE CRANIOSACRAL TREATMENT OF CHILDREN

5

Holistic craniosacral treatment of children involves these elements:

- professional and social competence as well as practical experience in Craniosacral Therapy, including its use in children, infants, and newborns
- openness, sensitivity, and intuition
- empathy
- resource-oriented verbal and nonverbal dialogue
- solution-oriented and interactive support of the process
- promoting understanding of the function and the wisdom of the body
- support of the child's mother, father, siblings, and other family members or trusted individuals and caregivers

How does healing occur? What are the other factors, apart from the actual Craniosacral Therapy, that contribute to the release of the physical, emotional, and spiritual imbalance? The following enhance the healing process:

- the practitioner's personal, nonjudgmental contact and attentive care for child and parents
- the gentle, noninvasive body contact, which communicates support and security
- social inclusion, interaction, and fresh opportunities to learn in a neutral space

- "letting go" and relaxation in a situation of trust
- contact, respect, care, and love

KEY POINT

When treating babies and children it is vital to understand them holistically in their present situation on the physical, energetic, emotional, and psychological-spiritual level. By means of empathy and tuning in to a child's world of experience, we support them in a way that frees them of stress instead of adding further to their stress. Particular attention should be paid to this point when treating children with a disability.

Physical growth and psychological-spiritual growth are sometimes accompanied by pain and sadness. Children's craniosacral treatment can reduce this; it provides caring, resource-oriented support by standing alongside them in difficult situations and phases and enabling children to better bear these burdens. The craniosacral practitioner offers a reliable and secure context in which children can reflect and express the current situation and experience something new. Mothers can also be treated if they want. One way of doing this is for the child to lie on or next to the mother, enjoying the mother's relaxed presence. Sometimes, instead of relaxing, the child may become restless or loudly demand attention. On the whole, however, the experience of resting contentedly in the center in togetherness has a regenerating and healing effect, and it provides a counterpoint to the opposite extreme of activity and being excited. This psychosocial accompanying process helps both mother and child to relax.

The therapeutic interaction between practitioner and child takes place consciously or unconsciously on several levels: the bodily structures, the emotions, and the immaterial energies. Craniosacral practitioners listen with their hands to the structure and to the dynamics of the motion of primary respiration. Their fundamentally open, receptive, meditative attitude with its confidence in the process can also give them access to levels beyond the structure, emotions, and thoughts. This is a sign that a deepening of the neutral has occurred and a strong connection has been established with dynamic stillness.

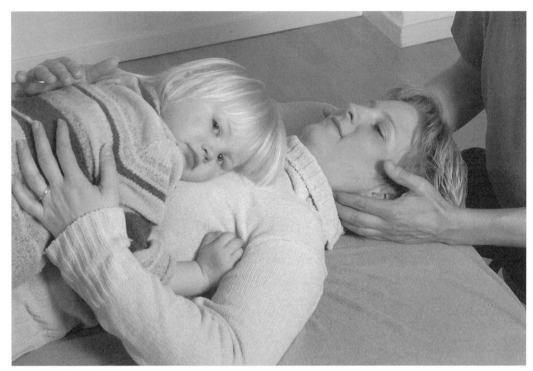

Figure 5.1. Treatment of the mother: relaxing the sternocleidomastoid muscle.

WHAT IS THE PURPOSE OF CRANIOSACRAL TREATMENT FOR CHILDREN?

6.1. Areas of Application

Craniosacral treatment promotes the capacity for self-regulation and so greatly aids self-healing. This book explains how it can provide support across the whole field of pregnancy and birth and the development of the child from infancy through the school environment. A number of different solutions and treatment possibilities will be introduced. See chapter 30 for a discussion of selected indications with pointers for Craniosacral Therapy.

FREQUENT AREAS OF APPLICATION AND INDICATIONS

- unfulfilled desire to have children
- emotional and organic support of the mother during pregnancy, especially in the case of a problem pregnancy
- following the birth, for the newborn and the mother, especially after a difficult birth or cesarean delivery (C-section)
- care of the mother during her recovery following the birth
- in babies with asymmetries of the skull, spinal column, pelvis, or sacrum; torticollis; irritation of the cranial nerves; digestive problems or colic; sleep disturbances; squint; problems of tonus; disturbances of perception; and in children with growth disturbances
- in infants and children of school age with unelucidated developmental disturbances

- in children of school age with learning or speech difficulties, dyslexia, concentration disturbances, ADHD, and autism
- for all children: to boost immune defenses, especially in the case of frequent colds, coughs, or chronic inflammation such as sinusitis or inflammation of the middle ear
- for children of preschool and school age to avoid or to accompany orthodontic treatment
- for children and parents following falls, accidents, emotional shock, and trauma
- to facilitate making contact with the environment
- to support health, happiness, balance, and composure, and to improve ease and lightness in life

---

Every birth is a transition, and in some sense a process of death and becoming. Even a healthy baby will have experienced compression and constricting narrowness at various stages of the birth process, and even for healthy newborns it is a challenge to adapt following birth and to acclimate to the new circumstances of life. This adaptation is made easier by respectful and loving craniosacral treatment. A baby that feels secure and protected is better able to come to terms with the major changes involved in breathing, feeding, and digesting as well as encountering a novel environment than a disturbed baby. A vaginal delivery can also be seen as the first stimulation or "treatment" that the child experiences, because all bodily structures are moved and the whole child is stimulated to a considerable degree. Some births occur quite slowly, others quickly, and at each stage difficult situations can arise for the child, so it is ideal if a midwife can give the infant a craniosacral assessment and brief treatment a few hours after the birth or the following day. This will also help the ability of mother and child to bond.

Depending on the course of the birth, craniosacral practitioners accompany mother and baby with a few treatments. They may accompany them through a birth that is proving to be a difficult experience, helping it to reach its conclusion in a more satisfactory way. Also, they can release any restrictions in the head, neck, and trunk regions, enabling more balanced functioning of the body as a whole. This helps the child in its arrival here on earth and aids its physical and psychological development. The earlier this help is given, the more effective it is.

Pregnancy, birth, and the postnatal period are more often attended by stress factors today than in the past, and these have their effect on mother and child. Even a few craniosacral treatments provide support to mother and child on the physical, psychological, and energetic levels and give the baby the best foundation for the intensive growth that will take place over the coming months and years.

Seen overall, probably more than half of all newborns could benefit from craniosacral treatment. The increase in C-section deliveries always means some degree of trauma for mother and baby. Even in normal vaginal deliveries, there is marked compression of the baby's head, neck, and trunk. In infants the vital forces are very strong, so that just a few craniosacral treatments are sufficient to release factors causing restriction. In the words of Sutherland, "as the twig is bent, so the tree inclines":[1] if prompt assistance is not given and the newborn remains untreated, the effects can lead to restrictions, pain, and syndromes years or even decades later. This is not to spread the impression that the prognosis is poor or to unsettle parents, as has occasionally happened with some allopathic medical pronouncements to justify a particular treatment. However, positive conditions and events that occur during Craniosacral Therapy to strengthen resources create pleasure in the child, and these things are ideally suited to promote development and growth, enabling that to happen relatively unhindered.

In my practice, I regularly treat children and their parents. The clients who visit me are mainly worried or exhausted mothers with babies who cry a great deal, suffer from colic, and scream for long periods, often after a difficult birth, as well as schoolchildren with hyperactivity disorder or specific learning disabilities (SLD). Diagnoses are important and concepts matter, but there is sometimes the risk that the diagnosis itself will have the effect of making the child into a problem child. The parents' concern is, of course, something I take seriously, and the diagnosis from conventional allopathic medical physicians and neurologists is very helpful. It gives an important insight into the psychopathology of the child. This provides me with indications as to the kinds of structural treatment I might be able to use when giving Craniosacral Therapy. Equally important in my view is the fact that the mobility of the structures, and the way in which primary respiration is developing in the young patient, together with the force it embodies, are an expression of health. It is health that I want to promote rather than taking the one-sided approach of combating disease. As a practitioner of holistic and gentle bodywork, I am confident that the body knows the answers to resolve problems. Experience confirms this. When I approach problems using more than just techniques and seek the way forward in concert with mother and child, I find that the problems are resolved in a few sessions. Even the causes are resolved, and comprehensive healing can take place.

I was once asked by a participant at an evening seminar whether it was really important for every child to receive craniosacral treatment; since nature takes care of us, why should concerned mothers bring their children to have Craniosacral Therapy? My answer then, as now, was to agree that sometimes we do rush too quickly to make a diagnosis. Treatment is then ordered, and sometimes the child's condition is made worse rather than better by concern and pressure on the part of the parents. I am also in general of the opinion that we should not overtreat our children and so place them under additional pressure. At the same time, there are parents—sometimes just one of the parents—who go to the opposite extreme. They maintain that things are not so bad and will improve as time goes on; the child will "grow out of it." They may sometimes categorically question whether gentle therapies are of any use at all and insist that hyperactivity or post–traumatic stress disorder are new and invented diseases. The fact that they did not previously exist, were not recognized, or were called something else does not mean that they do not exist now. The lesson to be drawn is that of course not every child needs craniosacral treatment, but it would be of benefit to most.

6.2. Contraindications to Treating Children

A number of different contraindications exist because of the variety of treatment approaches in Craniosacral Therapy. Various factors determine whether a treatment is indicated or contraindicated. Other questions also influence the decision: the techniques chosen and the form in which they will be applied; the experience of the practitioner in treating adults and in particular babies, young children, and adolescents; and the time factor. The aim in all this is to address what is appropriate and lead the therapeutic process to a rounded conclusion. The intensity and length of a technique and the time gap between one treatment and the next also play a part in the effects of the Craniosacral Therapy. We can see from this that it is not so much the gentle method itself that is contraindicated; rather practitioners can be lacking in care, uncertain or inexperienced, or may not listen sufficiently with their heart and sensitive hands. Touch should be applied slowly; it should be tuned as accurately as possible to the needs of the child and adjusted at any time to match changes in those needs. This demands a great deal of empathy on the part of the practitioner, who needs to be fully present and to work with respectful attentiveness. If there is any lack in these areas, the context of protection and security that the child needs to have in place during the treatment can quickly fall away. If practitioners fail to recognize this and do not give the child and themselves sufficient space and time, the child will react to an inappropriate situation with increased stress, or may even "freeze" or "act dead." That would be neither resource- nor solution-oriented.

This is an appropriate point to mention another precautionary measure that I apply when there has been a previous difficult birth, such as miscarriage or preterm delivery: it is advisable not to induce a stillpoint at the occipital bone (the CV4 technique) during the pregnancy.

Contraindications sometimes give rise to discussion, even among teachers of Craniosacral Therapy. Contraindications are:

- severe or open head wounds in the acute stage
- acute inflammation
- brain tumor
- acute cerebral edema, hematoma (effusion or collection of blood as a result of injury), cerebral aneurysm (widening of a blood vessel as a result of changes in the vessel wall), and intracranial bleeding

Midwives and pediatricians know the difference between caput succedaneum, cephalhematoma, and intracranial bleeding and can assess whether and to what extent Craniosacral Therapy can or cannot be used.

The very greatest care is advised in the case of epilepsy or other conditions involving discrete episodes in the neurological realm. It is advisable not to perform any manipulation in the head region in such cases. A helpful approach in this situation, instead of treating the symptom, is to touch the child in regions that feel pleasant; appropriate gentle touch increasingly encourages a general physical and emotional release of stress. This usually happens without applying a specific technique. To act in this way is to use the functional treatment approach and above all to encourage those parts that are healthy. Trained craniosacral practitioners or osteopaths who have many years of experience with such clinical conditions will be better able to assess when direct therapeutic assistance is helpful, for example in the case of hydrocephalus or epilepsy, and provide treatment following diagnosis from a conventional physician. My advice to untrained individuals presented with patients with the any of the conditions listed above is to refrain from giving craniosacral treatment in all instances on the grounds of duty of care.

Frequently, palpation in the abdominal, pelvic, and sacral region or on the feet of a child is in itself effective in relaxing tension without giving rise to symptoms. Taking this approach means that the affected person can, as necessary, calmly "rest in the center" while the slow rhythms help to balance various structures and strengthen the immune system.

WHO SHOULD GIVE CRANIOSACRAL TREATMENT TO CHILDREN?

7

Craniosacral treatment of children is a specialized area of Craniosacral Therapy. It is performed by midwives, pediatric nurses, teachers at special schools, remedial teachers, consultants for lactation and nursing mothers, nursery school and other teachers, speech and language pathologists, physiotherapists and occupational therapists, practitioners of complementary and alternative medicine, movement therapists, homeopaths, and other trained specialists. Parents and family members can use craniosacral touch as an aid to relaxation, to help the child go to sleep, to ease cold symptoms, or to help the child to feel contented and calm, if the child allows it. It is advisable for those who want to use craniosacral touch to have attended a number of courses and to have gained sufficient practice treating adults before working with children.

In children with physical symptoms or other problems, my advice is that they should be treated by a craniosacral practitioner specialized in treating children. A practitioner who is detached and not involved in the family circle is often able to take a freer and more neutral view than parents or other family members, who are more directly affected. An experienced craniosacral practitioner is probably better able to assess how much or how little is appropriate in terms of touch. If treatment is given by someone close to the child, there is a greater tendency for them to identify with that person; they are already affected themselves and may perhaps unconsciously overlook important factors, or fix on certain other factors because they place too much significance on them.

This book outlines a great many principles and techniques that may be combined as appropriate to meet the needs of the individual child. As a general guide, section 28.1.1 illustrates how to get started in a pediatric craniosacral session.

7.1. Combination with Other Methods

In Craniosacral Therapy, the whole locomotor apparatus and craniosacral system, as well as the organs, in the case of visceral treatment, become relaxed. Craniosacral treatment of infants, young children, and school-age children can also be combined with other methods of complementary medicine. Of course, if methods are combined, it becomes less easy to decide which therapy is working or how well it is working, or to see whether invasive manual methods have led to restrictions, for example. Overstimulation by using too many therapies is not advisable.

PARENTS AND CHILDREN AND THEIR CHANGED ENVIRONMENT IN THE TWENTY-FIRST CENTURY

8

I would like to revisit the question of whether and why children's craniosacral treatment is necessary for healthy children. Our society has changed a lot over the last century. The stories told by my one-hundred-year-old grandmother and my 102-year-old neighbor about what life was like in the old days reflect the enormous development that has taken place from the industrial era to the information age. Yesterday's new inventions are already being updated today; tomorrow the pace of change is likely to be even faster. We have less and less time to reflect, relax, and be calm. Everyone is constantly on the move, and to rest for a moment is to get left behind. Children watch violent cartoons on television instead of hearing stories at their grandmother's knee. Needs are created, and synthetic satisfaction is supplied in the form of brand-name clothing, fast food, and luxury goods. Overburdened teachers are under pressure and bullying and violence are on the increase in schools while timetables and class sizes mean that there is often neither time nor space to attend to children's individual needs. There are situations where the involvement of parents and teachers consists more in sorting out and organizing schedules than in the kind of direct personal contact that is needed if they are to deal in any detail with the abilities of the child as an individual. This sometimes difficult state of society is to the disadvantage of mothers and children, with results such as:

- bleeding during pregnancy, caused by stress
- increase in the number of premature births and deliveries by C-section
- an unsettled environment, which disturbs the rhythm of mother and child
- diminished capacity to forge relationships
- an agitated, hyperactive atmosphere at home
- agitated, hyperactive children, for example under treatment with pharmaceutical drugs to moderate their behavior so as not to be sent to a special school

If an individual is overstressed, it produces a reaction on the part of families and entire social groups. They behave in a hectic, agitated way and lack any time to rest to establish order in their lives. It should hardly surprise us, then, that there is disorder, aggression, and violence in many parts of society. Treatment with Craniosacral Therapy creates calm in a natural way and provides a counterpoint to this tendency.

PART TWO

Conception, Pregnancy, Birth, and Development

THE UNFULFILLED DESIRE
TO HAVE CHILDREN

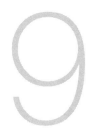

The following tips and possible treatment options are of value where there is the desire to have a child. If the woman has a healthy balanced diet and enjoys plenty of exercise, it can be assumed that her pelvic organs, diaphragm, and pelvic floor are free of adhesions, torsions, tensions, and restrictions. Following falls, emotional trauma, or surgical operations, or if scars are present, Craniosacral Therapy prior to pregnancy provides ideal preparation. Appropriate elements of the techniques described in the following chapters can be used.

9.1. "We've Wanted to Have a Child for So Long"

Before moving on to the subjects of conception and development during pregnancy, the first issue is the unfulfilled desire to have a child. It is a situation that approximately one in six couples has to confront.

When I have stated in a lecture or during a course that craniosacral and visceral treatment can help those with an unfulfilled desire to have a child, the reaction has sometimes been one of disbelief. Why is that be possible, and how? From the viewpoint of Craniosacral Therapy, there are several things that could cause a woman's desire to have a child to remain unfulfilled. The first is stress, which can have a negative effect both on the vitality of the man's sperm and on the hormonal system and fertility of the woman. Studies have demonstrated this. For many people in Western-style civilizations, the stress factor in our professional lives and leisure is constantly high. For men, this can lead to diminished sex drive and infertility. In women, it can cause the menstrual cycle to become irregular or cease altogether and so disrupt the possibility of conception.

Both in my practice and among my friends I have often seen how much stress is felt by a woman who does not get pregnant despite wanting to. The man shares in this unhappy situation; as part of the partnership, he too suffers stress. In some partnerships, the issue of children and managing to have children has even destroyed relationships.

In the case of impotence or lessened sexual desire, Craniosacral Therapy can produce better balance of the ANS. If the parasympathetic system is strengthened and more active, this assists the man's erection, and activated elements of the sympathetic system enable ejaculation.

Other possible reasons for the failure to conceive include an inadequacy of the sperm, or that fertilization may not be happening because of some organic or hormonal problem on the part of the woman. Causes include, for example, reduced secretion in the fallopian tubes or reduced flow of fluid, first to the ovary and then as the ovum travels through the fallopian tube to the uterus. Or it may be that the fertilized egg does not implant successfully.

Clearly, then, pregnancy depends on many factors that have to be organically in harmony with one another. It is a gift and a miracle that cannot be taken for granted. Nor can it, by natural means, be forced. The following favor the achievement of pregnancy:

- freedom from restriction of the pelvis, especially the sacrum and symphysis, hip and sacroiliac joints, and transition from the lumbar vertebrae to the sacrum (L5–S1, lumbosacral joint)
- balanced muscle tension in the abdominal and pelvic regions
- balanced tension of the numerous ligaments in the abdominal and pelvic regions
- connective tissue free of restrictions, which gives support to all structures and contributes to their flexibility
- uterus, left and right ovaries, fallopian tubes, bladder, and urinary

tract free of restrictions and in optimum position, perfusion, and functioning

- good overall function of the entire hormonal system, especially the hypothalamic-pituitary-adrenal axis (sphenoid–third ventricle)
- optimum interaction of all these structures

9.1.1. Specific Structural Treatments

Treatment should relax the connective tissue as a whole, including the fasciae and muscles. The joints, especially the ankle, knee, and hip joints, should also be freely mobile, and the tone of the muscles and ligaments of the abdomen, pelvis, and thigh should be even. The abdominal and pelvic organs should also be freely mobile. This applies both to their intrinsic motion (motility) and optimum ability to move along with other structures (mobility). Restrictions can press the ovary and fallopian tube against each other, or temporarily block the fallopian tube. These restrictions can be reduced using visceral treatment and by relaxing the connective tissue through fascial glide. Unilateral tensions and adhesions can also begin to release with a few craniosacral treatment sessions from a practitioner. This can be supplemented by regular craniosacral self-treatment.

The sacrum should move without restriction in the craniosacral rhythm; this indicates that the sacrotuberous ligament is fairly free. The release of the sacroiliac joints and lumbosacral transition zone, the CV4 technique at the occipital bone or sacrum, and other release techniques are helpful here. This can be supplemented by gentle mobilization using the manual pump technique with the patient prone: place one hand on the patient's sacrum, and with the other hand on top of the first hand, perform rhythmic pumping movements in various directions. Then follow the spontaneous unwinding, or reorganization of the structure, at the sacrum and in the pelvic region.

In the region of the uterus, cysts can delay or prevent conception. Cysts can be treated externally by means of gentle yet definite touch.

In the case of one patient, her appointment for surgery to remove the cyst was canceled because the cyst resolved within a few weeks. This happened after her third treatment session with me. However, if there is any suspicion of growths or tumors, the patient should undergo extensive medical examination.

Release of restrictions of the pubic symphysis eases the movement of the bladder. Specific treatment of the symphysis can be given, for example, by spacious touch combined with gentle fascial glide.

Place your thumbs to the left and right of the two parts of the symphysis, with your thumb tips touching each other. Then invite both parts of the symphysis to move laterally, away from each other. If you include the respiratory or craniosacral rhythm in your field of consciousness, these rhythms can help the symphysis become more mobile. The symphysis can also be treated at the thigh, combined with various minute movements of the hips with the patient supine. To do this, place one hand across the symphysis, touching both pubic bones. Grasp the patient's hip from below with the other hand and perform slow, gentle movements from time to time. Then treat the other side in the same way.

The normal position of the uterus is inclined forward (anteverted) onto the dorsal half of the bladder, supported by numerous ligaments. The broad ligament of the uterus attaches the uterus laterally to the internal walls of the pelvis. The round ligaments of the uterus hold the uterus forward in its anteverted and anteflexed position. These ligaments are about four to five inches long and one- to two-tenths of an inch in diameter. Pain can occur along these ligaments during the pregnancy, called round ligament pain, which is caused by the growth of the uterus and it assuming an upright position. The pain can radiate as far as the labia. The sacrouterine ligaments provide an attachment between the internal surface of the sacrum and the uterus and rectum.

Scars in the abdominal and pelvic regions can lead to restrictions in the pelvic region. The scar tissue can be treated and the restrictions produced by them released.

If craniosacral treatment is combined with visceral treatment, it is possible to address all of the structures described above, individually and as a whole. By improving the balance of these structures, the effect is more favorable for pregnancy.

Balancing the hormonal system is aided by cranial treatment, especially by harmonizing the motions of the sphenoid, which influences the hypothalamus and pituitary via the third ventricle, and the occipital bone, which influences areas of the brain stem via the fourth ventricle.

Balancing the ANS: the deep relaxation brought about during craniosacral treatment sessions can help reduce the high levels of cortisol produced by stress. Cortisol not only reduces the appetite, it also leads to reduced production of sex hormones in males and females. Excessive psychological stress reduces the amount of the male hormone testosterone, and in men this leads to disturbances in the sex drive or fertility. In women, permanent stress can cause cessation of monthly periods and reduced ability to conceive. A number of studies have shown an increased risk of premature birth in cases of prolonged stress.

After performing these treatment sequences, you should listen to the craniosacral rhythm and spontaneous stillpoints. Include other regions of the body, as these usually act in a compensatory way and may even be the origin of restrictions in the pelvic region. Then evaluate the craniosacral rhythm at the head, harmonize it using specific techniques, and compare its new quality with the quality of the rhythm at the sacrum or sides of the pelvis.

During craniosacral treatment sessions, emotional themes can arise. For example, what it means to be a woman and the theme of receptivity, consciously welcoming the pregnancy and the child, giving time to oneself and to others, trusting in the right moment, and letting go and allowing something to happen. The dialogue accompanying the treatment enables the client to better access conscious and unconscious themes that may make pregnancy more difficult or easier. Valuable insights, together with the craniosacral and visceral treatment, can bring about changes in the woman's body and biochemistry within one or two menstrual cycles to increase the possibility of pregnancy.

Other possible causes for nonfulfillment of the desire to have children:

- Infections, for example chlamydia, which can lead to problems affecting the fallopian tubes; vaginal fungal infection; and other STDs.
- Uterine tissue damaged by an abortion.
- Anxiety on the part of the patient leading to tension and reflexive spasm in the fallopian tubes and elsewhere in the pelvic region. A number of different triggers and emotions, including the fear of being infertile, can affect conception.
- Location of the patient's home or sleeping area that may be unfavorable, for example over an underground watercourse or near a power line.

Additional factors to consider:

- Sexual intercourse: the time of maximum fertility is between the seventh and seventeenth day following the onset of the menstrual period. Regions of the uterus expand or contract during various phases; at orgasm, the uterus rhythmically assumes an upright position and the cervix opens, facilitating conception.
- A diet rich in folic acid, with foods such as leafy vegetables, tomatoes, oranges, and whole-wheat products, is favorable to pregnancy.
- Bathing in a warm bath with warming natural essences or herbs is beneficial, as is drinking lady's mantle tea, which has an opening up effect, both physically and spiritually.
- Addictive substances: nicotine and smoking should be stopped immediately, and alcohol and too much coffee should be avoided.
- Food intolerances.

Examples of emotional themes:

- Unconscious defensiveness based on the woman's own experiences in childhood, with her own parents, or with other family members.
- Unconscious or unacknowledged motives: the woman's desire to compensate for something in her own life, to bind her partner to her, or to find fulfillment and meaning in life by having a child.
- What it means to be a woman, personal and societal images of femininity, and the sense of self-worth.
- Anxiety or fear—women experiencing anxiety can describe the associations and thoughts they have in this regard.
- Hopes or desires—women can be asked to formulate their feelings, associations, and thoughts.
- Commitment, dependency, and restriction of freedom.
- Affection, love, eroticism, and sexuality all affect oxytocin levels in both men and women.

9.1.2. Oxytocin: Hormone of Love, Affection, and Desire

The hormone oxytocin—the name means "rapid birth" in ancient Greek—has an important role in the birthing process and stimulates cells of the mammary glands. Today, the practice of obstetrics seems almost unimaginable without its use. Scientists such as Sue Carter, Kerstin Uvnäs Moberg, and Candace Pert have discovered and described further functions stimulated by this hormone: oxytocin not only stimulates labor but also produces contractions of the uterus during orgasm. In the brain it stimulates maternal behavior and above all promotes bonding and emotions. Oxytocin levels rise in people sharing a meal together, for example. Polygamous behavior changes, and monogamous altruistic behavior takes its place. Michel Odent, one of the most important proponents of gentle birth, describes the neuropeptide oxytocin as "the hormone of love."[1] In both men and women, oxytocin levels rise during the experience of sexual pleasure and orgasm. In the man, it helps stimulate the contractions of the prostate and seminal vesicles during orgasm; in the woman, the contractions of the uterus help the sperm travel upward to reach the ovum. For a couple trying for children, the chance of achieving natural pregnancy is increased if they allow themselves more stress-free time together in a loving, sensual, pleasurable atmosphere.

THE PREGNANCY

This chapter discusses questions relating to a pregnancy from the point of view of the mother and sets out appropriate treatments during pregnancy.

Pregnancy is calculated from the first day of the last menstrual period and lasts 280 days, or ten lunar months. Depending on the cycle, this is approximately thirty-nine to forty-one weeks. Around ninety-six percent of babies arrive between two weeks before and two weeks after the calculated birth date. The mother experiences many physical and emotional changes during pregnancy as her body adapts in a variety of ways to new needs and circumstances. Existential questions, marked mood swings, and spiritual experiences often arise and can set in motion transformational processes in the mother. This is a time to recall what is of essential importance. The mother-to-be needs to adapt her external environment to her new situation and focus to a greater degree on her internal environment.

Today, we know that the fetus is not just some growing clump of cells, as in the view of experts in the past. Even the mother's physical and emotional condition creates a hormonal state that has some effect on the fetus. Craniosacral Therapy can provide support to the mother during pregnancy on the physical and emotional levels as well as preparing her for the birth.

Questions relating to the pregnancy:

- Does the woman feel happy to be pregnant? If so, where does she sense this joy, and how does it feel?
- Is this a wanted or planned pregnancy, or an unwanted one?
- What changes will come about in the coming months as a result of

the pregnancy, after the birth, and in the coming years? Spell out the perspectives along with mental and emotional preparation for the new situation.

- Does she have any anxiety or fears about the pregnancy? What are they?
- Are there any signs of a high-risk pregnancy?

Pregnancy and motherhood bring about major and utterly new situations. Often these represent a challenge to set out a clearer life plan and to order it to suit the new circumstances. Pregnancy presents the need to take responsibility for one's own life and that of the child—a catalyst for personal development.

10.1. Avoiding Stress, Anger, and Anxiety

Pregnant women should try to ensure as stress-free an environment as possible. A number of studies have shown that stress hormones pass into the amniotic fluid. British researchers demonstrated that higher levels of stress hormones in the mother's blood were matched by greater amounts of cortisol in the amniotic fluid. Cortisol is a hormone produced in increased quantity when the gene for corticotropin-releasing hormone (CRH) is activated in the brain. In situations of psychological stress and danger, the CRH gene is activated within minutes, causing a rise in cortisol via the hypothalamic-pituitary-adrenal axis. This can produce a state of inner unrest, raise blood pressure, and reduce appetite. Interpersonal relationships as well as partnership and sexuality influence whether the "stress genes" are switched on or off.

The changes that take place during pregnancy also offer an opportunity for the child's father to help. He can aid and accompany this significant change actively by participating in joint "nest-building," for example, or in the background by reflecting on the condition of his own emotions.

10.2. Prenatal Testing: The Lure of the Possible or Just Stoking Fear?

Pregnant women should ask a midwife about prenatal testing. What are the possibilities? How many and what type of tests are appropriate? By no means are all the possible tests necessary, and none of them have one hundred percent certainty. It is more helpful to strengthen the woman's confidence in herself and in natural pregnancy and birth than to suggest seeking excessive reassurance, and there is a risk that this will foster fears of birth defects. The selection and number of tests and the announcement of results often cause pregnant women considerable stress (see section 12.2).

Research offers many new options. For example, stem cells can be taken from the umbilical cord immediately after birth and frozen to provide a means of curing future diseases. In a way this is yet another demonstration of an enticing dream: full control and certainty. It is quickly placed in perspective if we make a historical, cultural, and ethnological comparison; this opens up instead the mythical, archetypal, and spiritual aspects of pregnancy and birth. Another point to bear in mind is that if we encourage joy and confidence instead of fear and doubt, our hormonal systems produce happiness hormones that have the effect of reducing stress.

10.3. Delivery Interventions

C-section can be a lifesaving measure if the size of the baby's head is considerably out of proportion to that of the mother's pelvis, or in cases of emergency. In other situations it represents an unnecessary intervention in the natural course of the delivery and has an effect on mother and child. Any stressful situation causes the release of epinephrine and norepinephrine, commonly called adrenaline. These inhibit labor and the birth process. Large quantities of epinephrine are released in the last minutes before birth. The importance of the mother withdrawing into an intimate space during birth is recognized in societies that live close to nature. A pleasant atmosphere of trust and individual attention from a companion are valuable to the mother and help avoid unnecessary stress and complications.

For most of today's mothers, the choice of where to give birth is fortunately self-evident. However, the real risks are often overstated in informational brochures, and this promotes anxiety. Other problems in the past have included the idea that the first breast milk, called colostrum, was impure and harmful to the child; modern biology now understands it to be very valuable.

10.4. Structural Treatments during Pregnancy

Craniosacral Therapy is almost always appropriate during pregnancy, and the woman can be given support through both structural and biodynamic approaches. Where there are problems, for example premature opening of the cervix or severe bleeding, I advise only giving treatment on the recommendation of a midwife or gynecologist.

10.5. Treatment with the Client Lying on Her Side or Seated

Craniosacral treatment during pregnancy can be performed with the client lying on her side or seated. After discussion with the pregnant woman, treatment can also be given for short periods with the client supine. The length of time taken for these treatment sequences in the supine position should become shorter as the pregnancy becomes more advanced so as not to compress the mother's major blood vessels. The inferior vena cava collects blood from the whole of the lower half of the body and transports it to the right atrium of the heart. In the inferior and middle regions, the inferior vena cava is immediately to the right of the abdominal aorta and follows a similar course as it runs upward close to the lumbar vertebrae. The pressure of the uterus can bring about compression of the inferior vena cava, called vena cava inferior syndrome, causing a reduction in the venous return to the heart and the heart rate.

As a consequence of the lowered blood pressure, perfusion of the uterus can also decline to a critical level, severely reducing the supply of oxygen to the fetus and its heart rate. Mild forms of this syndrome occur in the supine position in around thirty percent of pregnant women during the last trimester. Signs include pallor, nausea, sweating, hypothermia, and breathlessness. As early as the sixth month of pregnancy, a fifteen-minute treatment in the supine position is no longer advisable. The decision depends on the size and weight of the fetus and on how the mother feels; ask and observe the client and request feedback from time to time. It then becomes necessary either to shorten the length of treatment when supine or to stop treating in this position altogether, replacing it with treatment in which the client is lying on her side or seated.

10.5.1. Position

It is recommended that treatment be given on a padded surface. For short treatment sequences with the client supine, it is necessary to have adequate support material, for example knee roll bolsters of various sizes, perhaps a robust support wedge, and sufficient blankets and cushions. When the client is supine, place a cushion under her right buttock to incline the pelvis slightly to the left and relieve pressure on the inferior vena cava.

When the client is lying on her side, it is recommended to place cushions to support her head and cervical spine as well as between her knees and feet. It will help her feel comfortable if a fairly large cushion is placed by her rib cage, as support on which to rest the uppermost arm. This is especially helpful when the pregnancy is advanced. As an alternative to this, blankets can be rolled around a support bolster to provide a comfortable support for the weight of the arm. In the photographs in this book, the rolled blankets that support the client's arm have been removed to provide a better view.

10.6. Protective Space for the Fetus

The guiding aim when treating the mother during pregnancy is to provide protective space for the fetus. Out of respect for the developing baby, I personally hardly ever give direct treatment to the mother's abdomen, the fetus's immediate home. In traditional Chinese medicine, it is appropriately described as the "child's palace." Since the body is a unity, I am able to relieve stresses on this region indirectly by treating the bone structure and peripheral tissue structures. I avoid any direct influence on the unborn child using manual techniques. However, I am convinced that freer and more mobile structures, improved blood flow, more even and slower craniosacral rhythms and tides, and the general physical and emotional relaxation of the mother-to-be also support the child in its being and its growth. For the mother, this time provides beautiful opportunities to make contact with her child.

If difficulties arise during the pregnancy, the midwife or craniosacral practitioner can accompany the mother to support her in achieving relaxation.

10.7. Treatment of the Pregnant Woman

Many of the treatment principles described in detail in my textbook *Craniosacral Rhythm*[1] can be used to treat pregnant women, and therefore I won't outline any basic craniosacral treatments in detail here but will assume that they are already sufficiently well understood and that the practitioner already has plenty of practice in applying them. Some basic possible methods of providing support for the pregnant woman, followed by some more specific treatment methods:

- Evaluation of the craniosacral rhythm at the feet or knees, sides of the pelvis or sacrum, shoulders, and head region, for example at the occipital bone.
- Relaxing transverse connective tissue: diaphragm or inferior thoracic aperture.
- Shoulder girdle or superior thoracic aperture.
- Cranial base or atlanto-occipital joint.
- Craniosacral rhythm: listening at individual cranial bones and supporting the rhythm, followed by listening across the entire head using the cranial vault hold.
- Effleurage of the sternocleidomastoid and the masseter and temporal muscles.
- Relaxation of the mandible.
- Deep relaxation of the region of the diaphragm, solar plexus, and kidneys.
- Evaluation of the dural tube (spinal dura mater) and relaxation by gentle traction via the occipital bone and, if comfortable for the

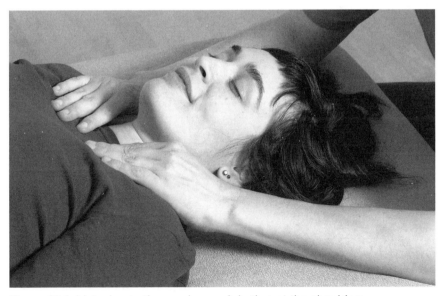

Figure 10.1. Listening to the craniosacral rhythm at the shoulders and relaxing the lungs.

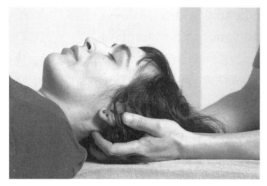

Figure 10.2. Effleurage of muscle attachments.

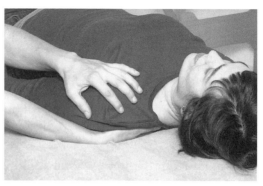

Figure 10.4. Relaxing the shoulders.

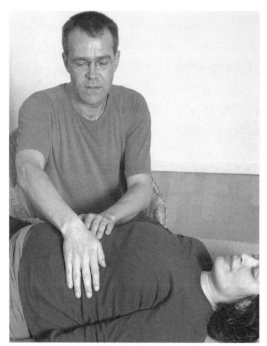

Figure 10.3. Relaxing the diaphragm and costal arch.

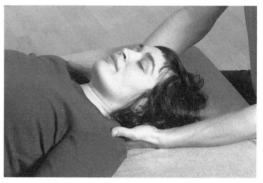

Figure 10.5. Relaxing the muscles of the nape of the neck using two-by-four fingers and palpating the shoulders with the thumbs.

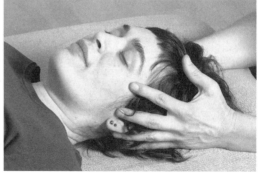

Figure 10.6. Cranial vault hold, listening to the craniosacral rhythm.

client, via the sacrum. Alternative: relaxation of the dural tube with client lying on her side and balancing the craniosacral rhythm (see section 10.8.6, below, and figs. 10.13 and 10.14).

- Compare craniosacral rhythm at the beginning and now.
- How does the client feel now compared to how she felt at the beginning?

When evaluating and treating a pregnant client, craniosacral practitioners should make use of all the avenues known to them: how free or restricted are the locomotor system, craniosacral system and rhythm, and organs? With specific regard to the pelvis, you should evaluate whether there are any signs present such as a difference in leg length, pelvic torsion, marked pelvic tilt, and motion restriction of the lumbosacral joint, symphysis or sacroiliac joints, sacrum, and coccyx. Attention should also be paid to the level of the fasciae, muscles, and bones surrounding these structures, which should also be assessed and treated. Once you have carried out the local assessment and treatment, you should, of course, evaluate and harmonize the craniosacral system as a whole and its rhythm. If possible, this should be done on the bony, membranous, CSF, and fluid levels.

In the first months of pregnancy, it is also helpful to assess the pelvic floor and neighboring muscles and organs for mobility and freedom from tension, and to give treatment as appropriate. The whole pelvis is then freer of dysfunctions, and the craniosacral rhythm is more even. This eases the pregnancy and encourages an easier delivery. Pay particular attention to freedom of movement of the pelvis and sacrum, a relaxed coccygeal region, and free flow between segments.

The following specific treatments are also performed gently. Apply the touch slowly, calculating it in such a way that the connective tissue or bone level, for example, receives definite touch and the invitation to adjust in a more relaxed direction. Do so without exerting pressure and in no way mechanically. You should allow the bodily structure sufficient time to react to your treatment invitation in a relaxed way

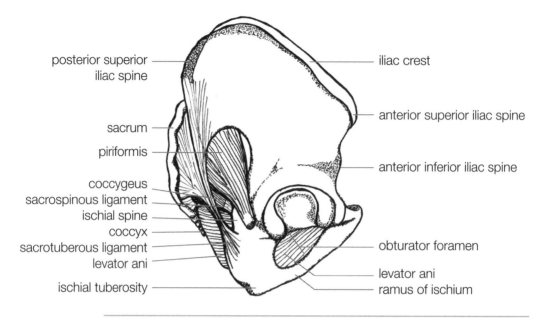

Figure 10.7. Lateral view of the pelvis, showing muscles.

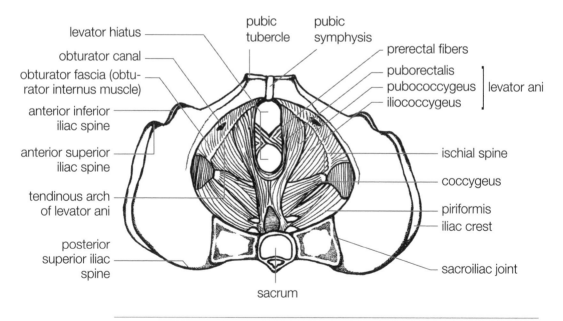

Figure 10.8. Muscles and fasciae of the pelvic floor.

and to find a more balanced position; the aim here is to enable an increase in mobility and rhythm and thus vitality.

10.8. More Specific Treatments That Can Be Used in Combination

I recommend that these techniques not be used in isolation but introduced by first treating a pleasant part of the body as brief preparation. If you start by asking, "Which part of your body feels most pleasant and comfortable at the moment?" the client becomes involved in her treatment. The well-being at that location is then established more deeply in her body awareness. Following this, you should apply one or more of the following release techniques and perhaps round off the treatment at another location, for example at the occipital bone, shoulders, or feet.

10.8.1. Peripheral Relief of Stress in the Pelvic and Abdominal Region (Patient Supine or Lying on Her Side); Relief of Stress on the Trunk via the Thighs

- Apply touch on the front of both thighs, your hands taking up contact with the muscles of the thigh through the client's clothing and skin. Then, slowly and without sliding, exert a definite pull in the direction of the knees. This also relaxes the neighboring structure on the ventral side of the pelvis, for example the groin, pelvis, and lower abdominal region (see fig. 10.9).
- Apply touch to the back of both thighs and slowly apply a slight hint of a pull in the direction of the knees. This stretches and relaxes the neighboring structure on the dorsal side of the pelvis, such as the sacroiliac joints, sacrum, and lumbar region.
- Slowly, raise both of the client's thighs slightly, from the back of the thigh, and then, just as slowly, administer a gentle downward traction. This has the effect of relieving stress on both hips, the

bony structure of the pelvis, and the vertebral bodies and disks of the lumbar vertebrae. It stretches and relaxes the entire pelvic and abdominal region. It also slightly stretches the psoas major muscle, running from the thigh through the pelvis to below the diaphragm, with attachments of the various parts of the muscle on the lumbar spine.

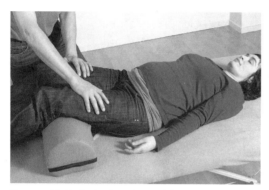

Figure 10.9. Relaxing the pelvis via the thighs.

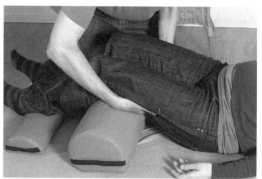

Figure 10.10. Hand position at the back of the thighs.

- Take a position beside the treatment table, approximately level with the client's pelvis. Place your cephalad hand sideways relative to the lumbar region; you can allow your fingertips to touch the lumbar vertebrae, but do not exert any pressure. With this hand, and all the fingers, make touch contact with the tissue and mold them to its tone. With your caudal free hand, relieve the stress of one leg by lifting the thigh as before. What do you sense with one hand, and with the other? What is happening in the tissue between your hands? Listen with the hands for a few moments and then slowly begin gentle traction on the thigh toward the feet. As you do so, continue to listen with the hand on the client's lumbar region. You may sense the traction or an individual reaction by the tissue of the client's body. What happens in the tissue between your hands during the gentle traction? What is the client's breathing like? Can she sense this traction, and if so, does it feel right? What does the client feel? Ask her. Change to the other side of the treatment table and administer relief and relaxation to the other side of the client's body in the same way.

10.8.2. Relief of Stress at the Shoulder Blades

The client should be in the supine position. The practitioner sits at the head of the treatment table.

If using a soft massage table, push both hands down into the soft surface and position them under the client's shoulder blades. If using a hard treatment table, put your hands under her upper arms, either side of her rib cage, and ask her to assist by raising one shoulder to enable you to place one hand under that shoulder blade, and then the same with the other. Spread your fingers and grasp the whole shoulder blade. Adjust your position so that you are sitting at the table in the most relaxed possible posture. You may want to move your head slightly to the side to avoid breathing into the client's face.

Let the weight of your hands and the client's shoulder blades as well as all the weight pass down onto the padded surface and onward to the table itself. Allow your hands to be carried as if floating like corks in water. Your hands are free, moving in concert with every slight motion of the tissue. Also observe the client's breathing and sense her respiratory

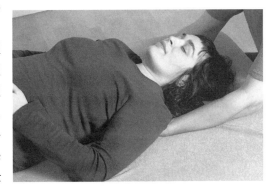

Figure 10.11. Relaxing the shoulder blades.

movements in this position from time to time with your hands. After a while, your fingertips around the shoulder blades can make more definite contact with the tissue and muscles so that you sense the muscle tone around the shoulder blades. With the warmth and softness of your touch, tensions begin to resolve. At this point, listen to the micromovements of the tissue, respiratory movement, and, if it can be sensed, the craniosacral rhythm or slower rhythms.

10.8.3. Treatments to Relieve Stresses of the Lumbar Region and Avoid Pronounced Lordosis

There is a simple and effective method of relieving stress in the muscles and spinal column in the lumbar region:

- Position 1: position your hands so that your fingertips touch the latissimus dorsi muscle. You should be touching the tissue over the broad surface of your fingers and hands. Use a definite but at the same time spacious touch so that you can sense the muscle tension of the lumbar region. Listen with your hands and sense how the tensions begin to release in response to your warm, soft touch.
- Position 2: position your hands so that as far as possible, your fingertips touch the regions between the transverse processes.
- Position 3: position your hands still further medially, so that as far as possible, your fingertips gently touch the regions between the spinous processes.

Even when using positions 2 or 3, you should not put any pressure on the vertebral bodies or the lumbar region, but touch in a manner that is at once encompassing, definite, and gentle. Here too you should wait until the vertebral bodies feel freer in response to your warm, soft touch—possibly also spontaneously performing dancing micromovements—and the lumbar spine and muscles of the region are freed of tensions.

10.8.4. Harmonization of the Craniosacral Rhythm at the Sacrum and Sides of the Pelvis

The client should be lying on her side. The practitioner sits to the side of the treatment table. Place one hand on the client's sacrum, with clarity and without pressure, and palpate the motions of flexion and extension. Meanwhile, with the other hand on the side of the pelvis that is on top, palpate the external and internal rotation of the hip bone. Tune in to the motions of the craniosacral rhythm. Taking the more balanced motion as your reference, invite the structure that is less free to become similarly free. Always work with the rhythm, never against it. Then harmonize the other side in the same way.

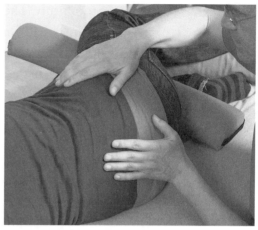

Figure 10.12. Position for treating the sacrum and sides of the pelvis.

10.8.5. Treating the Sitting Bones with the Patient Seated

The sitting bones or ischial tuberosities have attachments to several muscles and ligaments. The semitendinosus and semimembranosus muscles as well as the long head of the biceps femoris have their origin here. It is also the point of attachment of the sacrotuberous ligament, which runs from the ischium to the sacrum and from there to the posterior inferior side of the pelvis (see figs. 10.7 and 10.8). During pregnancy there is a change in the balance of static forces acting on the abdomen and pelvis. There is a loosening of the connections in the female pelvis through the effect of hormones. Various muscles and ligaments that have held the pelvis stably fixed for many years may remain very tense and can be painful. They play a part in producing back pain in the lumbar and sacral regions.

Before relieving these structures, I recommend beginning at the thighs or knees. Briefly apply touch and relax tensions there first. Beginning in this way provides preparation; without it, treatment of the sitting bones in isolation can have a very strong effect. This is especially true if the treatment is administered in a mechanical manner for too long or too firmly. The body is better able to integrate the release of tension in the pelvic floor region if it is preceded and followed by treatment of peripheral tissue and other sections of the body.

Place your hands under the sitting bones so that your fingertips can slowly sink in directly at the medial border of the ischial tuberosities. As they do, allow plenty of time for the tissue to yield and soften. Then you can perform slow, rotating movements in a semicircle two or three times around the tuberosities with your fingertips. After doing so, pause again to give yourself and the client time to sense the body once more. Finally, with your fingertips medially on the ischial tuberosities, slowly administer a sensitive hint of traction in the lateral direction.

This has the effect of making the inferior pelvic aperture and its muscles, fasciae, and ligaments, especially the sacrotuberous and sacrospinous ligaments, more flexible. For a pregnant woman suffering lower back pain, this relieves tension and is helpful for her and the baby at the time of birth.

10.8.6. Sacrum–Occipital Bone Technique

Position: the client should be lying on her side with appropriate support (see fig. 10.12). The practitioner should be positioned to the side of the treatment table, facing the client's back. Place your elbows or arms on the table to create a fulcrum. This will help you to palpate and treat in a relaxed way over the next three to ten minutes. Place one hand on the client's occiput and the other on the sacrum.

1. Cradle the structure, letting your hands begin to merge with these two key bones of the craniosacral system. The pleasant sensation of touch at the occiput and sacrum in itself encourages relaxation because a large number of parasympathetic nerves pass through these regions, and these are activated. Listen for a while at these two locations. You may choose from time to time to listen in a targeted way to the sensations and motions at the occipital bone, then at the sacrum, then once more equally at both key bones.

2. Listen to the slow motions of the craniosacral rhythm, around six to twelve cycles per minute. The occipital bone and sacrum perform an equal slow-motion rocking movement: in the flexion phase, the squama of the occipital bone becomes fuller and broader across its width and at the same time moves slightly caudally. The superior part of the sacrum tips posteriorly, and the inferior tip moves anteriorly. In the extension phase, both of these key bones move in the opposite direction: the occipital bone becomes slightly narrower across its width and moves slightly cephalad. At the same time, the superior part of the sacrum moves slightly anteriorly and the inferior tip glides slightly away from the pelvis in a posterior direction. Listen for several minutes to the slow rocking motions of the craniosacral rhythm, noting especially whether it becomes stronger and more even. Then, as appropriate, you can emphasize the motions slightly, always going with the rhythm, never against it. As you do so, you should not exert any pressure at the level of the bones but instead follow the motion that appears, supporting it in its upward or downward tendency and intensifying it. Having done so, listen in the same position to sense whether the craniosacral rhythm appears to be more even. Then slowly remove your hands.

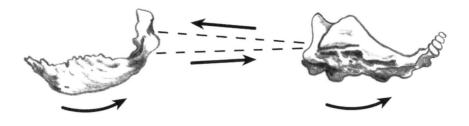

Figure 10.13. Simplified outline of the direction of motion of the occipital bone and the sacrum in flexion.

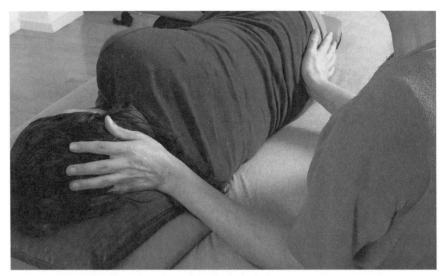

Figure 10.14. Position for the sacrum–occipital bone technique.

10.8.7. Relaxing the Trochanter and the Knees and Feet

The client should be lying on her side. It's important that if the client is suffering from severe sciatic pain, this treatment should only be carried out by experienced practitioners.

Stand at the side of the treatment table, facing the client's back, level with her hips. Relax each hip individually. More precisely, the area to be relaxed is the tissue around the greater trochanter. The client should be lying close to the edge of the table. Establish clear contact with the whole of the tissue at depth, without exerting pressure on the hip joint. If the client feels the contact is clear and pleasant, begin to relax as much of the tissue as possible by making slow circling movements without letting your hands slide. Carry out these relaxing movements alternately clockwise and counterclockwise. They may sometimes give rise to slight movements of the entire pelvis. Vary the strength of pressure and the movement, which should always be felt by the client as clearly relaxing and agreeably within the range of comfort.

The client should then turn onto her other side, and treatment of the other hip is carried out in the same way.

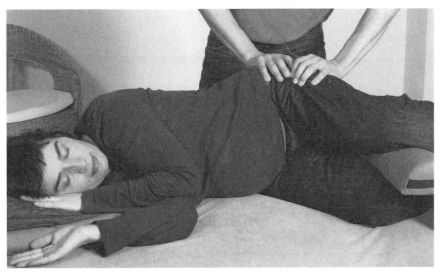

Figure 10.15. Relaxing the tissue around the trochanter.

10.8.8. Treating the Course of the Sciatic Nerve with the Client Seated

Method: as the practitioner, you have to be positioned sufficiently high, as in standing at the treatment table, to be able to use your body weight. This part of the treatment follows the previous section, once you have relaxed the tissue around the greater trochanter and helped to improve pelvic mobility. Place both of your thumbs and thenar eminences, parallel and touching, immediately beneath the hip joint with your thumbs pointing caudad. First, slide the broad area of your thumbs and thenar eminences into the depth of the muscle tissue. This spreads the tissue in both directions laterally and so relaxes it. Following this lateral stretching, return your thumbs to their initial position. Next, without losing contact at depth, slowly stretch the thigh muscles along their length in the direction of the knee and foot. Then, and not until then, slowly release the contact with the depths of the tissue. Work down the length of the lateral musculature of the thigh to the knee, applying the same method. This has the indirect effect of relaxing and stretching the sciatic nerve.

Omit the region immediately around the knee. Continue to apply the touch of both thumbs and thenar eminences below the knee, sinking in between the calf muscle and the shin bone, then relaxing the musculature, along with those sections of the sciatic nerve lying below it, laterally and stretching it along its length, in the same way as before.

The ankle joint, as with the knee, is omitted. However, the tissue around the ankle joint can be massaged on both sides.

Then massage the instep of the foot and spread the anterior part of the foot, where divisions of the sciatic nerve branch out. Ask the client for feedback from time to time as to the intensity of the massage. This should always be clearly relaxing and agreeably within the range of comfort.

The client should then turn onto her other side, and treatment of the other leg and sciatic nerve should be carried out in the same way to widen and relax the tissue.

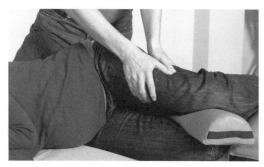

Figure 10.16. Relaxing the lateral thigh muscles.

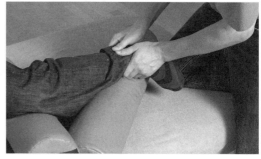

Figure 10.17. Relaxing the tissue around the ankle and Achilles tendon.

10.8.9. Visceral Treatment for Heartburn

Pregnant women often suffer from heartburn, especially in advanced pregnancy. In such cases, treatment can be given to the diaphragm, esophagus, stomach, duodenum, liver, gallbladder and spleen with the client in the side-lying position. If the client is supine, the upper body should be elevated and supported.

THE PRENATAL PERIOD: FROM CONCEPTION TO MATURE FETUS

11

The period of development of the embryo lasts until the tenth or twelfth week of gestation. From then on the unborn child is called a fetus. There are various ways of understanding the growth of the child in the mother's body: morphological, phenomenological, and spiritual; all are fascinating. Morphology is the study of the form and structure of the human being, of how the body is formed and built. Phenomenology can be seen as the understanding of being in the sense of the intuitive mental aspect as opposed to the rational.

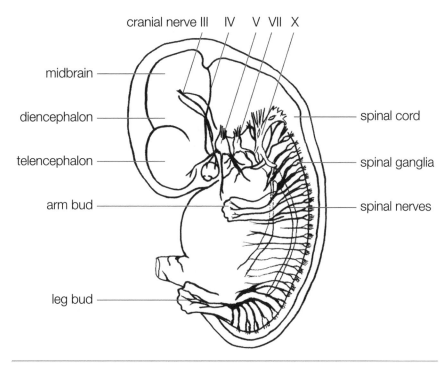

Figure 11.1. Embryo at around the end of the eighth week.

11.1. Biodynamic Metabolic Processes

The embryologist Erich Blechschmidt conducted decades of research into the development of the human embryo. He concluded that the differentiation and the associated molecular processes that take place in the embryo are biodynamically determined. Gene function is passive, since even the first processes in germ-cell differentiation occur in response to stimuli arriving from outside via the cell membrane. Growth and differentiation are an externally stimulated process that has a direction. The earliest functions and actions of the human embryo are its developmental motions. Differentiation then leads to motions of growth. It would therefore be wrong to think of the human body and the person as gradually becoming a unified entity; from the very earliest stage of development it is a united whole. This is true in several respects: a holistic entity in the process of becoming, a material reality, and a being that is growing, has a spiritual nature, and is spiritually active. Differentiation means development, and development means growth. This in turn is enabled by various formative forces, and various tensile and compressive forces are involved in the process. The tensile forces operate mainly on the surface, and the compressive forces act in the interior of the cells, producing a change in form. Blechschmidt identified three principles of embryonic development:

- The spiritual nature is practiced in advance.
- Developmental motions are actions performed.
- Nothing is performed without resistance.

Before we, as newborn babies, perform the actions of touch, breathing, and movement, we have already experienced and practiced growth movements—actual developmental gestures—as embryo and fetus. Jaap van der Wal, the anatomist and founder of holistic "embryosophy," quotes the philosopher Julien Offray de la Mettrie in this regard when he says that the human beings "do not have a soul; we are a soul."[1]

Various formative and regulatory forces exert a determining influence on the development of the embryo. These are assumed to include the capacity of fluid crystal structures to store information, electromagnetic fields, biophoton fields, and morphogenetic fields—which, according to Rupert Sheldrake, have a "morphic resonance."[2] All of these can either develop morphogenetic properties or be involved in them. The embryo develops among the immense forces of polarity and along with them. Differentiation and the creation of space are constantly taking place.

Movements that have a formative effect on the human body are generated by deep, organized motions in the cytoplasm. They function as a continuum in the human body, becoming oriented in relation to a functional midline. These movements are thought to arise from the potency of the Breath of Life, primary respiration. It is possible to sense primary respiration at the level of the Long Tide, with its one-hundred-second cycle. This is the level at which a life is conceived—the level of incarnation—and at this level the Breath of Life is thought to act on every living thing on earth, ordering and creating form with a kind of comprehensive building plan, breathing life into the living being. The Long Tide and mid-tide and their inherent potency exert a rhythmic and energizing influence on the protoplasm and cytoplasm.

11.2. Formation and Development of the Embryo and Fetus

In each menstrual cycle, ten to one hundred follicles begin to mature. After ovulation, the egg passes from the ovary into the fallopian tube. The conditions that exist prior to conception, meaning before the egg is fertilized, continue for several hours. The egg remains in the fallopian tube for up to twenty hours, waiting to be fertilized by sperm. Sperm take an hour or less to reach the fallopian tube.

On fertilization, the two cell nuclei fuse to create a new whole. One understanding of what happens is that the sperm does not penetrate the egg, but rather the surface tension of the cell membrane changes so as to open the egg to one particular sperm. Powerful metabolic processes occur inside the egg cell to enable the sperm to move onward toward the center, where it has to pass through a second, thinner layer for fusion to take place. Fertilization occurs when the sperm reaches the central nucleus of the egg. The nuclei of both cells fuse, forming a cell with a complete chromosome set. Fertilization therefore produces an entire organism in which differentiation and division then take place. There is a change in relative surface, volume, and proportions. Construction of the greater organism is not the work of the cells but of the whole—the work of the organism by means of division, differentiation, and organization.

Shortly after fertilization the cells begin to divide, producing an assembly of cells called a morula, which travels down the fallopian tube for about four days toward the uterus. A fluid-filled cavity develops in the center; it is now a blastocyst. Around seven days after fertilization there is a change in the membranes, which become looser and ready to implant in the wall of the uterus. The inner cells are now around 150 in number, and it is from these that the baby will develop. The outer cells will form the placenta and amniotic sac.

In the second week of gestation, it develops a two-chambered form with a germ disc, and complete implantation begins. Around fourteen days after conception, the fertilized egg is strongly embedded in the wall of the uterus and continues to grow quickly. The amniotic cavity and the yolk sac take shape, with the double-layered germ disc between them. A "primitive streak" appears on the surface. Soon after this, a third germ layer forms, and the neural tube, gut, and circulatory system begin to develop. The ectoderm of the disc folds inward, and the three-chambered form takes shape. A field develops around the head of the embryo, and the primitive human heart takes shape. Around the twentieth day, the earliest brain activity is already thought to be present, and three weeks after fertilization, the embryonic heart begins to beat. The closing of the neural tube and the development of the brain vesicles develop. Shortly after this, two brain hemispheres are already present. Segmentation into head, neck, and trunk begins in the fourth week, and the ventral abdominal wall closes. The embryo's head, trunk, eyes, and the first indication of hands and feet become evident. The major organ systems develop: brain, spinal cord and nerves, gut, muscles, and skeleton. The tip of the nose can be distinguished; nerves run to the muscles, and the embryo reacts to stimuli by making movements.

From the seventh week, the network of the brain begins to take shape, and after eight weeks of life the sense of smell and taste, the trigeminal nerve, and the spinal cord begin to develop. All the primordial structures are formed after eight to ten weeks, including the heart, with atria and ventricles, and the liver, with both lobes. The eyelids and palms of the hands are sensitive to touch. Soon, the eyelids close, and the eyes do not open again until the sixth or seventh month. The umbilical cord is formed. The skeleton is still mainly cartilaginous and slowly begins to ossify. The first reflex movements of the embryo's muscles of facial expression are seen. In the third month of pregnancy, around ten to twelve weeks after ovulation, the embryonic phase comes to an end. The embryo is about one inch long. The upper part of the head is relatively large, and the facial region small. The embryo has thin limbs. Its form and organ system are already present, and the remaining twenty-eight to thirty weeks in utero are devoted to maturation and growth. In the embryo, the red blood cells have the role of "workers," carrying all the materials needed to build the body, proteins, fat, amino acids, calcium, and phosphates. The cells then begin to order these materials in molecular layers to form three-dimensional structures, for example, according to the instructions from the DNA.

The first cranial bones form from the third month onward at the border of the cartilaginous cranial base. At the end of the third month the fetus can move its lips and turn its head. Its hearing and sense of balance begin to develop. Sucking, swallowing, and breathing reflexes are present, and the fetus can kick with its legs, curl and spread its toes, make a fist, and wrinkle its forehead. The fetus is now around five inches long and weighs just four ounces. It will soon begin to suck its thumb. The differences between males and females become visible. In the fourth month the fetus can stretch and bend, turn, and perform somersaults. The first reactions to sensory stimuli become evident—for example, the fetus might move toward the place where a hand is stroking the abdomen. The cochlea of the inner ear has reached its definitive size. In the fifth month the fetus is around eight inches long; it floats in the amniotic sac within its mother's body and is already beginning to develop good hearing. By now, if not earlier, the mother can feel her baby's first movements. Brain-wave activity can be demonstrated, and the fetus is capable of feeling pain.

In the sixth month, the unborn child weighs about eighteen ounces and is around thirteen inches long. It appears to alternate between sleep and wakefulness, with sleep predominating and accompanied by periods of dreaming rapid eye movement. The primordial teeth develop. The length of the nasal septum increases sevenfold between the tenth and the fortieth week. When a boy is sucking his thumb, at this stage he may even have an erection, which suggests that oxytocin is being released. In the sixth or seventh month, the eyes open, and the fetus is able to orient itself spatially. The amniotic sac contains a great deal of fluid, enabling the fetus to "float" freely. The baby's body weight doubles within a period of about six weeks. The mother may experience practice contractions or prelabor pains—a sign that her body is preparing for birth. Ultrasound examinations have shown that twins may be active inside their mother's body, playing together and displaying tenderness. During the eighth month, the maturation of important organ systems, such as the lungs, is almost complete. The baby's weight is now increasing by around seven ounces each week, and its head may already be positioned downward toward the pelvic aperture.

In the ninth month, the baby has rounded out and continues to accumulate fat stores, with a weight increase of around 3.5 ounces per week. Brain activity increases again, and eye movements are well coordinated. Hormones prepare the uterus and cervix for the birth. Hormonal signals from the fetus and from the placenta trigger the birth.

11.3. The Germ Layers and the Development of the Nervous System

From the second week of gestation, a special differentiation and transformation takes place. Three different layers of cells, the three germ layers, are formed, and it is from these that the individual bodily structures will develop. The outer germ layer, the ectoderm, will form the brain and sensory organs; the middle layer, called the mesoderm, forms the cranial base and vault; and the inner layer or endoderm mainly forms the mucous membranes and digestive organs.

11.3.1. Germ Layers and Regions Formed from Them

Ectoderm, Outer Germ Layer—Amniotic Epithelium:

- CNS: brain and spinal cord
- the entire nervous system, parts of the eyes, lenses, ears, nose
- skin: epidermis, with hair and glands
- mesectoderm, ectomesenchyme, and paraganglia, including adrenal medulla

Mesoderm, Middle Germ Layer—Cranial Base and Vault, Notochord, Somites, Lateral Plates:

- support tissue: connective tissue, cartilage, tendons
- muscle tissue: smooth and striated muscle, including heart muscle, which is also to some extent from neural crest material

- lymphatic and blood vascular system: blood, vessels, heart, spleen, lymph nodes, bone marrow
- genitourinary system: kidneys, urinary tract collection system as far as the bladder, gonads without gametes, ductus deferens, ejaculatory duct, uterus, fallopian tubes
- adrenal cortex

Endoderm, Inner Germ Layer—Yolk Sac, Allantois:

- mucous membranes of the digestive tract, respiratory system, and investment of the organs below
- gastrointestinal tract, including associated glands of the liver, bile ducts, and pancreas
- esophagus, posterior third of the buccal cavity
- thyroid, parathyroid glands, epithelium of the palatine tonsils, mammary glands, auditory tubes, and epithelium of the tympanic cavity
- respiratory organs: epithelium and glands of the lungs, bronchial tree, trachea, and larynx
- lower urinary tract: bladder, urethra, urachus

The notochord is the primitive axial rod, the axial mesoderm or central axis of the embryonic body in the process of formation. It does not differentiate further into organs but induces the development of the first major organ system of the embryo in the overlying ectoderm; this is the primordial nervous system.

11.4. The Importance of the Prenatal Period for Our Lives

The outstanding medical research of recent decades and the imaging procedures developed during this time have enabled us to discover a great deal about the biological development of the embryo and fetus.

In comparison relatively little is known about the world of the emotions and the mental and spiritual dimension in the prenatal and perinatal period. The research and publications of Otto Rank, Thomas R. Verny, Peter Nathanielsz, Alessandra Piontelli, Ludwig Janus, and Stanislav Grof, along with other courageous pioneers, have played an important part in building a comprehensive understanding of the prenatal and perinatal period.

By no means is the information contained in the parental genes the only factor that determines the growth of the embryo and fetus. Its cells and genes are influenced by other factors, above all the inner attitude and emotional state, nutrition, and everyday life. Genetic information is then activated and read, or not. Another influence that seems to me to be at least as important is one that has been demonstrated in numerous experiments: according to Thomas R. Verny, the child is constantly attuned to its mother's every action, thought, and feeling, regardless of whether the child is awake or asleep. The child's experience in its mother's body influences the growth of the brain and nervous system. Stress in the mother activates stress hormones for a fight-or-flight reaction. These signals produce reactions in the same organs in the fetus as in the mother. In response to stress, therefore, blood supply to the hindbrain, arms, and legs increases to enable protective reflexes to be put into action instantly. This inhibits the development of the forebrain and reduces blood supply to the viscera.

These early experiences remain a lifelong presence, so it is always a very touching experience to be allowed to follow prenatal and perinatal experiences in adults. Warm water rebirthing, in which the client, accompanied by appropriate support, breathes underwater through a snorkel, opens up memories from the world of prenatal experience. The water is at body temperature. It represents the nourishing female element, and it enables a weightless experience of dimensions like those experienced for so long during the time we spent inside our mothers' bodies. The intention in this case is not regression or return to the protection of our mothers' bodies but rather to enable a retrospective link to be made with our prenatal and perinatal roots. As adults we can reexperience the ancient and fundamental trust that may have become diminished or lost through our personal histories. We can then integrate it into our present-day lives. We can also consciously experience difficult prenatal and perinatal situations in the security of the here and now. The practitioner accompanies the therapeutic process in a resource-based manner. This resource-oriented approach is particularly helpful in the unburdening of high trauma energy from the nervous system and cell memory. Embryological and prenatal experiences can also be accessed in craniosacral treatments, especially the Breath of Life principle, which works with the fluid body. This surrounds us even as an embryo.

Experience with breathwork therapies such as Rebirthing and conscious breathing, established by Leonard Orr, and holotropic breathwork, established by Stanislav Grof, have proved helpful to many people to enable them to process prenatal and perinatal trauma. Grof's definition of transpersonal psychology enlarged psychotherapy by giving it an archetypal and transcendental dimension. The chanting of mantras and the integration of the elements of earth, fire, water, and air, as in Rebirthing, were also used, thus including the spiritual dimension rather than considering only the physical or psychological level.

Something that has been very helpful to me personally has been the way that various therapeutic methods of humanistic psychology have opened up prenatal and perinatal worlds of experience, usually unintentionally. I discovered biographical connections that I found to be operating through to the present. This has helped me in my therapeutic support of groups and patients. I know feelings of helplessness or anxiety just as I also know powerful and joyful feelings or the boundless ocean, and as a therapist I am able to tune in to them.

The contact with our earliest prenatal experience can become a conscious link back, enabling greater trust in our lives and a greater ability to experience things on a spiritual level. It brings the sense of being supported and securely held in worldly reality as well as cosmic reality. In this way the experiences that were ours in the period before birth are integrated into our lives as adults, and we can know them in the form of bonds with other people, animals, nature, and the cosmos. We experience a transformation of that all-embracing and nourishing placenta, that place within our mothers' bodies that was our constant home; now, as human individuals, we feel at home on mother earth. We know ourselves to be supported, surrounded, and perhaps cared for by this great and nurturing primeval mother, Amba. Consciously or unconsciously, where our confidence may perhaps have been fragile, we regain that ancient trust.

BONDING DURING PREGNANCY

12

The close emotional relationship between mother and child begins to form during pregnancy. While the child is still in the amniotic sac, it can already sense protection or threat. It can hear the mother's heartbeat, slow and relaxed or accelerated and tense. The mother's emotional state influences the secretion of pleasure or stress hormones. When she feels stressed, this instantly causes increased production of cortisol, a stress hormone. If this is present in her bloodstream, it also reaches the fetus. Some of the cortisol is absorbed and affects the development of the nervous system. The unborn child both hears and senses whether its mother is singing, crying, or angry. Especially during the second half of the pregnancy, the unborn child also senses whether its mother is constantly active or agitated, or whether she is allowing herself enough time to rest, be calm, and turn her emotional attention to the child, talking to it and reaching out to it with a loving touch. During the prenatal period of its life, the child knows itself to be peaceful and protected, effortlessly receiving nourishment.

The child's development as an individual, the influences that form its character, and the process of bonding therefore begin before birth. The fundamental existential conditions during our early development determine the way we perceive and experience the world today. The child in its mother's womb is sensitive and can feel and react to its environment from a remarkably early stage. Although the fetus has its own independent circulatory system, it is highly dependent, for example for an adequate supply of oxygen. From the sixteenth week on, the unborn child reacts to acoustic stimulation with a change in heartbeat; in the sixth month it can display a shocked reaction in which it raises its hands. Parents need to remember, when using cell phones or in an environment full of ringtones and other sources of noise, that sound affects the fetus. The unborn child is highly sensitive to sound, in addition to the fact that these devices generate electromagnetic fields.

Appropriate stimulation is, of course, important for brain development; however, stimulation should be as pleasurable and balanced as possible: neither too little nor too often, neither too hectic nor too monotonous, and with anything that could be frightening kept to a minimum. Remember the importance of the limbic system—the "emotional brain"—in the fetus. Before the child is born, the amygdalae are already storing emotions such as fear and fright. Of course, it is not always possible to avoid stress, and the unborn child learns to deal with it and react to it, but the effects of excessive stress while still in the womb are hardly beneficial, either on the growth of the child or on its later equilibrium. The effects can be felt as a baby, as a small child, or as an adolescent, and problems can be expressed in the form of hyperactivity or a greater tendency to violence.

The sense of touch, sense of smell, and sense of hearing are all important for the baby's ability to recognize its mother before and after it is born. A newborn recognizes languages and melodies that it has heard previously while still in the womb. Gentle, loving touch to the mother's abdomen also stimulates the unborn child's rapidly developing brain. Even before birth, the child develops all kinds of skills that it practices during the prenatal stage and which continue to develop further after it is born. Today, it is accepted as an established fact that prenatal and perinatal experiences influence the psyche, development, and health of the individual.

12.1. Prenatal Stress and Trauma: Occurrence and Effects

The development and birth of a child are a gift of existence, with a background of evolutionary development and biodynamics. In all living processes, however, there can be certain situations or phases in which development does not proceed lightly and easily but with difficulty and even with some risk to life. Consumption of alcohol during its early developmental stages can harm the embryo, although this is not an area where I want to moralize or expand on the various pathologies, which are fully dealt with in the medical literature. I do, however, want to make readers, especially parents and practitioners, more fully aware of the spiritual and emotional world of experience of the unborn child. We know that prenatal trauma can affect the brain and nervous system. The resulting states vary in duration, but their effect can be life-threatening, and this gives the unborn child the sense that it is going to die. Examples of these influences are difficulties in the implantation of the embryo, hemorrhage or inadequate supply of oxygen during pregnancy, and a sense of constriction and hunger during the birth. The last of these produces marked activation of the child's entire nervous system, and this is stored in the cell memory.

In one case known to me, a pregnant woman experienced severe bleeding because she was subjecting herself to too much physical stress building a new house. The unexpected bleeding caused her anxiety about the unborn child and stress during the emergency hospital examination. The doctor performing the examination was helpful, but he was a nonnative speaker with a poor command of the language. This led to communication difficulties; he did not understand whether the woman wanted an injection to end the pregnancy or not. In the end the child survived, but later the birth was a traumatic experience. Existential fears in the prenatal period cause stress to the unborn child. These can be reactivated during the next existential threat—birth—which can intensify the power of shock and trauma on the physical level as well as the mental and spiritual level.

The "vanishing twin" is a phenomenon that has been increasingly recognized. It occurs in the first three to four months of fetal development. It is estimated that as many as thirty percent of pregnancies begin as twin pregnancies, but in the early months one of the twins may not even be seen in ultrasound scans. This may be because no one is looking for a twin, or because the twins do not have the same placenta and are positioned differently. Sometimes, however, both twins are seen, but later on, only one child is present.

Observations made by the conventional medical physician Alessandra Piontelli in her studies of twins were both touching and tragic.[3] From a certain stage of development onward, twins behave in a loving way toward each other; they are gentle and play together, or they have conflict and fight. There is a close connection between them as early as the embryonic stage and during the first three or four months. However, during this period the twin pregnancy often goes unnoticed, and it often ends with the loss of one twin. It may be expelled together with vaginal bleeding, or if the fetus is dead it may become compressed and remain only as an insignificant appendage to the placenta. One way of looking at the vanishing-twin phenomenon from a spiritual angle is to think that sometimes, one twin has the companionship of the other for a little while, like a kind of guardian angel. It is as if the angel companion is there for a time to give help in finding the way, and having completed this task, takes its leave. For the surviving sibling, the vanishing twin is felt as a loss that can continue to have a mental and spiritual effect on all stages of development into adulthood. Emotionally, an experience of this kind that has been incompletely dealt with can cause the person to feel incomplete as a child and as an adult. Individuals may have the sense that something is lacking and may subconsciously replay the scene of losses experienced in early life, or the effects may take the form of loneliness and grief, fear of loss, and unsatisfactory relationships.

Usually unresolved issues are reflected in everyday life unconsciously. These problems are resolved not by regression but by working with the themes and associated bodily sensations that arise momentarily as they occur. This is another situation where Craniosacral Therapy and other methods of trauma healing offer ways of processing the problem using resource-oriented means. In this way the stressful situation can become an opportunity for growth and transformation.

Athanassios Kafkalides developed the idea that the mother's body can be "accepting" or "rejecting."[1] In a pregnancy that is unwanted, the result of sexual assault, or the outcome of a failed abortion, the child may later feel unhappy, unwanted, constricted, blocked, or rejected and may be at risk of suicide.

The psychologist Stanislav Grof, founder of the International Transpersonal Association (ITA), defined the psychological and physical experience of the individual stages of the birth process from the point of view of the child in terms of four birth matrices,[2] described in section 14.4. Critical situations representing a threat to the survival of the unborn child can arise in the embryonic, fetal, prenatal, and perinatal stage.

In that timeless period of its nine-month gestation, the child undergoes many metamorphoses. At the end of the journey, it bids farewell to its familiar surroundings and makes the transition to a new world. It is a kind of death and rebirth. If life-threatening situations arise, this can produce intense feelings of separation, isolation, or destruction. The prenatal and perinatal processes leave their mark in individual ways on the biological, neurobiological, emotional-spiritual, and social levels. Conditions and experiences around the time of birth make a lasting mark that helps to form the child's character.

When encountering difficult topics, however, parents and family members—as well as the practitioner—can establish contact with the client's sources of strength and should remember that those affected have in most cases survived. There is no longer the risk to life that there was in the past, even if the body and the subconscious still remember it. There is the chance for those involved to seek out the energy and the themes associated with the birth trauma, free themselves from them, and thus integrate them.

During the great growth phases that take place in childhood, the child repeatedly experiences times of transition and threshold events and assesses these on the basis of past experience. If the child can free itself from difficult prenatal and perinatal experiences early on, there will be fewer conscious or unconscious fears to weigh on it. There will be much more confidence in life, and the child will have greater freedom to experience, to learn, to make strategic choices, and so on. During the stages that mark the milestones of development— including weaning, learning to walk, relating to siblings, starting day care or kindergarten and then school, and especially puberty—earlier stressful experiences can be reactivated, but they can also be integrated. The relief experienced and the new options for decision-making greatly assist the child's development, bring greater joy, and strengthen resilience.

12.2. The Benefits and Limitations of Prenatal Diagnosis

With prenatal diagnosis, potential diseases, disabilities, and malformations can be recognized early. The risk of Down syndrome, for example, or other serious chromosomal abnormalities can be assessed. Testing can help allay an expectant mother's fears, but it can also exacerbate them and present parents with the anxiety of a difficult decision. Some parents and midwives believe that about three ultrasound exams and a blood test for the mother should be sufficient during pregnancy, as long as there are no indications of serious risks. However, many expectant mothers face pressure from physicians, friends, colleagues, in-laws, and others to undergo as many precautionary tests as possible. These additional tests include ultrasound exams for malformations, nuchal translucency screening, amniocentesis, chorionic villus sampling, ultrasound exams, and triple screening. A mother-to-be who does not take advantage of all the tests available may be accused of not doing everything possible for her unborn child. She may even find her suitability to be a mother being questioned. Instead of encouraging confidence and joy at the prospect of motherhood and supporting her natural intuition, there is a disregard of her gut feeling, and worry and anxiety are stirred up in its place. The effect can be so extreme that the woman is no longer able to enjoy her pregnancy because fears and anxiety have taken over. Worry causes stress for the mother, and that in turn can affect the pregnancy and perhaps the timing and course of the birth.

It is increasingly the practice for women over age thirty-five to have an amniocentesis between the fourteenth and sixteenth week of pregnancy, especially if there is a specific risk factor. The gynecologist uses a hollow needle, with ultrasound monitoring, to extract amniotic fluid through the abdominal wall and the uterus. The fluid contains fetal cells that are then examined in a laboratory for any chromosomal abnormalities. Alternatively, chorionic villus sampling is used to extract placental tissue. Both procedures are invasive, and for the baby they mean an invasion of the protective barrier that surrounds it and represents its home. The fetus often reacts with a faster heartbeat, by moving to avoid the needle, or striking out against it with a hand. These reactions all show that this kind of test is experienced as a great threat or that the effect is trau-matic. There can be complications, such as loss of amniotic fluid and injury to the uterus or placenta, as well as an increased risk of later miscarriage (0.5–1 percent), especially if the amniocentesis is carried out before the fourteenth week.

Ultrasound instead of amniocentesis: it would be better to offer every woman the alternative of first-trimester screen-ing, as it is a gentler procedure. It can be done from the eleventh week. The

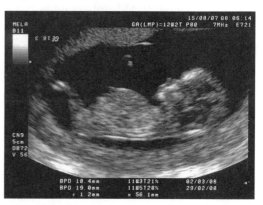

Figure 12.1. A baby in the eleventh week of gestation.

physician, using ultrasound, measures the nuchal fold of the fetus, among other elements. Other general screening tests are also carried out. Together with the maternal blood test, this combination of tests enables a number of important tests to be conducted with ninety percent certainty.

12.3. Gentle Preparation

During her pregnancy the mother will sometimes have had several Craniosacral Therapy sessions with a practitioner, who may also have given her some self-treatment methods to use periodically. The free flow of the breath, for example, creates changes in pressure that help the better return of oxygen-depleted blood to the heart from the lower half of the body, as the mother performs breathing exercises during pregnancy. These are helpful for her and the baby during the birth and can be an important resource. Prelabor pains, which are practice contractions, during the final weeks of the pregnancy prepare the baby for birth. The baby's whole body, including the head, is prepared for the stage when the baby emerges through the birth canal.

Around one-third of pregnancies last beyond the expected delivery date, which need not be cause for alarm. A birth is regarded as post-term if the pregnancy continues beyond forty-two weeks. The midwife may decide to strengthen the natural stimulation of labor using the CV4 technique and acupuncture and may recommend abdominal massage with natural essential oils such as ginger, cinnamon, clove, or vervain; stimulation of the nipples; or more physical movement by the mother. The midwife might demonstrate CV4 using soft juggling balls to be used as a self-help technique, or may suggest that the woman speak kindly to the child, explaining what is happening and inviting it to make its own effort to come into the world.

PRESENTATION AND
THE BIRTH PROCESS

13

In approximately the thirty-fourth to thirty-sixth week of the pregnancy, many fetuses turn to be head downward, lying longitudinally. This is the head or cephalic presentation (see fig. 13.1). It can happen later, however; the baby can still rotate before birth so that ideally the head engages first. In the initial stage it lies in the mother's superior pelvis. The position of the head is important, as it should be fairly centered in relation to the uterus and the pelvic inlet. Otherwise it would press against the pelvis, and this could cause intraosseous lesions of the cranial base or neck region. The chin rests closely against the chest. The most common presentation is vertex, also called occipital presentation, in which the baby's occiput leads. Other variations are median vertex presentation, with the head straight; brow presentation, with the chin raised more than in median vertex presentation; and face presentation, in which the head is extended backward into the nape. The opposite is breech presentation, in which the baby's buttocks or feet are positioned in the pelvic inlet. This occurs in about one in twenty births. In about one in two hundred cases, the presentation is transverse, a more difficult situation. Transverse lie makes a normal delivery impossible, and a C-section becomes necessary.

Birth assistants have several methods to enable the baby to turn and adopt a head-down presentation in order to provide the best starting position for birth. One method, from Chinese medicine, is moxibustion, warming the body using mugwort. Another is craniosacral touch, combined with a mental and verbal invitation to the child. These can enable spontaneous repositioning, even shortly before birth. Craniosacral treatment has a relaxing effect that can also influence uterine tonus. The baby responds by moving more, and may turn to adopt a better position for birth, making a C-section unnecessary.

The pelvic inlet is oval in shape, wider in the transverse direction, and in a normal delivery the baby's head aligns itself to match. The position of the head is named with reference to the position of the baby's occiput relative to the mother's pelvis. Around two-thirds of babies make their arrival in the world in the left occiput anterior position.

The following account of the birth process begins with a general description, followed by a description from the point of view of the child and a section giving details specific to Craniosacral Therapy. In the next section are the birth matrices outlined by Stanislav Grof to provide a psychological and spiritual component; together these accounts offer the craniosacral practitioner comprehensive insight into the birth process on several different levels. Awareness of the levels involved helps the practitioner understand and recognize their dynamics during the craniosacral treatment of the child as well as to accompany the process: the practitioner will perhaps see the motions associated with birth occurring in the child and support them in an appropriate way. More detailed accounts are given in the literature for midwives and in courses on craniosacral treatment of children.

Birth is a process in which the baby is expelled from the uterus by the contraction and relaxation of specific muscles. At the same time, the child is making its own way and aiding the process—not only because the space has become too confined and does not allow further growth but also because of a hormonal exchange between mother and child. This cocktail of hormones also has the effect of causing reabsorption of the amniotic fluid from the infant's lungs. This is assisted by the massaging effects of labor and the narrowness of the birth canal. It seems as if a primordial biological and spiritual program "knows" how the birth process should proceed and conclude.

Labor is a complex event governed by the interaction of the hormone-producing glands and the nervous systems of the mother and the child. These processes are being prepared weeks before the

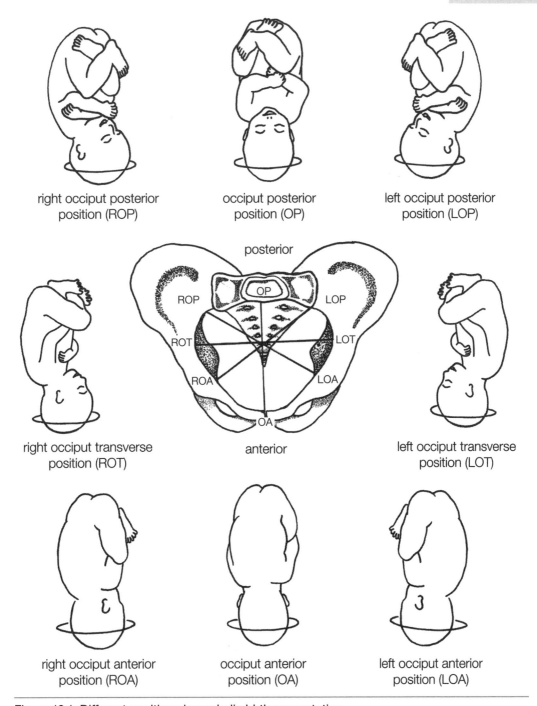

Figure 13.1. Different positions in cephalic birth presentation.

birth. Many women experience prelabor pains, strong contractions lasting ten to thirty minutes. In the paraventricular nucleus, a central part of the hypothalamus, oxytocin is synthesized and released into the bloodstream of the mother and the baby via the posterior lobe of the pituitary. The unborn child also plays a part in the onset of labor because this hormone stimulates the myometrium, the muscles of the uterus, to contract and causes the cervix to soften and dilate.

The first signs of birth are the thinning of the lower part of the cervix as the muscle fibers soften ("ripen") and the plug of mucus that had sealed the cervix drops out. There is a discharge from the vagina that looks like blood. Expulsion of bowel contents becomes more frequent. The amniotic sac that surrounds the baby in the uterus may break, releasing amniotic fluid. Each birth develops along its own individual lines and has its own individual rhythm as the labor pains become stronger and more frequent.

Childbirth is divided into three stages:

- dilation, followed by a transitional phase leading to
- expulsion of the baby, and
- the placental stage.

Each contraction spreads down from the upper region of the uterus toward the cervix. When the whole uterine muscle has contracted, relaxation occurs, again spreading downward from top to bottom, followed by a recovery phase. This is followed by a fresh contraction, with the gaps between them becoming shorter. The rhythm of labor is governed by the hormone oxytocin. In addition, the brain releases endorphins, which are natural opioids produced by the body. Their effect on both mother and baby is to ease pain and produce euphoria. With each contraction the superior and lateral muscle walls of the uterus push the baby toward the cervix.

The dilation stage lasts longest. During the early stage of dilation, the cervix opens by less than an inch, and in the middle stage 1.5 to 3 inches. As the stages of dilation become more advanced, the phases of contraction become longer and the contractions themselves stronger until the cervix is fully dilated, measuring around four inches.

The later active phase of dilation is followed by a transitional phase with strong contractions occurring at short irregular intervals. The elongated oval funnel shape of the pelvis guides the baby's head to turn so that it can pass through the elongated oval of the pelvic outlet. When the baby has reached the pelvic floor and the contractions become longer again, the expulsion contractions of the second stage of labor begin. The baby's head is now flexed, resting on the pelvic floor with the sagittal suture lying straight and the occiput leading.

In the expulsion stage, the contractions last about forty-five to ninety seconds, occurring every two to three minutes. The mother can take deep breaths and push the baby strongly downward. The two levator ani muscles are tensed across the pelvic outlet, and these relax during the expulsion stage. Delivery through the perineum involves an arching movement around the pubic symphysis: the baby's head, which was fully flexed, is raised briefly, hyperextending or deflecting so that at this point the nape leans against the inferior border of the symphysis. The baby works its way on through the final stages, aided by the mother's breathing and pushing and by the contractions. The head appears, and the baby's body now has to rotate to emerge from its mother's pelvis, the leading upper shoulder delivered first, followed by the shoulder behind or below, and then by the baby's trunk, pelvis, legs, and feet.

The first moments of contact between mother and child following birth are an important time of bonding. The newborn child takes its first breaths and hears, smells, feels, and sees its mother. The baby knows its mother's voice. It lies on its mother's abdomen as the cord gradually ceases to pulsate, then reaches for her breast and begins to suckle. This suckling is important as it stimulates the further production and release of oxytocin, which leads to the next stage of contractions to detach and expel the placenta.

The placental stage: following birth, the contractions of the uterus and muscles come to a halt, but the birth process is not yet over, even if the umbilical cord has been cut. After about fifteen minutes, the contractions of the uterus build up again in order to detach the placenta from the internal wall. It has to be completely removed. Finally, the afterbirth is expelled and the uterus can return to its original position. If this does not happen successfully, delivery of the placenta is prompted by, for example, injection of oxytocin. In some countries, Methergine is used; but this is not a substance synthesized by the body, and it can affect milk production and breast-feeding. For this reason it is increasingly being replaced by prostaglandins. In some cases, curettage may be needed to scrape away any remaining placental tissue from the uterus and prevent life-threatening hemorrhage or infection.

The umbilical cord is best cut only after it has stopped pulsating. This transitional phase is when the baby has to regulate its supply of oxygen and its temperature, among many other needs. The cutting of the cord is a fundamentally decisive moment, as it marks the end of the child's biological dependence on its mother's body.

The birth reaches its conclusion during or following the period of bonding when the baby falls asleep at its mother's breast.

13.1. Craniosacral Therapy during Birth

Craniosacral Therapy, kinesiology, acupuncture, and homeopathy performed by a fully qualified practitioner can assist the birth process by reducing pain and by providing recovery intervals in which the woman can renew her strength. In the specific case of Craniosacral Therapy, a stillpoint can be induced where appropriate, for example by means of the CV4 technique. Other approaches that can be used for pain reduction are affirmation, suggestion, hypnosis, and breathing exercises, and the woman can be helped to access reserves of strength by establishing contact with her own resources. If some of these measures are practiced sufficiently early and regularly applied before the pains begin or become too severe, they can make painkillers unnecessary, or at least allow lower doses to be used. Birth is a stage of initiation for the mother and the child. Surrender and trust in the power of nature can transform doubts and fears into joy. The pain of giving birth leads to the increased production and release of endorphins; even the woman's mental attitude, which determines her ability to accept and allow the pain, is fundamentally important.

For the woman who is giving birth, it is important to have secure surroundings and a safe retreat because disturbances cause stress and so affect the birthing process. People living close to nature are more inclined to know and respect the mother-to-be's instinctive need for a retreat and an intimate environment. Fortunately, the value of an undisturbed atmosphere and natural delivery is increasingly being recognized again, even in some technologically equipped maternity hospitals. Nevertheless, there are still some birth assistants and physicians who try to take an active role in influencing labor, or who intervene in that first contact between mother and baby.

A midwife working at a Swiss university hospital who also has experience in craniosacral work told me that in cases where there was difficulty administering epidural anesthesia, she was able to help the woman giving birth using the arm-bridge technique. This brought better relaxation of the sacroiliac joints and also of the L3–L4–L5 region. The midwife exerts gentle pressure with the palm of the hand on the superior iliac wing. The woman should meanwhile bend her head forward so that her chin rests on her chest. This can sometimes provide enough help to enable the anesthetist to administer the epidural successfully and spare the woman further injection discomfort and stress.

HOW THE CHILD EXPERIENCES BIRTH

14

The child's experience is preverbal. Every birth is unique, and it is an individual experience that the child is unable to put into words.

14.1. The Physical Experience of Birth

Before birth, in the eighth and ninth months of gestation, the baby has already felt occasional contractions, so they are already familiar. It seems that hormones from the baby's as well as the mother's pituitary glands are already stimulating the increased production of oxytocin and triggering labor pains. This is an interactive process of intensive nonverbal communication between two individuals, and it is part of prenatal bonding.

If the birth takes place in a hospital or birthing center, the fetal heartbeat is audibly monitored. The course of the delivery is determined by parameters such as the relationship between the fetal head and the mother's pelvis and the position and attitude of the fetal head. During the dilation stage, the fetus continues to be supplied with oxygen and nutrients through the placenta. The strengthening contractions regularly massage its body. In most cases, the baby's head is positioned in the pelvic inlet, dropping downward and rotating as it moves through the birth canal. It feels the pressure of the dilating cervix. If the amniotic sac is still unbroken, the amniotic fluid will help cushion the pressure on the head; if it breaks, the fetal head exerts direct pressure on the cervix and helps it to open. The baby also helps the process by moving its head, twisting, and turning. Normally the baby's cranial bones have not yet fused; they can be compressed and can even slide over each other by four- to eight-tenths of an inch, which reduces the circumference of the head during the birth process, adapting its shape to that of the pelvis.

During the dilation stage, the contractions produce an effect on the cervix, drawing it tautly over the fetal head. The baby experiences the strengthening contractions, the pressure of the cervix, the solidity of the walls of the pelvis, and the movement away from the placenta.

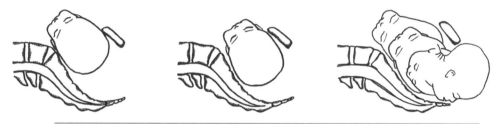

Figure 14.1. Simplified illustration of the stages of delivery.

The transitional phase at the end of the dilation stage may last from a few minutes to several hours and occurs between the complete dilation of the cervix and the spontaneous pressure of the expul-

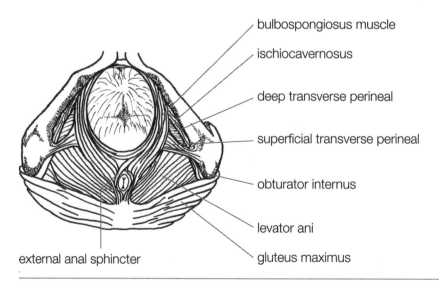

bulbospongiosus muscle

ischiocavernosus

deep transverse perineal

superficial transverse perineal

obturator internus

levator ani

gluteus maximus

external anal sphincter

Figure 14.2. Emergence of the head through the muscles of the pelvic floor.

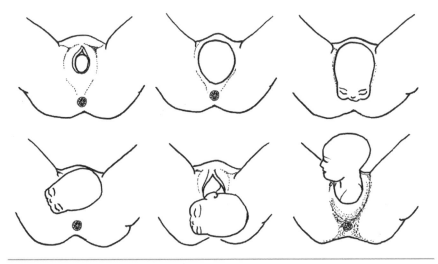

Figure 14.3. Emergence of the baby through the floor of the pelvis.

sion stage. The contractions are long lasting and powerful while the gaps between them are very short; their downward force drives the baby's head onward, helped by its twisting and turning motion, and it descends into the pelvic canal. The head moves on past the symphysis and pubic bones and then the mother's sacrum. When the cervix is fully open, the baby's head is surrounded by the walls of the vagina.

The expulsion stage begins when the head rotates ninety degrees and has dropped deeper to the pelvic floor and the cervix is fully dilated. This stage can last a few minutes or up to a maximum of one to two hours; any longer is considered a prolonged expulsion stage. The duration is usually shorter for a second delivery.

14.2. The Mechanism of Delivery for Occiput Anterior Presentation

As the baby emerges from the vagina, it encounters a host of new sensations: the air, the sensations of its skin, the difference in temperature, gravity, and the sounds of its surroundings. Until this point, oxygen-rich blood was supplied through the placenta, but now this supply is decreasing and pulmonary circulation is beginning to operate. The air sacs of the lungs, the alveoli, expand like tiny balloons; the surfactant on their surfaces is responsible for the expansion of the lungs and first breaths. The breathing reflex is also stimulated by the cooler temperature of the surrounding air. The newborn takes its first breath, the blood vessels in the lungs open, and blood flows through the lungs to take up oxygen from the inhaled air. The sudden opening of the blood vessels and the coolness of the air in the baby's lungs can be a powerful experience for the baby. The newborn begins to move; lying on its mother's body, it begins to find its way, recognizing her smell and her voice. The baby opens its eyes and experiences light for the first time. In many cases the baby undergoes an examination immediately after it is born for respiration, pulse, muscle tone, reflexes, and perfusion judged by the color of its skin. There is sufficient time later for these examinations; they should be done once the first contact between mother and child has been made and the vital initial bonding has taken place.

14.3. Details of Birth Relevant to Craniosacral Issues

The birth canal consists of the pelvic inlet (superior opening), the mid-pelvis, and the pelvic outlet (lower opening). In at least two-thirds of vaginal deliveries, the fetal head is in the left occiput anterior position. This presentation will therefore be described here, with brief references to the effects of other presentations.

The baby's head moves deeper into the pelvis, flexing slightly and turning to pass through the pelvic inlet. By flexing in this way, it adapts its position to the roundness of the pelvic cavity, and the baby's chin is pushed down onto its chest. The occiput, which has a rounded shape, is the leading part.

In the left occiput anterior position, the occipital bone lies toward the anterior and to the left as the baby's head passes through the pelvic inlet, with the baby's back aligned toward the mother's left flank. The two parietal bones should, as far as possible, enter simultaneously, with the sagittal suture lying across the oval of the pelvic inlet. This eases the physiological rotation as the baby descends into the mid-pelvis. The occiput experiences the greatest stress. Resistance in the pelvis causes the squamous part of the occipital bone to turn forty-five degrees toward the anterior left as the head descends, and at the same time the head flexes downward to the chest. During this descent, the left posterior part of the parietal bone encounters resistance as it reaches the superior inner border (the promontory) of the sacrum. The increasing intrauterine pressure has the effect of molding the baby's head to conform to the pelvis; the inner border of the left parietal bone often slides under the border of the right anterior part of the parietal bone, which is moving behind the pubic symphysis more quickly than the left. The occipital bone and the two parts of the frontal bone slide very slightly under the parietal bones, which reduces the circumference of the head.

Head volume is also reduced by the fact that there is a smaller quantity of blood and CSF; to some extent this is pressed out of the head. The degree of flexion or extension of the head as the fetus descends, called deflexion, determines the type of vertex presentation. It may be median vertex presentation, with the region of the sagittal suture–bregma or anterior fontanel leading; brow presentation; or face presentation. These are very unfavorable for mother and child: in the median vertex or brow presentations, the diameter of the presenting fetal head is greater, so the bones of the cranial vault tend to be pushed over each other more than if the occipital bone in the lambda region is leading. In face presentation, the frontal and facial bones are compressed, distorted, and displaced.

As the baby descends, its chin flexes onto its chest, its parietal bones come into contact with the mother's sacrum and coccyx, and its occipital bone receives counterpressure from one of her pubic bones. This pressure and counterpressure, along with the spiral circular contractions of the uterus, force the baby onward, turning as it advances. In the mother's mid-pelvis, its head turns forty-five degrees, rotating as the base of the occiput passes under the pubic symphysis.

During the expulsion stage, the baby's head becomes hyperextended (flexed backward) as it passes under the pubic bone on its way through the pelvic outlet. Its frontal and facial bones, nose, mouth, and mandible slide past the sacrum and coccyx of the mother; the occipital bone, lying anteriorly, has to turn to pass the pubic symphysis. This is another moment that imposes stress on the baby's head and cervical spine, especially the occipital bone, the occipital condyles, and the foramen magnum. As the head emerges, the shoulder girdle begins to turn toward the pelvic outlet. In left occiput anterior presentation, it is usually the right shoulder that leads, with the left following; these are referred to as the posterior and anterior shoulders. The neck emerges turning forty-five degrees to the left; in this way it aligns with the right or anterior shoulder, which works its way out anteriorly under the pubic symphysis. Further spiral twisting movements deliver the rest of the trunk and pelvis.

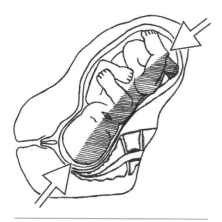

Figure 14.4. Compression of the longitudinal axis mainly affects the same side as the birth position.

The baby experiences forces of traction and propulsion, compression and turning at every stage of birth, affecting not only the fetal head but the cervical spine, further sections of the spinal column, and the entire trunk, including the shoulders and pelvis.

In addition to putting pressure on the cranium, locomotor apparatus, and organs, the birth process can also affect the intracranial membranes, spinal meninges, and cranial and spinal nerves, imposing excessive stretching, twisting, distortion, or compression. These regions all interact and affect each other.

Vaginal birth should not be seen only from the point of view of the pressures it imposes, however. The natural birth process also provides a kind of massage for the baby at every level of its body. It is the first sensory, motor, and neuromuscular stimulation that it receives on its way into its new surroundings outside the protective environment of its mother's body. Some craniosacral teachers see this stimulation and compression of the cranial sutures as rather like the ignition signal in a race, as they prompt the primary respiratory mechanism into action. Certain stages of birth have a stimulating and energizing effect. It is also interesting to note that the flexing and extension of head and neck that occurs during the birth process is in fact something experienced and practiced in advance, during the development of the embryo.

The adaptation of the baby's body to the mother's pelvis before and during birth should resolve within a few days. The action of crying helps expand the baby's head circumference and helps correct the compressed cranial and cervical region. As the baby suckles, the sucking motion works through the vomer to bring the SBS further into flexion, relieving the stress on the cranial base and the tension on the intracranial membranes. The tension of the dural tube is eased by the baby's various body postures while being carried by the parents and by them supporting the spontaneous spiral twisting movements of the baby's trunk and neck. Craniosacral practitioners can give targeted support to these regions in their treatment of the child.

Birth is an existential physical, mental, and spiritual event, and the effect that it has on the child involves powerful pressure and high energy. These experiences are stored not in the subconscious but in the cell memory, and therefore in the body. They can be reactivated by situations in life or by certain types of therapeutic touch by the practitioner. It is possible to defuse this charge and resolve the vital energy bound up in the trauma of birth in the course of a few sessions of therapy given in infancy or childhood. This releases it from the physical, energetic, and emotional body, after which symptoms spontaneously resolve and the child has greater vital strength for its development and greater joy in life.

14.4. Grof's Birth Matrices

The physician and psychiatrist Stanislav Grof is today considered one of the major figures in transpersonal psychology. He has researched expanded states of consciousness, including through the use of LSD, over more than forty years and has published many books on the subject. He later developed breathing techniques, in particular holotropic breathwork, which enables people to arrive at a state of deeper consciousness. In these states, individuals can, for example, recall suppressed childhood experiences to their consciousness and then reintegrate them. Grof discovered that the birth experience as well as biographical issues influence physical and psychological illness and health.[1] During the birth process, archetypal aspects of the collective unconscious, as described by the psychologist Carl Jung, can be experienced. An encounter with the existential transitions of birth and death can open up mystical and spiritual dimensions.

Each stage of birth activates specific physical and emotional sensations in the child, and these exert a marked influence on the child's life and perception of the world. The experience of birth involves powerful stimulation of the child's whole being. Grof identifies the stages of this experience in terms of four basic perinatal matrices. The period immediately prior to birth is basic perinatal matrix I, and the three clinical stages of birth correspond to matrices II, III, and IV. The experiences of each child are highly individual.

In basic perinatal matrix I, one of the experiences is limitless oceanic consciousness. The child is held and nourished as it swims dolphin-like in the ocean or cosmos. This experience corresponds to a "good womb." Archetypes that represent this are states felt to be "like paradise" or heavenly visions. In contrast, prenatal complications such as attempted abortion or the threat of miscarriage may produce experiences of a "bad womb." These experiences are dark, eerie, and existentially threatening. They may be represented by states such as all-encompassing destruction or "the end of the world."

Unpleasant bodily sensations include a feeling of cold, nausea, or the sense of being poisoned.

In basic perinatal matrix II, which corresponds to the first stage of the birth process, in which the uterus is contracting rhythmically, the child may have the sense of being drawn into a whirlpool or of being engulfed. The transition from matrix I to matrix II and matrix II itself bring a sense of enclosure and mistrust, mortal danger, and fear. Visions of hell or the sense of being shut in a cage with no way out correspond to this matrix. The sense of close confinement and the contractions of the uterus produce physical and spiritual pain, helplessness and hopelessness, and perhaps even existential despair. Archetypes representing this are a situation of desperation, eternal damnation, or the "dark night of the soul." Unpleasant bodily sensations include palpitations or a sense of pressure.

In basic perinatal matrix III, corresponding to the second stage of the birth process, which is expulsion through the dilated cervix, the child feels itself in the power of contradictory forces of pressure and propulsion. Every part is activated, and the child feels unavoidable pain, but also causes pain. In this life-threatening situation the child is in mortal fear; it cannot breathe, yet still makes its way onward. There may be simultaneous joy and pain. These experiences have their archetypal equivalent in such situations as murder and violence, where the child is alternately victim and perpetrator and the suffering is great. These are moments of death and rebirth in which we are confronted with the dark side of ourselves—we face the shadow. The intense physical sensations that can accompany them include the threat of suffocation, the jerky release of muscle spasms, nausea and vomiting, and cardiac pain.

Basic perinatal matrix IV, corresponding to the final stage of expulsion in which the child enters the world, begins with symbols of fire, according to Grof. This may take the form of a sense of heat, the purifying flames of purgatory, or a phoenix rising from the ashes reborn. The child is unable to express its powerful feelings and sensations during the birth process. The death of all that was and the battle to be reborn, an all-or-nothing struggle, can give the child the sense that everything vital to it has been utterly destroyed. At the same time, however, this is an elemental spiritual new beginning; the child has freed itself of the folds that separated it and has made its way into the world. Instead of the pressure bound up with the birth, the child now feels the breadth of the space that opens up around it. The sensations that greet the newborn baby are positive and strong; this is birth into a world of light. The only risk to these conditions is if the birth has been too exhausting or clouded by high doses of anesthetics. This fourth matrix can blend into certain elements belonging to the first basic perinatal matrix. However, the pleasant sensations can be interrupted if the umbilical cord is cut too soon. This can often cause breathing to stop and lead to fear of death.

14.5. The Cocktail of Hormones during and after Birth

A number of morphine-like opiate hormones called endorphins are released during labor and delivery. Secretion of epinephrine, commonly called adrenaline, by the mother is at its greatest during the final contractions of the uterus before delivery. The woman is then highly alert, and the fetus-ejection reflex kicks in. Often both mother and child are flooded with endorphins immediately following birth to ease the stress and pain of the process. One effect of the copious release of epinephrine is to enable the mother to be fully alert as she meets her baby for the first time and to defend it if necessary. The unborn child also secretes adrenaline during the last expulsion contractions. The norepinephrine, also called noradrenaline, released at this point enables the baby to cope better with the lack of oxygen and to be alert, eyes open, as it makes contact with its mother.

DIFFICULT BIRTHS

This chapter explains some of the potential complications that can occur around the time of the birth along with the interventions they require.

15.1. Interventions

Vacuum extraction with a ventouse is often used in difficult deliveries. It usually produces changes in intracranial pressure and deformation of the head, with some parts being stretched and others compressed. The method involves working in synchrony with the contractions to pull the child out of the mother's lower pelvis. The vacuum in the ventouse device is released gradually. The purpose of this is, as much as possible, to prevent hemorrhage caused by tearing blood vessels between the bone and the periosteum. Any swelling of the scalp should resolve within a few hours. The senior physician at a hospital in southern Germany told me that in his advice to parents, he always recommends that babies delivered by ventouse receive craniosacral treatment.

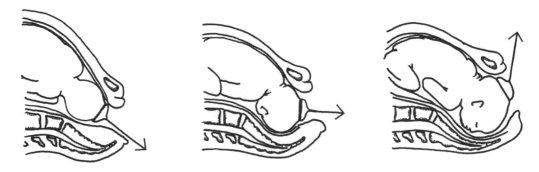

Figure 15.1. Stages of vacuum extraction.

Forceps are another method of delivery used in difficult births. However, the use of forceps can lead to injury of the mother, for example tearing of the uterus, vagina, or perineum. The risks to the child from forceps delivery and ventouse are from the forces of pressure, tension, and torsion, which make injury to the cranial base, cervical spine, and spinal cord more likely. Forceps can leave an imprint on the soft skull or cause skin abrasions; they can cause skull fractures or put pressure on the facial nerve, resulting in facial paralysis. Pressure can also produce subluxation of the atlas and damage to the cerebellum, since the atlas is still quite small in comparison to the foramen magnum. Tensile forces are hazardous to the baby's cervical spine and can cause injury to the spinal cord, spinal nerves, and vessels of the CNS. For example, they can cause ruptures of the middle cerebral artery and venous sinuses, which can lead to intracerebral and subdural hemorrhage. The resultant narrowing of the spinal dura mater and constriction of the spinal cord often cause damage to the spinal nerves. The turning or rotation brought about by the devices used to assist the birth can injure the cervical spine and upper regions of the spinal cord, which can cause pareses of the brachial plexus, hypotonia, and breathing difficulties. Twisting is the most dangerous kind of manipulation, because this can overstretch vessels, including the basilar artery, or even cause them to rupture, resulting in hemorrhage.

15.2. Birth Complications

15.2.1. Delayed Delivery of the Shoulder (Shoulder Dystocia)

Shoulder dystocia is when the baby's head had been delivered but the shoulder is held back because it has impacted on the pubic symphysis. It is more frequent in births where the weight of the fetus exceeds nine to eleven pounds. Shoulder dystocia is less common when the mother gives birth in the upright or squatting position or on all fours.

Shoulder dystocia involves an abnormal position of the fetus in which the shoulders are aligned in the anteroposterior direction prior to descent, or in the transverse direction at the later point of delivery. In the first instance, the shoulders are not aligned side by side as they need to be in order to enter the pelvic inlet. As a result, the baby's anterior shoulder lodges against the mother's pubic symphysis and cannot move farther. In the second instance, the delivery of the shoulders is delayed at the pelvic outlet. The shoulders may, for instance, come to lie across the urogenital hiatus, and one shoulder may lodge in the mother's pelvis on one side.

The mother should continue to breathe steadily while the midwife or physician carries out the necessary measures, for example mobilizing the pelvis in a specific way or exerting carefully directed pressure and vibration to the region of the symphysis. A still more helpful approach is for the mother to adopt a different posture. Shoulder dystocia can lead to birth injuries such as fracture of the baby's clavicle or brachial plexus injury, which may result in pareses.

15.2.2. Breech Presentation, Transverse Lie, and Oblique Lie

Breech presentation occurs in different forms. The terms used to describe these categories are frank breech, complete breech, and footling breech. In a breech birth, a great deal of work is performed by the baby's pelvis, since the pelvis instead of the head is the first part to make its way through the birth canal. Thorough craniosacral assessment and treatment of the pelvis, joints of the lower limbs, and spinal column in particular are therefore important following a breech birth.

A transverse or oblique lie is more common in early pregnancy—the first fifteen weeks—when it presents no problem; the fetus is often changing its position. It is also more common in multiple births. A transverse lie is when the fetal trunk lies across the uterus with the head and the buttocks at the same level. An oblique lie is when the fetus lies diagonally across the uterus with the head and the buttocks at different levels.

In cases where the fetus is in a transverse or oblique lie, spontaneous turning can be induced during the period from the thirty-fifth to the thirty-seventh week by craniosacral touch combined with verbal accompaniment of the process, expressed as an invitation. This can help induce the fetus to turn and adopt a longitudinal lie. Moxibustion and physical exercise can also encourage a change in fetal position. Later than the thirty-seventh week, a midwife, gynecologist, or maternity hospital should be consulted to avoid the risk of complications. The effect of uterine contractions after the amniotic sac has ruptured could lead to a transverse lie with a prolapsed arm as well as impaction of the baby's shoulder in the pelvis.

15.2.3. C-section

Cesarean section, often abbreviated to C-section, involves an incision to open the mother's abdomen and then the uterus. Primary C-section is a planned C-section, decided on before the time of the birth, before contractions have begun, or before the membranes have ruptured. It may be carried out because the fetus is in a transverse lie; because of placenta previa, in which the placenta is abnormally low and causes an obstruction; or in a multiple birth, where the first fetus is positioned in such a way that it would prevent a vaginal delivery. Other risks to the fetus, such as genital herpes or maternal HIV infection, are also reasons to consider an elective primary C-section.

A secondary C-section is one that becomes necessary during a difficult birth. Reasons would include a long and exhausting labor, labor that has been delayed or brought to a halt and has become life-threatening, disproportionate size of the fetal head in relation to the mother's pelvis, prolapse of the umbilical cord, or various abnormalities in the attitude of the fetus. For example, an arm may be delivered and block the way for the head. There may be severe bleeding due to detachment or abruption of the placenta, the risk that the uterus may rupture, or the risk of inadequate oxygen supply, called intrauterine hypoxia.

C-sections today are performed around ten times more frequently than in the 1960s. Prevalence varies by country and region; it also depends on the level of access to medical care, health insurance, and social status. The general picture today is that, depending on the hospital, from ten percent to over forty percent of births take place by C-section. However, all the midwives I know believe that the advantages of vaginal delivery are far greater. It is much easier for the baby to adapt to its surroundings and to suckle after a vaginal birth than a C-section. Bonding is usually more difficult after a C-section because the mother and the child are still flooded with anesthetics and in no state to communicate. The operation is also associated with more injury and pain for the mother.

C-section does save lives, of course, when the fetal head is clearly disproportionate in size in relation to the mother's pelvis, when a prolapsed cord threatens to deprive the fetus of oxygen, or when fetal heart sounds indicate distress. When a gynecologist advises a C-section in the absence of any apparent risk factors, however, it can cause much anxiety about complications during a natural birth. The resulting doubts can then make the course of the birth more difficult. Another issue is the timing of the birth: it should mainly be determined by the internal clock of mother and fetus, not by such considerations as the gynecologist's plans for the weekend or staff overtime pay.

It matters whether the mother has planned the C-section in advance, in which case she is to some extent prepared for the procedure, or has to undergo a secondary C-section unexpectedly in an emergency situation. The physical procedure of incision and delivery may be the same, but the actual experience for the mother and the child is quite different. An emergency C-section is a much greater shock to the mother's nervous system, and this affects both the mother and the child.

Other aspects of delivery by C-section are the time factor as well as the amount of pressure experienced. The sudden change in pressure produces considerable compression on the skull and its fragile membranes, including the falx and tentorium, blood vessels, and nerves. A baby delivered by C-section has not experienced the stimulation of its head and lungs on its way through the birth canal. Despite the different mode of delivery, there can still be dysfunctions present, caused, for example, by lying on its side in a single position during the final weeks of the pregnancy. From the psychological point of view, the baby as well as its mother feels the lack of the natural birth experience that it was biologically designed to have. This lack deprives the child of the experience of enduring and overcoming barriers.

15.2.4. Multiple Births

Multiple babies are usually born before the thirty-eighth week of pregnancy. They have a much lower birth weight than single babies and need intensive care. Today, practically half of the twins born as well as a high proportion of triplets are delivered by C-section. There are several reasons for this: the membranes are more likely to rupture early, increasing the likelihood of a prolapsed cord; the attitude of the fetuses may delay the delivery and cause exhaustion to the mother and the babies; and the unsuccessful use of a ventouse or forceps may result in the need for a C-section. Hypoxia is usually caused by insufficiency of the placenta. The contractions may weaken after the birth of the first twin, or the half-empty uterus may contract in such a way that the placenta detaches too soon and fails to supply the second twin adequately.

15.2.5. Preterm Birth

A baby is defined as preterm if it is born before the thirty-sixth or thirty-seventh week of pregnancy. The usual causes are premature labor or premature membrane rupture. Another reason is the recent increase in artificially assisted pregnancies, which often produce multiple births. Infections, previous uterine surgery, or stress can also trigger a preterm delivery. A premature infant is very susceptible to hypoxia, birth trauma such as intracerebral hemorrhage, and infections. It is true that improved medical care gives preterm babies a much better chance of survival than in the past, for example enabling maturation of the lungs. Nevertheless there is a danger of infections and intracerebral bleeding, which can lead to severe disabilities or death.

Preterm babies born from the thirty-second week on have a very good chance of a life without disabilities. In the period up to the end of the twenty-fourth week, however, the difficult ethical question is whether to resuscitate a fetus—for example, a twenty-one-week-old fetus with a body weight of around ten ounces that is incapable of survival—in order to give it a life with a high risk of lasting damage.

Preterm babies suffer the premature loss of the nurturing environment of the womb. In addition to the fight for survival, they lose bonding with the mother. Although technology and lifesaving medicine enable survival, the inanimate incubator and wires are no substitute for its mother and suckling at the breast.

Preterm babies need to have as much contact as possible with their mothers as early as possible. This has been recognized not only by bonding psychologists and neurobiologists but also by the staff of maternity hospitals. In an approach called "kangaroo care," the baby is placed directly on its mother's or father's abdomen or chest, covered with a warm blanket, and allowed to lie there for several hours a day. Body contact and nearness calm preterm babies, they breathe more easily, and their chances of survival are increased. Early physical contact between the child and its parents enables the important initial bonding to take place. Above all, its mother's touch, stroking and rocking, and the warmth of her body are spiritually nurturing to the preterm infant and help its initial orientation to life in the world.

I have given treatment to preterm babies born around the twenty-sixth week who survived despite the dire predictions of medical personnel and continued to make quite good progress. Their will to live testifies to a strong vital force that deserves to be recognized and valued.

When treating preterm babies it is important to remember how fragile they are. The parents help by regularly giving them warmth and affection, as described above. Your approach as the craniosacral practitioner should be to support their respiration and the growth of their lungs with visceral therapy, in particular to the thorax. If the child was fed by gastric tube, you should include the esophagus, diaphragm, and stomach in your perceptual field. Assess and support the baby's respiration, swallowing, and digestion. It is helpful to use biodynamic methods as well as structural and functional ones. Some months after birth you can move on increasingly to supporting the child's natural free breathing. This enables you to harmonize the ANS and nerve nuclei or the respiratory center in a more targeted way; their development and self-regulation will have been held back as a result of artificial ventilation, important as it was for the child's survival.

Both the baby and its parents need time to overcome the shock, despair, and suddenness with which bonding was snatched away from them. One way that these emotions are expressed and released is by crying and trembling. This gives expression to the associated sorrow and fear and eases them away. It may be right for you to address this in your craniosacral treatment and to support the parents by acknowledging the emotional situation rather than suppressing it. Sensitive care can restore trust, allow love to flow, and let healing take place.

15.2.6. Additional Perinatal Problems

- amniotic fluid problems
- amniotic infection syndrome
- weak contractions in a postterm pregnancy
- abnormalities in contractions
- chronic or acute inadequacy of placental supply

- green amniotic fluid (around ten percent of all pregnancies)
- size and shape of the maternal pelvis in relation to fetal position
- cessation of contractions
- precipitate delivery
- absence of heart sounds

15.2.7. Some Emergency Situations during Birth

- continuous sustained bradycardia[1]
- hypoxia caused by prolapsed umbilical cord, when, for example, the membranes have ruptured and a coil of umbilical cord lies ahead of the fetus, in front of the entrance to the vagina, or inside the vagina
- premature detachment of the placenta
- placenta previa, when the placenta is in the lower part of the uterus or even covers the cervix
- umbilical cord vessel rupture (bright red, acute bleeding)
- rupture of uterine wall
- maternal shock, reduced perfusion, in some cases cessation of breathing and heartbeat
- postpartum difficulties, severe or excessive bleeding

15.3. Epidural Anesthesia, Spinal Anesthesia, Caudal Anesthesia

From the results of studies in neurobiology and from prenatal and perinatal research, we know that the use of medication dulls the conscious experience of birth for both the mother and the baby. If the mother finds that the pain of giving birth is becoming too great, pain relief can be given. This varies by country and culture and also depends on the level of access to medical care. Methods used include painkillers given by injection; opiates; an epidural, which relaxes the muscles of the uterus; or "gas and air," a mixture of nitrous oxide and oxygen inhaled through a mask to relieve pain. Blocking the pudendal nerve, called a pudendal block, numbs the pelvic floor and helps relieve the pain when the head emerges, for example if a woman is having a ventouse delivery without an epidural.

Epidural anesthesia can be very useful during a long labor, when the mother is thoroughly exhausted or the pain is unbearable. It can also be used in a forceps delivery. Used during C-section, an epidural enables the mother to remain awake. Disadvantages are that a marked drop in blood pressure causes dilation of the blood vessels in the lower body, so that the blood drains slowly. This can reduce placental blood flow and lead to hypoxia for the fetus. This effect is ameliorated by having the mother lie on her side and using an intravenous drip to increase the mother's blood volume. The numbing of the pelvic muscles associated with the epidural reduces the mother's urge to push down. Catecholamines such as epinephrine as well as opioids are sometimes added to the local anesthetic to increase the effect. Uptake of local anesthetic by the fetus can produce marked changes that can be harmful. One risk is that it may depress respiration or even lead to cessation of breathing. This can affect the mother or the fetus. Consequently, obstetric intervention, such as forceps, ventouse, or C-section delivery, is considerably more likely following an epidural.

The epidural space lies between the ligamenta flava and the spinal dura mater, so outside the subarachnoid space containing the CSF. The woman should lie on her left side or adopt a sitting posture, and then hunch her back. In a gap between contractions, a hollow needle is inserted between the spinous processes of L3 and L4 or L2 and L3, penetrating only as far as the epidural space. It must not pierce the dura; there are various ways to verify this. Local anesthetic is therefore injected not into the CSF but into the area surrounding the spinal nerves. In the fatty tissue of the epidural space, the effect of the anesthetic is very local, acting on the spinal nerves of a few segments. As the effect of the epidural wears off, the nerves are often very sensitive, and a C-section or perineal scar can be extremely painful.

Spinal anesthesia is used less often, usually in emergency situations such as an urgent C-section. It has a rapid effect, blocking motor nerve transmission to the pelvic floor and legs and numbing many spinal nerves at the same time. After lumbar puncture, local anesthetic is injected into the subarachnoid space. It mixes with the CSF and also numbs the surrounding nerve roots. The anesthetic is directed toward particular nerve root fibers by adjusting the position of the patient. This type of anesthesia can lead to headaches.

Caudal anesthesia is used in the expulsion stage of labor. It numbs the vagina and perineum and is often used for forceps or ventouse deliveries. As in an epidural, local anesthetic is injected into the epidural space; in this case, however, it is injected at the inferior tip of the sacrum.

15.4. Potential Effects of a Difficult Birth

When a mother has an epidural, her mobility is often very restricted, but unlike general anesthesia, she remains conscious. The initial bonding can therefore take place following the birth. Having an epidural is an option for a woman giving birth, and she should not feel guilty or inadequate for choosing it if the pain becomes unbearable. The regulations governing the use of general anesthesia differ from one hospital to another, but it is only indicated in an absolute emergency.

It is hardly surprising that many babies born by vaginal delivery involving the use of medication have greater difficulty with self-attachment, in which they establish a link with their inner self. The resulting lack of contact with resources can affect autonomic functions and their ability to orient themselves in the world.

In the uterus the fetal lungs are filled with water and have to fill with air soon after birth. If there are any problems with this change-over, the baby may feel fear of suffocation. Later, the child may possibly have a fear of water or an anxious need for more air.

Birth complications often impose harmful pressure or tension on the head, neck, shoulder, spinal, and pelvic regions. If two cranial bones are forced to overlap, it can lead to cephalhematoma, a collection of blood between the periosteum and the bone, or to cerebral hemorrhage. A study in Sweden found that the risk among women of later developing anorexia was several times greater when their birth had involved excessive mechanical intervention. Many interventions—drug-induced labor, deep forceps delivery, delivery under general or local anesthetic, or the need for resuscitation during birth—present birth-related difficulties that affect the structures and functions of the infant's body. If adequate treatment is not given, or if the treatment is not sufficiently holistic, the effects can later lead to problems that include autistic tendencies, hyperactivity, and an increased risk of addiction.

Difficult and traumatic experiences during birth and early childhood affect our development on both the physical as well as the psychological and spiritual levels. Prenatal and birth experiences can have a formative effect. They can be consciously or unconsciously reenacted later by the child or the adult. The child of a restless mother, for example, may later be hyperactive. Unwanted children may perhaps change residence more frequently than other people or feel that they must do so. If an infant is abandoned by its mother or experiences a lack of personal contact in infancy, as an adult that individual will sometimes be abandoned in relationships or choose a partner who lives at a distance or whose profession involves frequent travel. Everyday situations that perhaps involve great physical or psychological pressure—actual or symbolic—may cause the individual to subconsciously relive a traumatic birth. William Emerson, one of the best-known proponents of prenatal and perinatal psychotherapy, along with Raymond F. Castellino and David Boadella, reached the conclusion that forty percent of births are severely traumatic, and fifty percent of children experience moderate to slight birth trauma.[2]

There is no doubt that when the situation makes them necessary, interventions such as C-sections, the ventouse, and forceps delivery save lives. The actual experience varies greatly, but generally they interrupt the natural process of birth that human beings are designed by nature and biology to experience. They produce either extreme activation or draining of the nervous system. All this has neurobiological consequences for the infant and makes it more difficult for it to maintain its fragile homeostasis or to accustom itself to the new circumstances of its life. In a baby whose system is highly activated as a result of birth trauma, we usually find hypertonia, and the child is hard to pacify. In a baby whose nervous system is drained, on the other hand, we find hypotonia; the baby seems apathetic and hardly "present." For the woman giving birth, anesthesia is often a shock. The reason may be the loss of a sense of the body, for example, or loss of consciousness, or loss of control in general.

In prenatal and perinatal psychology, a link can be found between postterm continuation of the pregnancy, prolapsed umbilical cord, or a halt in the birth process and refusal to be born on the part of the child, in which the baby is unwilling to go through birth and enter the world. The cause is often associated with intrauterine trauma.

Practitioners of body therapy and psychotherapy providing treatment for babies and children need to be familiar with the dynamics occurring around birth, and they need to have explored the emotional aspects of their own births. This gives them the empathy and understanding to talk with parents about the circumstances of the birth. Also, faced with the great range of situations following a C-section or interventions in a natural birth, a sympathetic background of experience enables practitioners to find the right answers and respond appropriately to anything from shrugging off minor problems to tragedy and guilt-laden tales of misery.

15.5. Malformations

Externally visible malformations include Down syndrome, also called trisomy 21; malformations of the limbs; facial deformities; and spina bifida, a result of the incomplete closure of the neural tube, usually in the lumbosacral region.

In situations of existential crisis such as a stillbirth, the midwife or craniosacral practitioner can provide emotional and physical support to all those affected. Through their empathy and presence and by delivering agreeable touch, they can ease the pain and help healing.

Practitioners will recognize if they are deeply moved to an excessive extent by the pain of others; this is their own unprocessed grief. If this happens, it helps to seek support by talking with colleagues or supervisors, attending a grief seminar, trauma healing, Craniosacral Therapy, or other means to enable them to process the past and progress in their own development.

DEVELOPMENT OF THE CHILD FROM BIRTH TO AROUND AGE FIVE

16

The topics presented here have been chosen because they are frequently encountered in the holistic treatment of children, and practitioners are able to recognize them. The practitioner should give multilevel support to the mother and the child and seek to relieve stress. A number of themes can be addressed while doing this and can provide a way in to achieve change and possibly progress to ease and healing.

Children develop quickly, and the need for compensation is less in children than in adults. As a result, the impulses delivered in pediatric craniosacral treatment toward greater balance and wholeness are usually taken up more quickly. The first changes can be seen during the treatment, within a few days or weeks. It should be kept in mind that healing and development never occur in fixed steps but are an individual process. Time and a certain degree of regularity are needed to bring about comprehensive changes.

A baby weighs around seven pounds eleven ounces at birth, is around twenty inches long, and has a head circumference of twelve or thirteen inches. Its abilities include being able to turn toward something or turn away. At the age of two to three months a baby lying on its back can transfer an object from one hand to the other. Placed in a sitting position, the baby can hold its head upright. At three to four months the baby can fix its gaze on an object or a light. It makes different sounds, laughs when played with, and recognizes its mother's face and her touch. It grabs for its feet and plays with its fingers. From four months, a baby lying on its front can raise its head and shoulders and support both shoulders.

Over the first six months, the baby develops quickly, constantly acquiring new skills that also change the type of interaction it has with its parents. A newborn needs time to become accustomed to the situation outside its mother's body and cannot remain attentive for too long or too often. By around the third month of its life, however, the baby's basic regulation will have adapted to its environment. The baby becomes increasingly attentive and interested in its surroundings as it takes in its environment. It smiles, especially at its parents, giving them its attention and maintaining strong visual contact with them.

From approximately the third month on, the exchange between the baby and its parents becomes more intensive and varied. They love to play together and spend a lot of time doing so. Babies love games involving repetition and the same basic sequence of events; this reaffirms their belief that events around them are, to an extent, predictable. From four months on, the baby is able to grasp objects and begins to play with them and also plays more with toys. The baby's attention has developed to the point where it can include more than one person or object. Its ability to crawl around is increasing, and on its journeys of exploration it can discover objects of interest on its own—the baby is developing independence from its parents.

Most aspects of mother-child communication also apply to other caregivers that the baby knows well. Babies enjoy being carried, rocked, stroked, and rubbed by their father or grandparents. If they do become shy, the right approach is to accept it and to see it as a newly acquired skill. The security provided by their closest caregivers helps them realize that they have a safe refuge in their parents, even when strangers are present. This sense of security also enables the child to satisfy its curiosity by exploring the world around, and then to conquer it and embark on fresh learning processes.

The presence of too many caregivers would overwhelm the baby; however, the closeness of a few beyond the immediate family is enriching and very helpful to the child's life and development. Caution is necessary when introducing new care situations. It is important to recognize and accept the baby's natural fear of separation. This is just as true for new caregivers such as babysitters and day-care workers as it is for the parents.

At around six months the baby can turn over independently onto its back or its belly and can sit unaided. It can recognize and comprehend objects and grasp two things at the same time, and it can recognize faces. It weighs around fourteen pounds, is approximately twenty-four to twenty-six inches long, and has a head circumference of fifteen to sixteen inches. From seven months the baby begins to crawl on its belly, and from eight months it can crawl around and pull itself upright in order to stand. It starts to wave and clap its hands. At around nine months it can stand with help. It can distinguish different kinds of food and grasp things between its thumb and forefinger. Infants receive solid food in addition to breast milk or bottled milk from around the age of six months. Patience is necessary, and the range of foods needs to be built up very gradually; this takes time. There is no need for sweet, spicy, or fatty foods. Cow's milk, soft cheese, and eggs are not particularly suitable. Parents should not try to impose their own tempo when feeding their child solid foods or liquids; they must let the child dictate the pace. A baby very quickly senses the atmosphere in the room and the mood of the people around it.

The first year of life sees the greatest growth of the brain. At birth the baby's brain is around twenty-five percent its ultimate size; a year later, it is around seventy-five percent. Small head circumference is not usually due to the sutures but to reduced brain growth.

As discussed, the baby takes great pleasure in the movements it can make and enjoys discovering and exploring new objects. Parents and craniosacral practitioners should encourage the baby's movements in line with its aptitudes but should not force anything. Allowed to develop in its own way, the baby learns on its own to turn, roll, crawl on its belly or on all fours, sit, stand, and walk. It shows remarkable perseverance.

From age one, the child can walk unaided, pick up objects with its thumb and forefinger, say simple words like "mama" and "dada," and recognize other members of the family. It weighs twenty to twenty-two pounds, is about twenty-eight inches tall, and has a head circumference of about seventeen or eighteen inches. At this age the baby's brain has around twice as many neurons as its mother's. In the first year or two of life the child plays with every single action over and over again, and each movement has its own developmental history. This persistent, independent exploration and development of movement does more than teach the child how to roll, sit, walk, and stand; it also teaches it how to learn. By experimenting, it learns how to overcome difficulties. It also finds enjoyment and contentment, the result of its own astonishing independent effort.

At around eighteen months, the child is able to walk unaided and to bend to pick things up. At two years of age, it can climb stairs, run, turn the pages of a book, and speak sequences of two or three words. It is starting to be able to dress unaided. It weighs around twenty-six pounds, is thirty-one to thirty-three inches tall, and has a head circumference of about eighteen inches.

At three years of age, the child can run, hop, kick, speak a whole sequence of words, and almost never wets the bed; it plays with other children and can ride a tricycle. The child weighs around thirty-one pounds, is thirty-three to thirty-five inches tall, and has a head circumference of about eighteen to nineteen inches. For the most part the child's motor skills have matured by age four. It has a good sense of balance and is able to stop itself from falling over; it has the ability to play an instrument, turn a cartwheel, and so on. At five years of age the child can hop on one leg, draw, and recite simple verses. It is has a much greater interest in anything new. It weighs around forty pounds, is thirty-nine to forty-one inches tall, and has a head circumference of about nineteen to twenty inches. In the first five years, nutrition, sleeping habits, how to keep clean, managing jealousy, and independence are important skills; the list varies from one source to another.

Play provides another suitable vehicle that can also be used in Craniosacral Therapy to express the joy of living and for processing difficult themes. Approaches include play itself; play interaction; play therapy, or offering possible means of promoting development through play; role-playing; fairy tales; and storytelling. Humor helps, as laughter is a well-known medicine.

Depending on the child's age, I always focus on certain points during a craniosacral session with children: eye contact, reflexes, movements, crawling, turning around, learning to walk, and speaking simple words. Is the child's development within the normal range? Signs of normal development are social skills and the ability to adapt, including:

- the ability to maintain visual contact
- the urge to interact
- behavior that is essentially "socially positive," such as smiling, reacting to signs of affection, and making contact through gestures
- purposeful, structured performance of actions
- imitative behavior

Craniosacral practitioners need to recognize when the child needs a break or requires the undisturbed attention of its mother, foster mother, or family. This is a fundamental need for a child and forms part of the child's individual rhythm.

Babies communicate in a nonverbal way by look, sound, and touch. They make immediate and profound contact, and look away when they have had enough. How far can the child maintain a balance between its inward self and its outwardly directed attention? On one hand, it must maintain the link with its inward self, its flow and its pulse; on the other hand, it is interested in contact with the external world. Carefully observe the baby and the actions and reactions of the parents, especially in the period following birth. Together with your caring support, this will help give them the best possible start to their life together. It is especially important to assist if the relationship has been burdened by a difficult birth or by a separation following birth, and if the child is upset, cries a great deal, or is very introverted.

Most parents can instinctively recognize their baby's subtle signals, which tell them how the child feels and what it needs. Craniosacral practitioners should try to assess how able the child is to express itself and identify the possibilities for self-regulation. If necessary, they can help the parents to see how they can stimulate or calm their child by visual contact. They may also work with the parents to point out these signs and try to discover how best to communicate with a child who has problems. Together they can look for ways to support the child with individually geared opportunities to learn, which will enable it to make use of help from outside as well as improved self-regulation in order to recover.

Babies as young as four months begin to differentiate different emotional states in other people as they receive certain auditory and visual signals. At five months babies can begin to recognize other people's emotional states on the basis of purely auditory signals; understanding visual signals happens somewhat later, at around seven months.

When I am playing with an infant and offer various objects, I carefully watch the child's expression and impulses as well as the movements it makes. I assess how well the child is able to focus or grasp the object. At the beginning of a session, I offer my finger as a way of making contact. Later I can offer objects, choosing toys suitable to the child's age. I have a number of interesting objects for children available in my treatment room: toys designed to appeal to various ages, including rattles and dolls as well as small children's books and an anatomy book for children. We can also offer the child various stimulating activities that are not too demanding.

BONDING AFTER BIRTH AND DURING CHILD DEVELOPMENT 17

The first hour following birth is vital for bonding between mother and child. There should be as little disturbance as possible of the intimate contact between them, at the very least during the time before the placenta has been fully expelled. Otherwise oxytocin levels will not rise as much as they should. There will be plenty of opportunity later for the father to establish his relationship with the child. The level of norepinephrine is also high following birth, around twenty to thirty times higher than it will be later in life. The locus coeruleus appears to be very active at this point. There is close contact between it and olfactory bulb, with the effect of activating the sense of smell in the infant. This is also very important for establishing the bond between mother and child.

Initial contact following birth is usually made by placing the newborn on its mother's abdomen or chest while it is still moist with amniotic fluid. Under a soft warm covering, the baby senses its mother through skin-to-skin contact. At the same time, the baby is held and supported. Once it has had its first cry, the newborn usually calms down in its mother's arms because it feels secure. The newborn is held by its mother as it was held inside her body. As she welcomes it, the baby recognizes her voice. The baby is still fully alert from the epinephrine. It explores its senses and becomes aware of the world around it with every sense. At this early moment, so soon after birth, the newborn is already able to make its way to the breast, recognize the nipple, and begin to suckle. It tastes the colostrum, also called the first milk, and drinks it. The suckling causes the mother's pituitary to secrete more oxytocin, which stimulates the flow of milk and contraction of the uterus.

The placenta is detached and expelled after three to thirty minutes, preventing severe bleeding. At this stage, the baby has not yet developed into a conscious individual with a distinct and autonomous self, and its boundaries are not clearly defined. It is taking in impressions with all its senses; in a way, it is its senses. Mother and child must be given time and left undisturbed to take in and understand each other. They need to be in contact with each other, using all their senses. If there are no complications such as severe bleeding, the baby should be left in skin-to-skin contact with its mother for at least an hour so that it can truly arrive. It is during this first hour after birth that the first intensive bonding outside the mother's body takes place; it is a mutual experience of feeling, smelling, hearing, and seeing, of eye contact with its mother, caresses, and comfort. If time and space allow, this initial bonding phase can be allowed to last longer. Other tasks such as cleaning and measuring the baby's weight and size can come later.

Men also produce more oxytocin during this time. If the father is in a position to do so and is not shocked by the birth process, he can be close by during the initial bonding stage. The father may even be the parent who spends time with the baby during this time if, for example, the mother still has to recover from general anesthetic. Otherwise, it is more usual for bonding with the father to take place via the established bond with the mother, either directly or indirectly. The skin-to-skin contact between mother and baby immediately after birth helps to develop a deepening bond now and during the first year of the baby's life.

Midwives and hospitals with baby-friendly policies fortunately place great value on undisturbed bonding. They know that arrival is a process that takes time. They also know that the baby's mother, or the bonding between mother and baby, is the first and most important point of arrival. This is the baby's home, its safe haven. Newborns are sensitive in their reaction to stress and disturbances, for example while being fed and when digesting a feed. Undisturbed bonding and a well-functioning breast-feeding relationship have time and again proved beneficial. The bonding of mother and baby begins before birth, and the child develops a bond with its closest caregivers that will continue and deepen throughout its life. This process substantially relies on the sensitivity of the adult. It calls for the ability on the part of the adult to see and correctly interpret the signals and messages in the child's behavior and to react promptly and appropriately. The child in turn comes to know and value the reactions of its caregivers. The child's caregivers help determine the bonding pattern and the child's self-image and sense of worth.

The baby's bonding with its parents can be secure or insecure, depending on the parents' sensitivity and loving daily interaction with their child. Their gentleness, care, and reliability encourage the development of the child's fundamental confidence in itself, its surroundings, and the world. The interpersonal link began weeks before birth; on this new level after birth, it can now strengthen and deepen.

To emphasize: the establishment of a good bond during and after birth is vital for happy, healthy children, parents, and families. It provides the foundation on which individuals and society in general can build to achieve their full potential, form fulfilled relationships, and experience love. Socially, the effects are far-reaching: rather than existing in isolation and tending to react by withdrawal or with aggression, people who have a sound bond behave in a more social way, have a sense of common belonging, help each other, and so on. This has an effect on our mutual coexistence in society as a whole.

Michel Odent, a long-term advocate of gentle birth, reports studies showing that the combination of birth complications and inadequate bonding can lead to an increased incidence of violence and self-destructive behavior, including drug dependency or anorexia, later on in life. The way that contact is established in the first hours after birth and during infancy have a determining influence on initial character formation.

The oxytocin released by the pituitary has an important role to play, not only in the birth process and suckling but in promoting maternal behavior. The level of oxytocin may be higher immediately after birth than during labor. Together, oxytocin, the hormone that promotes love, and prolactin, the hormone involved in lactation and suckling, create a complex hormonal balance.

The British child psychologist and psychoanalyst John Bowlby (1907–1990) is regarded as the pioneer of research into bonding. His report on a study commissioned by the World Health Organization into the connection between a mother's love and spiritual and emotional health was published in 1951. Later, the research carried out by the Canadian developmental psychologist Mary Ainsworth found convincing proof of the importance of the early emotional mother-child relationship. Bonding or attachment theory, meanwhile, has become accepted and established in psychology. Phillip Shaver and Karl-Heinz Brisch have published impressive explanatory work on attachment theory.

Attachment theory assumes that a newborn is preconditioned from birth to bond to its caregiver. During the first year of its life, this person is the mother, father, or other close caregiver with whom the baby has intensive contact. This early bonding and close emotional attachment is expressed by such behavior as smiling and crying, by the child seeking its mother or other caregiver, turning to them and holding them tightly. Attachment behavior is enabled and strengthened when both child and caregiver are able and willing to interact and establish closeness on a physical and emotional level. This is a source of emotional nourishment for the infant and provides comfort and protection in threatening situations. According to Bowlby, the bond with the mother that the child builds during its first year of life is essential to its development. The particular system of attachment that a child forms in this way remains fairly constant throughout life.

Bonding occurs through the creation of an emotional relationship between parents and child. Emotional bonding is more than providing comfort and dealing with hygiene requirements; it is a matter of sensing the child's needs and being able to respond appropriately. Every shared happy experience causes the attachment to grow, and so the child develops a bond of love with its parents and others who are very close to it. This emotional attachment enables children to develop a sense of who they are. It is a point of orientation that helps them to develop and discover the world. A strong parent-child bond gives them security and trust, and this secure trusting foundation improves basic self-regulation and, more importantly, gives them the self-confidence and trust in their own abilities to explore and discover the world.

Bonding and attachment are processes that all close family members experience if they are prepared to engage emotionally with each other, learn to love, and form relationships. The findings of a Scandinavian study are no surprise: the study found the incidence of chronic or recurrent health problems to be rarer among children who already had good strong interaction with their mothers at the age of eight to eleven weeks. The situation was quite different for children of that age who had limited contact with their mothers and were affected by disturbed bonding. Bonding disturbances usually occur because of traumatic experiences of separation, loss, serious neglect, or other traumatic experiences. A person who has frequently encountered difficulties of attachment during infancy may form the view that the world is not a safe place and that no one can be trusted. Such a belief may persist into adulthood. The process of childhood bonding and attachment therefore establishes the foundations for the way in which the person will form relationships later in life.

Many educators and therapists find it hard to understand why children in Western societies are increasingly deprived of time with their mothers. The idea that fatherhood almost always involves going to work is generally accepted without question, but if it becomes the norm for the mother to work as well, and she spends a substantial part of every day away from home earning a living, children are deprived of something they need. This is especially true in the first year or two of their lives. In order to develop a sense of self-worth, they need the assurance that they are welcome in the world and that they are loved. During the first twelve months of its life, a baby not only develops a fundamental sense of trust; its emotions are also taking shape. The capacity to feel, the sense of self, and personal identity are formed through experiences such as the exchange of eye contact and being carried. For this, the child needs the nearness of its mother or other constant caregiver.

If a baby is apart from its mother for substantial periods during their first year of its life, and if the mother's place is not taken by another reliable caregiver, the child plunges into inner emptiness. Its fragile sense of self shatters, setting it on a downward path. When a child has experienced secure attachment in the first year or two of life, periods of separation lasting two to three hours seem to cause no ill effects as long as the child is well prepared and there are no other stress factors in the family. When the attachment is insecure, there may be no adverse signs at first. However, disturbances may begin to emerge at around age two or three, for example in language development.

Once the baby becomes mobile, it will begin to explore. It needs to find its own equilibrium as it does so; risk and anxiety are part of that process. Stable and secure attachment to its caregiver is an important asset in these explorations as it provides a safe haven of protection, affection, and comfort. Even during the first year of life, a child can begin to build emotional attachments to other people besides its mother, when these individuals are well-known and the process happens slowly and sensitively.

17.1. Rebonding

In suitable circumstances, the craniosacral practitioner can create a reenactment of various kinds of bonding situations. Bonding to the most important caregivers is built up over several months. The fresh experience of a more intensive bonding with her child can have a special existential significance for the mother. C-section deliveries, in particular, and births in which the mother and the child were separated too quickly often leave the mother without the sense of having been able to fully welcome and accept her child.

17.2. Bonding Assists Development

It is enormously important for a baby's early development for it to look at its surroundings and be looked at, and to recognize the people around it and be recognized by them. This need continues for some time. Careful observation of its parents' reactions also teaches the baby how to assess what it sees happening; a quick look at its parents shows whether there is anything to worry about—is what is happening dangerous or harmless? In the early stages, the baby shares the emotions that its parents are feeling, such as joy or anger. Later it learns to distinguish more clearly between its own feelings and those of others.

Seeing and hearing are especially important for communication, and harmonious communication between the parents and the child assists the child's good spiritual and emotional development. Body contact and attachment to the people close to it are vital for the health of the baby, and babies want to be touched, held, and moved. Touch and movement of the right kind stimulate proprioception and the sense of movement and balance. They help the child to develop a sense of self and explore closeness and contact with other people. The daily task of bathing can be used to conduct a dialogue with the baby; in fact, it is dialogue, as the skin is an important organ in terms of contact. Touch nurtures enjoyment of living and reduces stress. Especially during the first year of the baby's life, parents can communicate with their child by affectionately touching the skin, and touch can even be used to communicate before the baby is born. The message to the child is one of caring contact, affection, warmth, and love. Meanwhile, the parents note subtle signals from the baby and become aware of its needs. They respond to eye contact and enter into the exchange of glances, smiles, movements, and sounds; the baby crawls to its mother, and so on.

The newborn tries to communicate what it needs. If the signals are misunderstood, the baby's unease grows until it starts to cry and scream. The time to react is remarkably short, so parents or practitioners should not delay their response. They should maintain ongoing contact with the child and react quickly to show the baby that they have understood.

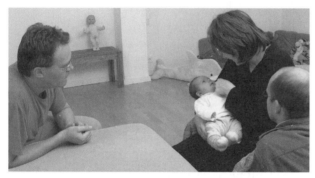

Figure 17.1. Mother-child bonding with father and practitioner present.

Parents' sensitivity to the child is significant in more ways than just showing that its needs will be met and its survival assured. This experience helps the baby begin to learn the connection between its actions and the reactions it receives from the world around it. Understanding how circumstances are connected teaches the child that it is not helpless but can achieve certain results. This enables it to develop goal-directed action later on, and it becomes the source of intentionality. On the emotional level the child increasingly experiences that it can rely on its caregivers and gains the assurance that it will be given or will be able to find all that it needs for survival from the world around it.

Parents assist their child's development by engaging with the child as an individual in the way they provide care, according to the situation, and in the way they communicate. Their behavior supports the child's capacity for self-regulation and its ability to express its needs. Parents and child are constantly adapting to the other, sensitively and on an emotional level, in verbal and nonverbal dialogue. As the parents see, hear, and understand the child's expressions of what it needs, they repeat them: expressing them in words and reflecting them in their facial expressions and movements. The parents provide the pattern by which the child will later be able to express its feelings, modulated and tuned in a suitable way. The act of orienting itself to its parents' reactions in unknown situations helps the child to estimate the importance of the situation, which reduces stress. This kind of social reassurance can only be successful if the child trusts the caregiver. An encouraging look, an expression of confidence, or supportive words will help the child in its discovery of new territory. If these are lacking, if the parents are overanxious or if they react with a look of criticism, rejection, or concern on their faces, a perfectly harmless situation can turn into an apparent threat.

Many parents whose own self-attachment is good have sound intuition and instinctively react in the right way to the expressions of the newborn. The less awareness parents have of their own state and their own immediate needs, the more likely it is that they will misinterpret the signals given by the child. This can create frustrating situations. Practitioners and parents need to realize that there is no such thing as wrong feelings; there are, however, wrong and inappropriate interpretations of signals and feelings. For example, newborns often pummel the mother's breast with their fists. Mothers might interpret this as refusal, but in fact the baby's actions assist the reflex that stimulates the flow of milk. It is therefore a healthy instinct, even if it can be a disturbance during breast-feeding. Parents sometimes underestimate or overestimate the baby's abilities.

Purposeful behavior tends to develop between three and nine months of age. Constant misinterpretation by the parents may have various causes: it may stem from their own fears and anxieties, they may find themselves overwhelmed by the situation, or they may be transferring fantasies or unconscious experiences from their own childhoods. If parents continue for some length of time to misinterpret the signals given by the child, the effect can begin to disturb the relationship between them. It can also have a negative effect on the child's self-image. Occasional misunderstandings are bound to happen, but upsets to self-regulation or early disturbances of the relationship mainly tend to occur in families where relationships are already insecure. Midwives and craniosacral practitioners should not reproach the parents or the child for misunderstanding. Practitioners can strengthen the resources that the child and its parents have available to draw on, and can give recognition to everything that is going well. By telling the parents what they have observed in a way that is as free of judgment as possible, practitioners can help parents deepen their capacity to recognize their child's signals.

Excessive crying, sleep disturbances, or feeding disturbances almost always indicate diminished self-regulation. One way that practitioners can approach this is to see whether the root of the problem lies in a disturbance in the relationship between the parents and the child—for example, do the parents view their child mainly in a negative way, as "difficult"? The child needs to be accepted and loved to ensure healthy psychological and emotional-spiritual development. It needs to experience recognition and trust from its primary caregiver. Parents who are overwhelmed by the situation over a long period of time often become less able to sense themselves. They too may then develop regulatory disturbances such as difficulties with sleeping or digestion, like their child. They then come to need professional help themselves.

In primates, especially humans, bonding behavior consists of such actions as smiling, crying, crawling up to the mother, embracing and holding on tightly, and seeking the caregiver. Outward expressions of bonding behavior are often evoked in alarm situations, for example when the caregiver goes away or is not near enough. However, it is also important to observe the type of bonding behavior when the caregiver returns—if the caregiver fails to recognize the child's signals begging for protection and security or refuses to respond to them. This can be seen in situations of uncertainty, when the child is anxious or ill, or when it feels ill at ease in any other way.

There is a complementarity in the development of bonding behavior and exploratory behavior. A child who enjoys secure attachment is more likely to dare to move away from the caregiver and more inclined to explore surrounding objects and encounter other nearby people. The child may seek reassurance from time to time from the caregiver that all is well. This exploratory behavior is very important for the development of the child's autonomy.

Bonding, then, is not a particular quality that the child possesses but an expression of the relationship between parents and child. It is an interpersonal quality held by everyone involved. During the first three months, the caregiver can change fairly freely among aunts, grandmothers, stepparents, or adoptive parents, but after that a firm bond is formed with one or more individuals close to the child. Bonding behavior is most strongly pronounced during the first six months. Once the child develops its motor capacities, which happens at the age of six to eight months, it can actively move toward its caregiver or independently explore its surroundings. From around age two, the child tries to influence the behavior of others in various ways.

17.3. Patterns of Attachment

Four patterns of attachment have been identified in the study of bonding: secure, anxious-avoidant (insecure), anxious-ambivalent (insecure), and disoriented or disorganized.

Children with a secure pattern of attachment maintain a suitable balance between closeness to their primary caregiver and exploratory behavior. If the caregiver leaves the room, they find this disturbing but are quickly pacified and play with the practitioner. When their caregiver returns, these children welcome them and again quickly settle down. The caregiver is the safe haven, the child's constant source of protection when needed.

Children with an anxious-avoidant pattern of attachment display pseudo-independence from the caregiver. To an outsider they do not seem to exhibit any problems, but separation causes them more distress than it does for children with secure attachment. If the primary caregiver goes away, the child appears unaffected and tends instead to play with the practitioner. When the caregiver returns, the child either ignores or rejects them. However, the rise in cortisol levels when the caregiver goes away is much greater in these children than in those with secure attachment. This is an indication of stress.

Children with an anxious-avoidant pattern of attachment lack confidence that their caregiver is there for them. They assume that their desires will generally be rejected and that they do not have a right to affection and love. This results in avoidance of relationships.

Children with an anxious-ambivalent pattern of attachment cling and behave in an anxious way. They are already disturbed and anxious before the caregiver leaves the room. When the caregiver does leave, the children's behavior is ambivalent. They are almost inconsolable. In the anxious-ambivalent pattern of attachment, the child feels that its caregiver is unreliable and unpredictable. The caregiver alternates between sensitivity and rejection, so the child constantly feels the need to find out what mood the caregiver is in. This permanent state of uncertainty involves considerable stress. For these children, their caregivers are often unavailable, even if they are actually physically nearby. That makes it difficult for such children to form positive expectations; with no expectation of positive change, they react to unknown situations with anxiety and stress.

Children with a disoriented pattern of attachment exhibit various combinations of the other attachment types, behaving in highly unpredictable ways that are impossible to classify. These children are disoriented and may seem paralyzed or frozen, turn around in circles, or behave in unusual and bizarre ways.

When a child needs protection and comfort, it is essential for it to make contact with its caregiver right away. If the child has not developed a coherent attachment strategy because the person who should be providing protection is also the cause of the attachment behavior, the resulting situation for the child becomes paradoxical and fairly hopeless. For children whose caregivers are behaving anxiously because of traumatic experiences of their own, the situation is similar. The child cannot understand the source of the anxiety on its caregiver's face. The caregiver is often insufficiently able to meet the child's need for care. The child may then experience the world as a constantly threatening place and see its fears reflected in the caregiver.

For children who enjoy secure attachment, the long-term effects on their development may be, for example, better and more open social behavior in day care and at school, more imagination, better concentration and attention span, and better sense of self-worth. Bowlby took the view that a child's pattern of attachment is formed and displayed in the first years of the child's life and remains fairly unchanged into adulthood.

The intensity of the attachment is no indication of its type or quality. Also, the quality of attachment of the adults affects that of the children. As caregivers, parents can be described in terms of the specific set of qualities they have: either capable of empathy and respect, self-confident, and able to tolerate frustration; more distant and disinclined to relationships, wrapped up in their own strong emotions; or ambivalent. The first set of qualities suggests adults who consciously reflect their attitude toward their own former caregiver; the second set suggests caregivers who deny their experience with their own parents and permit little emotion. They are often people whose own childhoods contained traumatic experiences and who have not sufficiently processed them. Adults in this category are themselves disoriented and dissociated to some extent and are thus unable to cope with the demands placed on them. As a result, they are less able to give the child the protection, security, and sense of safety that it needs. The child is then at greater risk, for example of being abused and living in a constant state of ambivalence or anxiety. This kind of primary caregiver becomes a source of fear and danger, and the permanent uncertainty produces constant and considerable stress. If caregivers with a traumatic background address their own themes, however, this immediately opens up the possibility of comprehensive healing. This can spread to benefit the entire family system. So parents whose own themes relate to difficulties of attachment need not have any sense of guilt; they can view it as a great opportunity to start the process of change that they need to deal with. With a degree of optimism and with professional help, they can look forward to the adventure of self-discovery.

Longer periods of separation from the caregiver can trigger a grieving process. Repeated breaks in the relationship can make children and adults unwilling to enter into any close relationships or cause them to transfer all their affection, for example to animals. Therapeutic help can enable them to live through the emotions brought up in the grieving process and be released from them.

17.4. Stable and Deep Bonds between Parents and Child

What determines the child's ability to develop true adult maturity and sound relationships, assuming that the model presented by its parents is a reliable one? Reaction to the child's behavior must come immediately in order to trigger a learning effect. Children love having the same sequence repeated over and over; it gives them a sense of security and predictability in an ever-changing world. The recurring rhythm of daily life helps them feel that they understand the way things work, and it gives structure to the passage of time. Through this experience, it becomes comprehensible to them. Events such as birthdays and cultural holidays are set points on the calendar that give shape to the year. In our era, marked by constant change and a high degree of mobility, such fixed points in life are what provide solidity and a means of orientation. The rituals or routines of everyday life are also firm markers to rely on. Children who grow up without them almost always tend to be rootless and lost. They need a great deal of continuity, clear structure, and reliability. Without them, children are continually on guard, feeling that they will have to defend themselves at any moment. In time this can lead to aggression and behavioral difficulties.

When dealing with slightly older children, the pediatric cranio-sacral practitioner should note whether the parents are allowing their child to do the kinds of activities that suit the child's individual development. Do they tend to expect too much of the child, or too little? Do they have too much or too little confidence in their child? To what extent do they allow the child space to explore and develop? Do the parents continually make suggestions to the child as to what to do, and do they one-sidedly direct the dialogue between them? The craniosacral practitioner is a point of reference, a fulcrum, during the treatment session

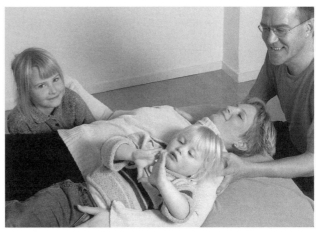

Figure 17.2. Bonding and sibling dynamics; brief treatment of the mother.

with the child. The more harmonious their interaction and the better the quality of the relationship between the child and the practitioner, the greater the effect of strengthening bonding behavior; after a number of sessions, the practitioner may even temporarily become a person with whom the child bonds.

17.5. Rituals and Routines

Rituals and routines are practices that happen regularly, for example, if the mother lies down for half an hour after lunch to rest while the children learn to play on their own. Rituals or routines in everyday life serve the purpose of setting boundaries and training in certain principles. Examples would be saying "please" and "thank you" as well as the bedtime routine. These not only provide a link to strength and stability but also help build fairness, sympathy, and mutual respect. Constant recurrence makes them part of a routine, and when they have special meaning, they become a ritual. The individuals involved need to relate to what they are doing, and the rituals need to be flexible and match the expectations of everyone involved. If the ritual is an obligation rather than a pleasure, it should be adapted to suit everyone. For example, as children's development progresses, they may outgrow the old rituals, and new ones will need to be devised. A creative and cooperative family approach to finding and observing new rituals can be a valuable experience for all. The visit to the craniosacral practitioner can itself be a ritual.

17.6. Sibling Dynamics

The child does not only interact with its mother; there are also interactions with other close family members, its father and siblings. Jealous behavior may be a cry for more love and attention. The child is afraid of being loved less and fears the withdrawal of love. When children receive less attention and less assurance that they are loved, they develop a sense of inferiority. They may compensate by inwardly steeling themselves or by self-resignation, all in an effort to be loved. Later in life, such individuals have a constant need to be successful and receive recognition.

One solution to the sibling problem might be to set aside certain times when the eldest has the full and undisturbed attention of its mother or father, when they can simply enjoy each other's company. Sibling rivalry can perhaps be defused by letting each child individually speak about the emotions caused by the tension between them and share its feelings. Forces are released when children feel that their feelings are sensed and taken seriously.

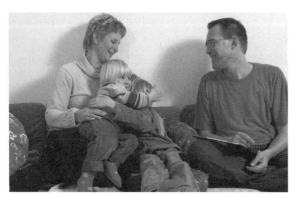
Figure 17.3. Sibling dynamics, with mother and practitioner present.

17.7. Pain of Separation

17.7.1. Pain of Separation Caused by Birth and Separation from the Mother

The undesired separation of the baby from its mother often leads to separation pain or trauma. The pain of separation at birth and during the initial weeks and months that follow is a considerable challenge for the child. It is fearful of loss and in need of protection, contact, and warmth. The baby adapts and learns strategies to try to avoid difficult situations. The infant pays particular attention on hearing the sound and rhythm of its mother's voice. A newborn baby is completely dependent on its mother; the way it experiences the world is mainly based on sensation, and it needs to feel assured that its mother or father is there and able to protect, feed, and care for it. The child's fundamental trust in its environment and life in general is established, and either strengthened or diminished, at that earliest stage after birth and during the time that follows.

17.7.2. Pain of Separation during the Early Years

Separation, with the pain that it brings, may be an inevitable part of life, but care should be taken during a child's early years to find a way of dealing with this important issue to minimize harm as much as possible. It is normal for children to have fears; they are part of healthy development and often occur at stages of transition. When faced with separation, the child screams, rages, and cries; it flies into a panic when its caregiver goes out of sight. When put to bed, the child is unable to go to sleep or cannot sleep through the night. Eventually autonomic symptoms such as stomachache or headache appear. There can be many reasons for fear of separation: the aftereffects of a difficult or traumatic birth, more frequent experiences of separation, smaller nuclear families living in isolated surroundings, or a loosening of social connections. If the parents are under stress—for example, stress at work or financial worries—this can affect the child, causing insecurity and vague fearfulness. Fear of separation is usually finished by age three. If a child of age five or older is still experiencing great fear of separation, professional help should be considered.

Motherless Child

Sometimes I feel like a motherless child
A long way from my home
Sometimes I wish I could fly
Like a bird up in the sky
Oh, sometimes I wish I could fly
Fly like a bird up in the sky
A little closer to my home

Sometimes I feel like a motherless child
A long way from my home
Sometimes I feel like freedom is near
Sometimes I feel like freedom is here
Sometimes I feel like it's close at hand
Sometimes I feel like the kingdom is at hand
But we're so far from home

These words are from a traditional gospel song[1] that dates from the days of slavery, when enslaved children were commonly sold and separated from their parents. The pain and despair it expresses are very clear and show the hopelessness felt by a child that has lost its mother. But there is hope in these words as well: the word *sometimes* suggests that there are at least some periods when the motherless child is not suffering those emotions.

ANATOMY, NEUROANATOMY, AND NEUROPHYSIOLOGY FOR CRANIOSACRAL WORK

18

Birth usually occurs around 259 to 287 days after conception. The baby weighs around seven pounds eleven ounces and is around twenty inches long. The baby's heart rate is 120 to 140 beats per minute, and its respiratory rate is forty-four breaths per minute. At birth the baby's brain has around one hundred billion neurons and weighs around twelve ounces.

Networks of neurons already exist for many functions of perception, and these networks are developed and extended if sufficiently stimulated. The infant brain has enormous plasticity; since the various functions are not yet firmly assigned to different regions of the brain, it is highly adaptable. At the end of the first year, the baby's brain weighs around two pounds. By the end of the second year, its size has almost reached that of an adult brain.

18.1. The Cranium: Growth and Ossification

The first cranial bones start to form from the third month of gestation at the border of the cranial base. At this stage the cranial base is still cartilaginous. At the time of birth the cranium of a newborn consists of forty-five individual bony components. Of these, thirteen small bones form the cranial base. The skull or cranium is the most complicated skeletal structure, with more connections than any other. Cranial growth is also a highly complex process. Seen from the structural point of view, it takes place on three levels:

- Sutural growth occurs in the cranial sutures, at the borders of the cranial bones.
- Chondral growth originates in the synchondroses (cartilaginous joints).
- Periosteal growth originates in the periosteum of the bones.

At birth, all the cranial bones are joined by cartilage. There are six fontanels. The size of the cranium doubles in the first year, and the sutures begin to form. At the end of one year, almost all the fontanels have closed except the anterior (large) fontanel, which closes in the first to second year.

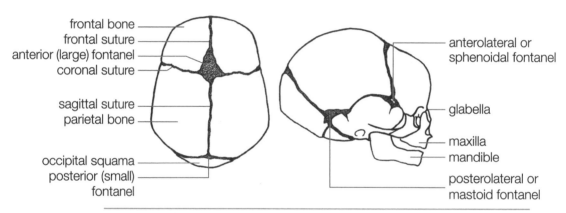

Figure 18.1. Cranium of a newborn.

At birth the **occipital bone** consists of four parts: the occipital squama, two lateral parts, and the basilar part, at the end of which is the SBS. The occipital condyle is still in two parts, around two-thirds of it consisting of the lateral part and one-third the basilar part. The connections between the condyle and the squama close by the third year of life, and by the sixth year they are completely ossified. Around the sixth year the basilar part ossifies with the lateral parts of the occipital bone. This can have the effect of enlarging the foramen magnum during the first six years of life. The SBS is almost completely ossified by age fourteen to eighteen.

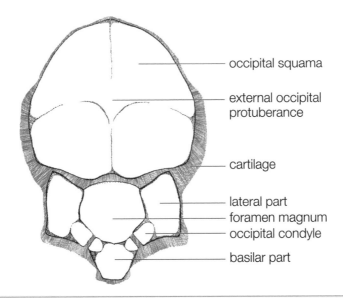

Figure 18.2. The occipital bone at birth.

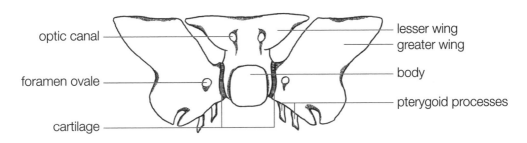

Figure 18.3. The three parts of the sphenoid at birth.

At birth the sphenoid consists of three parts: the body, the lesser wings along with the right and greater wings, and the pterygoid processes. The sphenoid ossifies in the first year.

At birth the **temporal bone** has three parts: the squamous part, the petrous part, and the tympanic ring. The temporal bone ossifies in the first year. The petrous part attains its full size by the sixth year. The mastoid process begins to form from the first year and is fully formed by around age four or five.

At birth the **frontal bone** consists of two parts, a right half and a left half linked by the metopic or frontal suture. This suture begins to close in the second or third month and is completely ossified by around the fourth to sixth year.

Regarding the **parietal bone,** after birth the interdigitations of the sagittal suture begin to form and are fully formed in the third year. The **ethmoid bone** consists of two lateral parts at birth, separated by a third part, the perpendicular plate. This forms the superior part of the nasal septum. The **vomer** ossifies completely by age sixteen. The **maxilla** is separated from the incisive bone at birth by the incisive suture. This suture can persist into adulthood, until middle age.

Ossification also occurs in:

- the palatine bone from the forty-fifth day of gestation
- the zygomatic bone from the fifth month of gestation
- the nasal bone from the third month of gestation

The **mandible,** which consists of two hemimandibles joined by cartilage at birth, ossify in the first year. The **lacrimal bone** develops in the third month of gestation.

The **atlas,** which is the first cervical vertebra, consists of three parts at birth: the anterior arch and two lateral parts, joined by cartilage. The posterior arch ossifies in the third year of life. The atlas is completely ossified by age seven to nine. **Vertebrae** consist of three parts at birth: the body and the two parts of the vertebral arch. The two parts of the arch fuse posteriorly in the first year, and the body fuses with the arch in the third year. In the lumbar region, the body fuses with the arch in the sixth year. The transverse process grows between age ten and age twenty-five. The **sacrum** consists of five sacral vertebrae at birth, joined by cartilage. The ossification of the sacrum is complete by around age twenty-five.

The **cranial base** develops over a period of five to seven years, changing from an initial thirteen parts to a total of four, or five if the ethmoid is included.

18.2. Cranial Growth

The growth of bones with a membranous origin is aided by external stimuli such as the force of expansion of the brain, primary respiration (the craniosacral rhythm, mid-tide, and Long Tide), and variations occurring during sucking and swallowing. Muscle contractions and the intraoral vacuum created when breast-feeding stimulate the development of the cranial base. The activity of the tongue influences the SBS. Suckling is even thought to reduce extension dysfunctions of the sphenoid and inferior vertical strain of the SBS, at least to some extent. Nevertheless, the release of lateral or vertical strain dysfunctions still requires the additional help of a craniosacral practitioner or cranial osteopath. This is because the occipital bone is stabilized and held in balance by a number of muscles during sucking. It is therefore necessary to balance as many structures as possible from at least the rib cage upward. The action of the lips when sucking stimulates the growth of the facial skeleton. The facial muscles all have their attachments close to the sutures, and the stimulation during sucking leads to a decrease in sutural dysfunctions. The intraoral vacuum and the movements of the tongue stimulate the growth of the intermaxillary and interpalatine sutures; this is important for the transverse growth of the cranium. The action of sucking, both during the fetal period and especially after birth, also helps the development of the mandible, for example. Its growth is also determined by perception of the position of the tongue in relation to the lips, dental arcades, and the soft and hard palates. It is therefore influenced by the way the sucking and swallowing motion is carried out.

18.2.1. The Cranial Sutures

The cranial sutures have an important role as the skull of the newborn develops. They function as growth centers for the cranium. The cranial sutures link the borders of the cranial bones. At birth, the sutures are about 0.04 to 0.4 inches wide. From the age of six months they can no longer be felt as clearly. The three most commonly occurring types of suture:

- plane suture: a smooth, flat meeting of two bones, for example between the ethmoid and lacrimal bones
- squamous suture: an overlapping scalelike joint, for example the suture between the temporal and parietal bones
- serrate suture: a jagged, deeply indented joint in which the bones interlink like the teeth of two combs

The suture tissue is highly elastic and consists of three layers or zones:

- the layer adjacent to the bone, the cellular or osteoblastic layer
- the fibrous layer, with many collagen fibers
- the middle layer, with many blood vessels and nociceptors (nerve endings), which links the two other layers

Sutures are highly nociceptive. Their mobility assists growth and form, so they contribute to skull growth in a fundamental way. The link they provide between the cranial bones is very elastic. During growth, the two edges of the bones concerned are joined by narrow plates of connective tissue, which are most marked in the region of the calvaria and viscerocranium. Reduced activity, which may, for example, be brought about by strong compression during birth, causes ossification to begin. This can lead to marked asymmetries of the head. Dysfunctions in the viscerocranium and neurocranium need to be corrected before the sutures have ossified. This not only promotes optimum development of the child but also preempts a variety of later symptoms in adolescence and adulthood.

The three largest cranial sutures are the coronal, lambdoid, and sagittal sutures. All the other sutures are named for the bones involved. The active growth zones of a cranial suture are at the bone ends. The osteoblastic layer gradually disappears until adulthood, which reduces growth activity. The size and number of vessels in the sutures also decreases once the cranium is fully grown.

The typical interdigitating joint of the cranial sutures begins to take shape around the fifth year of life. Formation is complete around age eight to twelve, and only then are the sutures fully joined. Ossification of the human body is mostly complete by about age twenty-four to twenty-eight, and at that stage the five sacral vertebrae form the single sacrum.

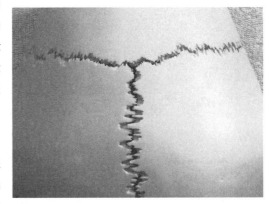

Figure 18.4. Sutures and the bregma, shown on an artificial model of a child's skull.

Suture systems and levels of growth:

- The coronal suture system, between the frontal and parietal bones, runs across the cranium and down each side to the cranial base. It promotes the lengthwise growth of the cranium.
- The lambdoid suture system forms the joint among the occipital squama, the parietal bones, and the mastoid process. It promotes the growth of the occiput.
- The sagittal suture system runs anteriorly from behind and across the calvaria (the roof of the skull) along the sagittal suture. In the newborn it continues down in the anterior direction via the frontal suture, nasal bones, and maxillae to the two halves of the mandible. It mainly aids the growth in width of the neurocranium and viscerocranium.

The craniofacial suture system links the anterior part of the neurocranium with the viscerocranium and maxillae. It helps enable the mid-facial region to develop anteriorly and downward through the growth of the facial bones.

The frontal suture closes between the second and third month and ossifies in the first years of life so that the frontal bone becomes a single unpaired cranial bone. This is one of the few sutures that has completely disappeared in most adults.

The partial ossification of the sutures occurs differently from one individual to another. This individual variation is both anatomical and a matter of timing. Isolated ossification centers can appear in all sutures and produce extra sutural or wormian bones such as the interparietal bones or the "Inca bone" in the region of the lambdoid suture.

The sutures retain a degree of flexibility even in their ossified state. The ability to sense the craniosacral rhythm results not only from the mobility of the cranial sutures but also from the relative intraosseous mobility of the cranial bones, changing membrane tension, fluctuation of the CSF, and CSF pressure.

18.2.2. Closure of the Sutures—Craniosynostosis

Premature closure of a suture, called premature synostosis, leads to deformities of the head. The growth impulse that determines the thickness of the cranial bones comes from the inner layer of the periosteum, and the impulse for growth in length and breadth comes from the sutures. This explains why their premature closure reduces or prevents normal growth of the cranial bones. The growth of the brain requires space, and if the sutures are closed, the head becomes deformed. If the squamous part of the frontal bone fuses too soon, it can lead to the formation of a wedge-shaped head, called trigonocephaly. If the sagittal suture fuses too soon, this leads to a scaphoid (boat-shaped) head; this is called scaphocephaly. Premature closure of the coronal suture, when symmetrical, produces a "tower head," called oxycephaly. Asymmetrical closure of the coronal suture produces a "slanting head," called plagiocephaly. Displacement of the four parts of the occipital bone can also lead to plagiocephaly. Increased cerebral pressure can in rare instances lead to drowsiness, vomiting, and convulsions.

Experience has shown that the subtle impulses delivered by Craniosacral Therapy have little effect on craniosynostosis. If the synostosis is causing increased pressure or restricting brain growth, a quick response is required. Surgical treatment should be arranged for around the third to sixth month, or at the latest by the age of nine months. In such cases, the purpose of craniosacral treatment should be to provide additional support, both prior to surgery and afterward. Before the operation, the purpose is to balance the whole surrounding area and entire craniosacral system on the bony, membranous, and fluid levels, or the fluid body. It is advisable to allow a certain amount of time between treatment and surgery. A few days after the operation, visceral therapy and peripheral treatment to the sacrum and trunk can be given. Cranial treatment needs to wait until some weeks after surgery. The aim of therapy at this stage is to reduce the physical, psychological, and emotional-spiritual effects on the child and to strengthen the self-healing forces.

The V-spread technique can be used, as well as the established release techniques for the cranium. In traditional Chinese medicine, the bones belong to the functional system of the kidneys and bladder; visceral treatment can support these.

18.2.3. Growth and Form of the Neurocranium and Viscerocranium

Craniosacral practitioners should include an assessment of the form of the viscerocranium and neurocranium in their evaluation. Slight lateral or anterior indentations usually disappear and only remain visible or palpable for about ten days after birth. If they last longer, the craniosacral practitioner should treat them, and as a precaution they should continue to be monitored by a pediatrician.

The sutures are often compressed by the birth process and even following a C-section. Craniosacral practitioners should evaluate the following items, and provide treatment if they are found:

- membranous and/or osseous dysfunctions of the SBS and cranial base as a whole

- membranous and/or osseous intraoccipital dysfunctions
- osseous sutural lesions of the roof of the skull, for example over-lapping of the sagittal suture and the coronal suture

Craniosacral practitioners should palpate the sutures for any abnormalities, such as unevenness, points of particular tenderness, or changes. The quality of the craniosacral rhythm, loss of mobility of one or more cranial bones, uneven tension of the dura mater, or reduced CSF flow are also important indicators. It is important to recognize these and provide accurately targeted treatment because problems originating as dysfunctions of the SBS can develop into other dysfunctions as the child grows.

An association has been found between the use of medication during birth and the frequency of compression of the SBS. Most of the children studied who had been delivered vaginally under epidural anesthesia were found to have compression of the SBS, usually membranous in nature; of those delivered by emergency C-section, seventy-five percent had compression of the SBS. Among those delivered naturally without the use of medication, only twelve percent were found to have compression of the SBS.

The dura mater plays an important role in the formation, shaping, and development of the cranial vault. Any impairment, for example

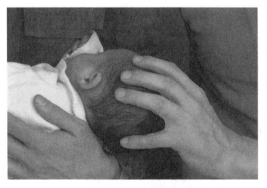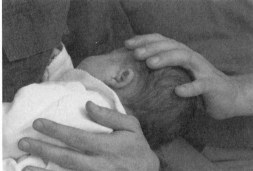

Figure 18.5. Palpating the parietal bones and listening to the craniosacral rhythm as appropriate.

because of injury or unbalanced membrane tensions during or following birth, can lead to disturbances of growth and regeneration processes in the sutures. It is possible that closure of a suture might occur in this way. Free mobility and a balanced state of tension of the meninges (the cranial and spinal dura) are important for the normal development of the CNS.

Sutural landmarks:

- bregma: the meeting point of the coronal and sagittal sutures; in newborns, the anterior (large) fontanel
- lambda: the meeting point of the lambdoid and sagittal sutures; in newborns, the posterior (small) fontanel
- pterion: at the lateral end of the coronal suture, at the meeting point of the frontal bone, sphenoid, and temporal bone; in newborns, the anterolateral or sphenoidal fontanel
- asterion: the meeting point of the lambdoid, parietomastoid, and occipitomastoid sutures, where the occipital, parietal, and temporal bones meet; in newborns, the posterolateral or mastoid fontanel
- inion: the external occipital protuberance, the most pronounced outward-protruding point of the occipital bone
- nasion: the most posteriorly situated point of the nose

The anterior fontanel is reduced in size shortly after birth, possibly due to displacement of the bones. It becomes larger again some days later. It can continue to enlarge during the first one to three months of the baby's life. It has an average diameter of one to two inches, and it closes between the fourth and the twenty-sixth month. Protrusion of the fontanel may indicate raised intracerebral pressure, and indentation can be a sign of excessive fluid loss; both should be monitored. If the situation does not show clear improvement, the practitioner should make a note of it, and the parents should mention it to the pediatrician on their next visit. For treatment, see section 27.7.

18.3. Some Examples of the Results of Disturbances at the Sutures

The occipitomastoid suture links the occipital bone and the mastoid process. When we consider the anatomical and functional structure of these two bones, the associated parts of the dura mater, the vessels in the region, and the surrounding parts of the musculoskeletal system, it becomes clear that the symptoms resulting from any disturbance here can be wide-ranging. The disturbances almost always affect the jugular foramen in the cranial base. The internal jugular vein receives venous blood from the brain from the anteromedial area and from the inferior petrosal sinus and sigmoid sinus in the posterolateral area. It drains this blood back to the heart through the jugular foramen. Around eighty-five percent of the blood from the brain is drained through these two foramina.

The frontozygomatic suture links the zygomatic process of the frontal bone and the frontal process of the zygomatic bone. Again, anatomy and function give an indication of the symptoms to be expected from disturbances at this suture. In newborns, disturbances at this suture are common as a result of facial trauma during birth and later as a result of falls onto the face when the child is learning to walk or during play. The zygomatic bone is often a "secret troublemaker" in the facial region, and one that receives too little attention. Compression or displacement at an angle can hinder the motion of the craniosacral rhythm in the entire hemisphere of the cranium. It often also influences the position of the frontal bone, sphenoid, maxilla, intracranial membranes, and the mandible, and can affect occlusion.

Just as these structures can be disturbed by effects operating from the zygomatic bone, the reverse can also occur. Therefore disturbances in the region of these structures can also affect the zygomatic bone and maxilla as well as the paranasal and frontal sinuses. The frontozygomatic suture is also connected to the temporal muscle and is situated close to the pterygopalatine ganglion. This ganglion is often compressed, leading to a number of different problems that include radiating headaches. It is then necessary to release all these sutures and the bones forming them, including the frontal and paranasal sinuses; the frontonasal, frontozygomatic, and pterygopalatine sutures; the maxilla, sphenoid, and palatine bones; and, intraorally, the vomer.

Structural craniosacral treatment is a gentle way to create more space fairly quickly. It achieves better positioning of the individual structures and the entire cranium, helping to produce a more balanced craniosacral rhythm. This in turn works from within to harmonize and vitalize the structures and vessels of the brain and membrane tension.

At birth the occipital bone consists of four parts, which fuse around age six to eight to form a single whole (see fig. 18.2). The birth process can adversely affect the four parts of the bone. W. G. Sutherland, Viola Frymann, and others discovered over many years of practical research that children with neurological problems also had structural changes or restrictions. Details of the research carried out by Frymann can be found in her *Collected Writings*.[1]

Abnormal patterns of motion or dysfunctions can quite often be palpated at the SBS, in particular, and in the region of the occipital bone. There is often strain or torsion as well as compression of the occipital bone (see fig. 28.5). The head then feels quite hard and immobile at the sutures. There can also be strain, displacement, or marked compression of the sphenoid and temporal bones, which consist of three parts at birth. The cause can be the position of the fetus in the weeks prior to birth, for example in the case of multiple pregnancies. The most common reason is a difficult birth or external physical trauma.

Restrictions of structure or function at the cranial base can have a variety of effects on a child's well-being and development. Asymmetry of the occipital bone and reduction in strength of the rhythms have an adverse effect on the growth of the cranial base, spinal column, and the child's general development. For example, these children tend later to become hyperactive or to suffer from learning difficulties or psychological and social deficits. The foramen magnum and atlanto-occipital joint are both important fulcrums of the craniosacral system and of central importance in the treatment of children. The external surfaces of the occipital bone provide attachment for fasciae and tendons of the pharyngeal and cervical musculature. The jugular foramen is situated in the cartilaginous structure directly next to the lateral parts of the occipital bone. The nerves and blood vessels that pass through it are also affected by the position of the lateral parts, via fasciae and cartilaginous tissue. The specific treatment of the occipital bone is described in section 28.4.

The lateral borders of the foramen magnum are defined by the occipital condyles. Together with the atlas, they form the atlanto-occipital joint, which allows the nodding movement of the head. The medulla oblongata passes through the foramen magnum, and cranial nerves emerge in this region. When there is more space for the basilar part, there is more space for the medulla oblongata.

KEY POINT

As a basic principle, improvement of the position and movement of all the bones of the cranial base should be considered. We should also consider the tension of the cranial and spinal dura mater. Achieving as balanced a state of tension as possible of the dura mater is just as important as the position and mobility of the bones and sutures. The dura mater surrounds the brain and spinal cord and is of central importance in Craniosacral Therapy. The thirteen components of the cranial base in infants are all linked to each other by cartilage and connective tissue, but it is primarily the dura mater that holds them together. Its outer layer forms the periosteum. In newborns, the bones are more membranous in nature and "float" on the dura mater. It is therefore mainly the dura mater that provides the required stability of the baby's head.

As craniosacral practitioners, we should assess and treat the meninges surrounding the whole brain within the cranial vault via the bones. We should also assess and treat the intracranial membranes that link the various regions of the brain. We should balance the membrane tension of the spinal dura mater and include the sacrum in this process. As a next step, we can encourage the overall balance of membrane tension of the cranial and spinal dura mater. Following bones and membranes, the third level to be considered is that of the fluids. Sutherland wrote, "Gently, gently, do not force anything—remember: the fluid in there is working for you."[2] We direct our attention to the fluids of the body, especially the flow and force of the CSF.

An experienced craniosacral practitioner will make a differentiated assessment of the three levels of this triad: the osseous, membranous, and fluid levels. The questions to ask are: which level is most accessible? Which is most responsive? Which has the greatest need of specific support? As one level achieves greater balance, this has an automatic effect on the other levels, since they are ultimately a unity. Having done this, the practitioner should encourage the integration of the new balance in the whole cranium and craniosacral system.

Note: it is important for the health of the child to attend to all abnormal findings—cranial asymmetry, torticollis, sensory or motor problems, and so on—in the course of the craniosacral treatment, and to monitor the further course of these findings. Examination by a pediatrician or neurologist should be considered and a referral made if necessary.

18.4. CSF, the Brain Stem, and CV4

Apart from water, the substances contained in the CSF are sodium, potassium, calcium, glucose, magnesium ions, and chloride ions, all important for CNS communication. The vitamin C content of the CSF is four times what it is in the blood; the pantothenic acid content is ten times higher; and the biotin content is many times higher. The

CSF contains hormones secreted by the pituitary, the pineal body, and the hypothalamus as well as endorphins, neurotransmitters, and substances involved in immune functions. The production of CSF amounts to around 0.7 to 1.4 ounces in one hour and seventeen to twenty-four ounces over twenty-four hours. The total volume of CSF, some six ounces, is exchanged four to seven times in a twenty-four hour period.

The two halves of the thalamus provide the lateral border on each side of the third ventricle in the middle of the brain. The ventral end of the ventricle is formed by the lamina terminalis; below is the optic chiasm and posteriorly the pineal body. Part of the floor of the third ventricle is formed by the hypothalamus. The thalamus is the control center for all incoming and outgoing information. The third ventricle is also seen as the "gateway to the consciousness."

The effect of the CV4 and the balancing of motions at the occipital bone is to stimulate the brain stem, the reticular system, and the locus coeruleus. In the brain stem, this stimulates nerve nuclei that control all physiologically important functions, such as heart rate, blood pressure, and respiratory function. It also produces an effect on the nuclei of the twelve cranial nerve pairs and their exit points. The reticular formation consists of a part ascending from the medulla oblongata, through parts of the brain stem to the midbrain and diencephalon, and descending connections running to the motor neurons of the anterior horn of the spinal cord. The reticular formation has several roles: the transmission of stimuli, control of autonomic functions, coordination of reflexes to produce motor sequences, and the processing of afferent information. It runs through the central core of the brain stem and the spinal cord as far down as its caudal end.

The neurotransmitters epinephrine, commonly called adrenaline, and acetylcholine are also present in the reticular formation in regions of the medulla oblongata. Serotonin and endorphins are found in the reticular system of the medulla oblongata, pons, and midbrain; norepinephrine, also called noradrenaline, in the medulla oblongata and pons; and dopamine in the midbrain and elsewhere. Stimulation of the reticular formation produces effects such as alertness to danger. Severe damage to it can lead to coma or death. The reticular formation is also important for the cycle of sleep and wakefulness, as it helps determine whether it is worth waking up. It operates in humans as well as primitive vertebrates, birds, and mammals as an instinctive control center that receives, evaluates, and processes millions of pieces of incoming sensory information. There are also interconnections with the cranial nerve systems: the trigeminal, optic, facial, and glossopharyngeal nerves.

The reticular formation warns us of danger signs received by various senses, such as the smell of smoke, sudden light at night time, and unpleasant tastes that might indicate the risk of poisoning. The brain stem and the reticular formation in particular date back many millennia to our distant ancestors, raising an instant instinctive alarm at signs of danger and thus saving the species. In the brain stem, the reticular formation also passes through the locus coeruleus, a blue-gray area at the ventrolateral border of the rhomboid fossa, which is the floor of the fourth ventricle.

Why do we need to know these anatomical details? One reason is that the information provides an important guide to location when we are treating breathing problems, for example following anesthesia, or when treating loss of the sense of smell and taste. It shows us how we can stimulate the appropriate structures of the brain by improving CSF fluctuation, as by using the CV4 technique. It also helps our understanding of craniosacral trauma healing: these are subcortical centers that are instinctively activated through neuroception in response to perceived danger, and they are often overstimulated following shock or trauma. Where there is a high degree of stress, shock, or trauma, more than one region is affected. Subcortical centers with different functions become involved and interact. These include the reticular formation, locus coeruleus, hippocampus, amygdalae, anterior nuclei of the thalamus, and cingulate gyrus. All operate in a subconscious, instinctive way, but their state is communicated to the cerebral cortex via plastic neural connections; in the cerebral cortex the subconsciously received impressions are experienced consciously and are understood and assessed rationally.

18.5. The Wonders of CV4

The neurophysiological connections described above show why the CV4 technique is so helpful in the treatment of so many symptoms. The temporary change in CSF pressure not only stimulates the brain as a whole; it specifically stimulates the areas mentioned above as well as the hormone system. Endorphins, which are morphine-like substances made by the body, are found in certain areas of the walls of the ventricle and the aqueduct of the midbrain. These areas are also stimulated by the CV4 technique. This has the effect of increasing endorphin production, which can be a natural way of reducing pain. Other effects of this fluctuation technique, its detoxifying function, and its many effects that create balance have been described in detail in my practical textbook *Craniosacral Rhythm*[3] and in Torsten Liem's *Cranial Osteopathy.*[4]

Another suggested effect that seems interesting here is that greater arousal of the sympathetic nervous system is thought to reduce CSF production by about twenty-five percent. On the other hand, greater arousal of the parasympathetic system is thought to increase CSF production by up to one hundred percent. Increased CSF flow operates like a lymphatic pump: the stronger longitudinal fluctuation increases the motility of tissues and fluids in the whole body, stimulating all the functions of the body.

The assistance provided by performing the CV4 technique can depend on the way it is administered. The technique is not applied by pressure; we invite or induce the stillpoint gently and carefully so that it can achieve wonderful results. The CV4 technique is both generally effective and helpful as a means of balancing in the treatment of many specific symptoms. It can therefore be used in hyperactive children, in those suffering from sluggishness, and in children with sleep disturbances.

The norepinephrine level in the blood of a newborn in the first hour after birth is about twenty to thirty times what it is later in life. The baby has already begun to secrete hormones of the epinephrine family during the last powerful contractions. The norepinephrine surge helps the baby adjust to the reduced availability of oxygen that usually occurs at this stage, as well as to be alert when first meeting its mother. One of the places where norepinephrine is produced is the locus coeruleus, an area in the brain stem that in evolutionary terms is the oldest part of the brain. This area is extremely active shortly before, during, and following birth. It is closely linked with the olfactory bulb. This is consistent with the observation that norepinephrine assists learning processes associated with the sense of smell, and also with the fact that recognition by smell is very important in the mother-child bonding process. The CV4 also stimulates CSF flow and the brain stem.

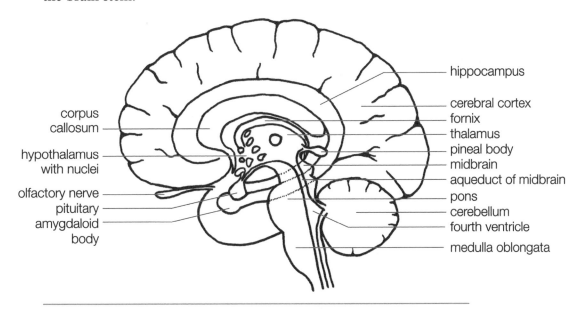

Figure 18.6. Median cross-section of the brain.

18.6. The Triune Brain

The human brain developed over millions of years of evolution. In simple terms we now see it as consisting of three active, integrated, functionally different parts:

1. The **reptilian brain**: its role is survival, and it is therefore responsible for fundamental regulatory mechanisms; it is reflected in instinctive and physical sensations (see also section 25.1).
2. The **old mammalian brain**: responsible for emotions and memory, it is reflected in the emotions.
3. The **neocortex**: responsible for rational thought and problem-solving, it is reflected in words and thoughts.

18.7. Cranial Nerve Reflexes

Parents can note these reflexes as they watch their child in the course of everyday life. Craniosacral practitioners will observe them during sessions and can support the function of the various cranial nerves as they treat the corresponding regions. If a reflex is found to be restricted over a period of time, the cause should be checked by a pediatrician.

18.7.1. Reflex Tests

- **Olfactory:** the baby gives a start when a substance with a strong, intense smell is held in front of its nose. The ability to smell provides a test of cranial nerve I.
- **Optic blink reflex:** the baby blinks when a bright light is momentarily shone directly into its eyes. The ability to see is a test of cranial nerve II.
- **Doll's eyes reflex:** this test involves turning the baby's head slowly to one side. Its eyes follow but move more slowly, like the eyes of a doll. This reflex normally continues to exist for only two or three

weeks after birth. The movement of the eyes tests cranial nerves III, IV, and VI.

- **Rooting reflex:** if the baby's cheek is stroked, the baby turns its head to that side. This reflex normally continues to exist for about the first year of life. Touching the cheek or face tests cranial nerves V and VII.

- **Yawn test:** when yawning, the baby moves the facial muscles of both sides symmetrically. Observation of yawning tests cranial nerve VII.

- **Moro reflex:** the baby has an instinctive fear of falling. Its startled response is to fling its arms out, then draw them back close to its body. Its fingers are flexed inward as if trying to grasp something. This startle response is very pronounced during the first two months of life and disappears after about four months. The function of balance or equilibrium provides a test of cranial nerve VIII.

- **Acoustic blink reflex:** the baby blinks in response to a sudden sound. Stand in front of the baby and clap your hands. The ability to hear tests cranial nerve VIII.

- **Gag reflex:** the baby reacts by gagging when the posterior wall of the pharynx or throat is touched. The function of the throat muscles provides a test of cranial nerves IX and X.

- **Swallowing test:** the baby completely swallows its milk, with smooth movements and without gasping or struggling for air. The ability to drink and swallow tests the function of the throat muscles and thus cranial nerves IX and X.

- **Neck turning test:** the baby turns its head easily and equally to each side with no restriction and without inclining its head. The ability to turn the head tests the function of the sternocleidomastoid muscle, and shrugging the shoulders tests the trapezius. These movements test cranial nerve XI.

- **Sucking reflex:** the baby begins a sucking action when its lips are stimulated. The function of the tongue muscles tests cranial nerve XII.

- **Tongue thrusting:** the baby is able to thrust out its tongue and draw it back completely. It may thrust out its tongue spontaneously in order to exercise the muscles and assist their development. The function of tongue movement tests cranial nerve XII.

These tests should be performed with great care and briefly. In my craniosacral treatment sessions, I do not begin by testing the reflexes and cranial nerves in isolation, as in an examination by a physician or neurologist. Our duty of care means that if any abnormalities or disease are present, medical examinations should be carried out first. Only then should the craniosacral practitioner begin a course of treatment, lasting three to nine sessions. I observe the kinds of function and the reflexes exhibited by the child from the beginning to the end of the session, particularly in the initial treatment sessions. I tell the parents and the child anything I have noticed, concentrating on the positive. If I notice anything abnormal, I observe it over the course of several sessions and record my findings. I then raise the subject with the parents when there is an appropriate opportunity. There is a list of the cranial nerves and their functions in the appendix.

18.8. Oxytocin, the Hormone of Love and Affection

For me, love is in the first instance an emotional state and a core experience; it is a primary condition rather than a fixed place; and love is not a hormone. Nevertheless, modern neurobiology can explain the biochemical reactions of different emotional states and can measure them. This research and the conclusions drawn from it provide fascinating insight into the interactions that take place in the unity of body, mind, and spirit. The spiritual-emotional level affects our body, which responds by producing its own endogenous drugs—or vice versa.

The physiological effects of the neuropeptide oxytocin in sexuality, its clinical use in midwifery, and its effects on lactation have already been discussed. I want to examine briefly the effect of oxytocin on behavior. Oxytocin has a calming effect on the nursing mother during breast-feeding, and this helps develop the intense emotional bond between her and her newborn child. When suckling, and in the act of sucking, the baby produces oxytocin, which helps it to feel an intimate bond with its mother. It then becomes tired and goes to sleep. The sight of a baby falling into blissful sleep is a delight.

Oxytocin is released in the brains of men and women during expressions of tenderness and sexual behavior. Like an opiate, it creates euphoria and calm. Following orgasm, oxytocin causes us to feel tired and to fall asleep more easily. It helps to cement interpersonal relationships and so is also seen as the hormone of faithfulness.

There are hypotheses suggesting that increased production of oxytocin before pregnancy encourages the increased formation of oxytocin receptors. This in turn is beneficial to labor. Another way for people to relate to one another is by eating together, which also raises oxytocin levels.

In 1973, Candace Pert demonstrated the existence of opiate receptors in the brain.[5] In 1979 it was shown that endorphins are released during labor and delivery. In Sweden, Kerstin Uvnäs Moberg has been researching the effect of oxytocin for more than ten years, showing that its regular release is helpful as a buffer against stress factors.[6] It has a beneficial effect on blood pressure and heart rate, and she found that oxytocin assists growth and healing. Touch and massage, and therefore Craniosacral Therapy, in a secure context can bring about a release of oxytocin, which works through the ANS to deepen relaxation.

Sue Carter has carried out research on the neurobiology of love for more than twenty years.[7] Definitions of human love are mainly based on the concept of social bonds. Our ability to engage in social behavior and form relationships, and to experience the associated hormonal changes, enables us to experience love; therefore falling in love is a neuronal activity. Stephen W. Porges discovered that oxytocin is released during positive social interactions and permits the forming of deep bonds without fear.[8] Social relationships also have a strong protective function. The sense of having social support improves recovery from cardiovascular disease, cancer, and psychological problems and can help to reduce dependency on medication and other drugs. A large number of studies in this area have clearly shown that social relationships and attachment are extremely valuable for the psychological and emotional-spiritual health of humans and other mammals.

Like all hormones, oxytocin forms part of a complex hormonal balance. Its effects depend on which other hormones are present and on the particular balance among them. One of these hormones is prolactin, which initiates and maintains lactation and also promotes nest-building and the aggressive defense of offspring. An elevated level of prolactin affects behavior by promoting loving care and reducing libido.

TREATMENT OF MOTHER AND CHILD AFTER BIRTH

19

19.1. Postnatal and Ongoing Care of the Mother

Craniosacral treatment can often help to restore strength following states of exhaustion, postnatal depression or "baby blues," and emotional-spiritual crises that may be the result of considerable hormonal changes. The position of the sacrum and all the pelvic structures should be assessed and corrected if necessary. The practitioner should then harmonize the craniosacral system, which will balance the endocrine glands in the head area and the entire hormonal system. Self-regulation and healing are assisted at all levels once membrane tension becomes more balanced; the dura mater, of course, forms the protective layers enveloping the CNS. The craniosacral practitioner can use visceral therapy to help relocate and restore the original position of the organs and musculoskeletal structures.

An episiotomy may be required if there is a risk of uncontrolled tearing of the tissue or if the heart-rate monitor presents serious concern during birth. In such circumstances the pelvic floor is usually under too much strain. If an episiotomy does become necessary, it should be done in zigzag form. Wound healing after a tear or episiotomy can be helped later by gently massaging the uninjured area with lavender oil and homeopathic treatment such as arnica globules and poultices. It is also important for rapid wound healing for the patient to take her time, avoid strain, and get plenty of rest. The mother's processing of the birth experience also helps to hasten wound healing. This can be aided by Craniosacral Therapy, psychological dialogue therapy, or art therapy.

Episiotomy scars and overstretching during birth often affect the urinary bladder, intestines, uterus, and vagina. This can cause restriction of function, sometimes years later when the association between the restriction and the scar may not come to mind. The incision and scar from a C-section can also cause a number of problems, such as bladder disturbances, backache, headache, hormonal changes, and pain during intercourse.

Treatment of scars: if the mother's resources are adequate and if she wants to receive this kind of assistance, one option is for an experienced female craniosacral practitioner to treat the fresh scar through the dressing without applying pressure. It is important to pay attention to the emotional level in this case and to accompany the process. The mother can also perform regular treatment of the scar resulting from a C-section or peritoneal tear herself, using techniques as instructed by the practitioner. In this regard I recommend the book *Effective Care in Pregnancy and Childbirth*.[1]

Mothers who had hoped for a natural birth but whose babies unexpectedly had to be delivered by C-section often feel great disappointment. The experience can be a shock for the woman, and she may later have feelings of guilt or failure. Sometimes mothers whose babies were delivered by C-section say that they feel as if they have not really given birth to their child because they did not go through the birth experience. In this case, it is possible to make up the lack of the experience of giving birth during Craniosacral Therapy. Choosing an appropriate time, it is possible, for example, to support the mother by reenacting the turning of the baby that happens during birth. Afterward, her baby is placed on her abdomen, deepening and completing the rebonding (see also sections 17.1 and 28.17).

19.2. Care of the Baby Following the Birth or After a Difficult Birth

From the outset, there are great demands on the baby: it is faced with the need to cope with nutritional intake at varying intervals, its mother's absences, and variations in temperature and noise.

As craniosacral practitioners, we try to balance the structure and function of the whole craniosacral system, the locomotor system that includes the joints, and the organs. It is also important to note carefully which parts of the body are hypertonic or hypotonic and which structures are storing prenatal and perinatal trauma and waiting to be given the ability to release this through sensitive support. The release of trauma energy from the nervous system assists the balancing of the system and so helps all autonomic functions. In the following days the baby often sleeps better. It is more ready to make contact, and homeostasis and immune defenses are strengthened. There is an interaction between all these areas; comprehensive craniosacral treatment balances a number of levels, and this potentiates the healing effect.

As trained craniosacral practitioners who recognize and work with prenatal and perinatal dynamics, we have a number of options available, such as playful methods of enquiry to apply during therapy. In this way opportunities for promoting healing can emerge on several levels, together with the Craniosacral Therapy and other elements such as the symbolic level and family systems therapy. A symptom often appears on several different levels, and release can occur on any of these levels. The mother may be able to process her earlier experience of powerlessness or worthlessness in this way. Giving Craniosacral Therapy to babies is especially beneficial in providing support at an early stage because somatic and psychological problems have not yet become entrenched.

19.3. Breast-Feeding

Breast-feeding is an essential interaction between mother and child. While suckling, the baby experiences the nourishing, symbiotic, and united relationship that it has with its mother's body outside the uterus. Just as the baby in the womb experienced the sense of receiving what it needed, now when suckling the infant has the sense of the goodness of its mother's breast. Being able to take in nourishment at its own speed is important in developing the child's capacity for self-regulation. After feeding, the baby slips into a trancelike state of blissful contentment. Sadly, babies are often torn from their state of deep relaxation by some physical interruption such as activity on the part of the mother or some outside disturbance.

Babies delivered by emergency C-section are often identified as having difficulty suckling. Trauma of all kinds can contribute to this, but even such influences as bottle-feeding with sugar water or a tea infusion in the hospital or nursery can have an effect. The baby opens its mouth but is unwilling to suck from the nipple. Possible solutions to this problem include expressing milk or bottle-feeding with infant formula, but these are a second-choice options. Breast-feeding has positive effects for both mother and child:

1. The female breast has a high density of myoepithelial cells. Stimulation of these cells prompts the milk-ejection reflex, which empties the alveoli of the mammary glands. The advantage for mothers is that breast-feeding reduces their risk of later developing breast cancer. For breast-fed babies the advantage is that they have a lower tendency to be obese later in life.

2. The birth process and the breast-feeding process raise the level of endorphins, bringing about a cascade of hormonal reactions. Beta endorphins stimulate the release of prolactin. When a mother breast-feeds her baby, the beta endorphins reach maximum level after around twenty minutes, and the baby takes in

endorphins with its mother's milk. These have a euphoric and pain-reducing effect.

Breast-feeding does, however, place a strain on the mother's thoracic and cervical spine. Craniosacral Therapy and self-treatment as well as postnatal exercises can reduce the strain on these regions and reduce or prevent pain.

In the past, breast-feeding was poorly regarded, and commercially manufactured infant formula was seen as the modern approach. Breast-feeding declined, although this trend is now gradually being reversed as the benefits are becoming recognized again. Breast milk helps the immune system and also has a positive effect on the child's development. The many complex activities of the muscles involves in suckling stimulate the development of the cranium. As an example of the effects, in breast-fed babies the zygomatic bone develops more than in bottle-fed babies, and a lower palate tends to encourage the development of a U-shaped dental arch. This enables better occlusion and alignment of the teeth later on. Assuming that there is no marked or multiple compression present, breast-feeding also reduces the occurrence of restrictions in the sutures, the membranous SBS, and the membranous and osseous structures of the facial bones.

Suckling teaches the child to use complex activities of the muscles of the tongue, lips, and face in combination with those of the palate and pharynx. The key muscle involved is the superior pharyngeal constrictor, which coordinates the muscles that are activated in sucking and swallowing. It runs from the pterygoid process to the pharyngeal raphe, which is a longitudinal tendon that suspends the pharynx from the cranial base.

Sucking at the breast requires a vacuum to be created. To do this, the nasopharynx and oropharynx need to be sealed. The mandible, hyoid bone and muscles, lateral pterygoid muscle, and superficial part of the masseter are all involved in creating the intraoral vacuum. The tongue performs anteroposterior movements, and sucking continues until the swallowing reflex is initiated. Although sucking at the breast may demand practice on the part of both the mother and the baby, the degree of activity and coordination in all these regions is much greater than when feeding from a bottle.

Swallowing involves contraction of the orbicularis oris, which is the sphincter-like muscle of the mouth, and buccinator muscles; the tip of the tongue presses against the dental arches and the root of the tongue descends, opening the pharynx. The soft palate prevents the milk from entering the nasal cavities. Raising the pharynx and larynx causes the milk to pass down into the esophagus.

The muscles around the hyoid and those responsible for movements of the tongue and for mastication participate in swallowing. The musculature of the palate is linked with the muscles of the tongue, pharynx, and cranial base. The three constrictor muscles are linked with the cranial base by the pharyngobasilar fascia. The key function here is that of the superior pharyngeal constrictor muscle. Because of its attachment to the sphenoid (the medial plate of the pterygoid process and the pterygoid hamulus), it affects the structure, function, and growth processes of the SBS. Its muscle loops lead, via other muscles, to the soft palate, tongue, face, and middle ear. The short, middle, long, and vertical loops are formed by the continuations of the superior pharyngeal constrictor. These are active in breathing, mastication, and articulation. These regions are therefore important in many respects, especially during growth, and also when considering symptoms relating to these functions. The muscles operate via their attachment to the styloid process to draw the pharynx, hyoid, and tongue in a superoposterior direction during swallowing. During sucking, the muscles use the temporal bone as a lever to draw them in the inferior direction.

During sucking, the infrahyoid muscles stabilize the hyoid. The suprahyoid muscles then use it as a fixed point to draw the mandible downward and mobilize the tongue. Therefore, active regular contractions of the superior pharyngeal constrictor occur during sucking. The fixed point or fulcrum for this is the occipital bone. The constrictor muscle in turn serves as a fixed point for its four muscle loops to enable the root of the tongue or the hyoid to be raised. All of this means that the baby is achieving a great deal: learning through sucking and swallowing to synchronize myofascial chains.

Most of the muscles of the soft palate and pharynx are linked with the bones of the cranial base, in most cases to points of attachment with a membranous origin. The key muscle of these muscle loops, the superior pharyngeal constrictor, is in contact with the cranial system, through its attachment at the medial plate of the pterygoid process and through the basilar part of the occipital bone, and with the mandible.

Breast-feeding can improve occlusion. For this to happen, it should be continued for at least six months, and as far as possible it should not be combined with bottle-feeding. However, where there is a risk of cross bite, extended breast-feeding is not found to achieve any reduction. In such cases there is often side-bending or lateral strain of the SBS. The craniosacral practitioner should therefore assess and treat these regions so as to achieve the release of these early patterns.

19.3.1. Disturbance in the Sucking Function

Disturbance in the sucking should be treated early and regularly. If there is any restriction or marked hindrance to the sucking function, it can cause a number of difficulties: feeding, the general capacity of perception, motor function, and later in speech acquisition and articulation. There is an interaction among these issues and the child's psychological makeup. The action of sucking moves the cranial base via the vomer, which moves further into flexion. As a result, it becomes easier to balance the traction and tension exerted on the intracranial membranes by the birth process.

On the psychological level, this can give rise to anxiety, problems in the interaction of the child with its environment, and difficulties in the interaction between mother and child. If this happens, the mother should also receive support. The situation can be an unhappy one for the baby too: it may feel the lack of emotional-spiritual nourishment in the form of deep stable contact, stress-free affectionate care, loving touch, and tenderness.

Compression or displacement of the atlanto-occipital region or cranial base is another possible cause of difficulty with sucking after birth. The use of a ventouse or forceps during delivery distorts the cranium and meninges and the suboccipital region through excessive traction and rotation. Babies delivered by C-section appear to suffer more frequently from disturbances of proprioception, which can make feeding more difficult. Preterm infants often have too little experience sucking because of their need for special nutrition. They need patient, loving help to learn, which will also aid their nutrition.

As craniosacral practitioners, we should work toward freer structure and more balanced functions in the infant, using gentle touch that delivers a very slight, subtle stimulus and enables better mobility.

The parents can assist their baby's proprioception at the superficial and deeper levels by regular infant massage. Massage of the face and neck region has a particularly marked stimulating effect when applied to the lips and mouth. Encouragement of the masticatory and swallowing function in the infant reduces the risk of problems in articulation or use of the tongue in childhood or adolescence. These dysfunctions can later lead to anomalies of the jaw or dental alignment.

19.4. Constantly Crying Babies with Problems in Sucking, Sleeping, Digestion, and Colic

Colic, also known as baby colic or abdominal cramps, infantile colic, or three-month colic, affects around one-quarter of newborn babies. The baby cries and screams for periods of at least three hours on at least three days and can become red and blue in the face with the pain.

The baby's eyes water, it sweats profusely, and the abdomen appears bloated. The pain may be eased by giving fennel tea, by gentle touch, and by massaging the baby's belly with a mixture of almond and caraway oil. Some sources say that the causes are unknown, that the problem is harmless and will soon pass, but that is little consolation for the parents and babies affected.

Constant crying is a problem that involves approximately one in every four babies. For no apparent reason, the baby cries for hours at a time, is difficult to console, and even when settled, soon begins to cry again. The usual pattern is for the screaming to build up over the first six weeks, to ease in the third month, and from the fourth month to stop completely. This does not mean that newborn babies are in no need of support. Quite the contrary; the supporting presence of the baby's parents, grandparents, or other family members through this painful phase often helps to relieve the tension.

Why do some babies cry so much? One reason is that crying and screaming help the baby to process the birth. Another is the extent to which the baby has to adapt after birth. It is a fundamental adaptation—the baby has lost its safe familiar home. Crying also helps the newborn restore the dimensions of its head following birth. Crying and screaming can mean many things: trouble with its sleep rhythm, with feeding or nutritional changes, or organic disturbances. By screaming, the baby may be trying to communicate that it is unwell or in pain, to express fear, or to express the need for quiet, more care and affection, body contact, or protection. There is even a hypothesis that abdominal pain or three-month colic might be caused by crying rather than the other way around.

Other possible reasons for the baby to cry and scream are a lack of emotional support from its mother or an atmosphere of conflict in the family. The child may feel a lack of emotional acceptance or support. Admittedly, if babies are left to cry, they do eventually give up and stop, but this is hardly helpful to either the baby or its parents. It is certainly unhelpful in the first six weeks of life, when the baby has not yet learned how to calm down. Distracting the child with a favorite teddy bear, for example, only helps for a short while, as children do not learn to occupy themselves independently until they reach toddler age.

Incessant screaming and the lack of sleep severely test the parents' patience and nerves. Rather than becoming so irritated by the noise that they shake the baby, parents need to keep calm. It helps if they can remove themselves from the stressful situation by letting other family members take care of the child while they recover. Babies and toddlers have weak neck muscles, and they cannot support their heads unaided when subjected to violent movement. Forceful shaking can kill or cause lasting damage to a child. A call to a parent helpline for professional help and advice provides a way forward for stressed parents. In this kind of situation, Craniosacral Therapy combined with emotional first aid to parents and child is important for everyone concerned. It aids relaxation for everyone and helps produce a relaxed atmosphere in the family system as a whole. Children can sense their parents' uncertainty, tension, and irritation.

Some tips for calming a crying baby:

- Give the baby your undivided, affectionate attention.
- Carry the baby around with you, lovingly rocking it slowly and gently.
- Talk calmly to the baby and show your acceptance of it in its pain.
- Sing to the baby from time to time.

Parents who want to carry their baby around with them frequently find a sling or baby carrier helpful. Choose one that enables plenty of direct body contact.

When treating a baby who cries persistently, I always assess the structural and functional situation and provide support as needed. The cause of the crying may, for example, be spinal scoliosis or slight torticollis with a dysfunction of the cranial base. There is almost always unbalanced tension of the intracranial membranes and dural tube. Following structural and functional treatment, I tune in to the mid-tide and support the fluid body.

It is not unusual for babies to cry during the treatment session, and this is not something negative. A baby sometimes cries when the practitioner touches a site where there is a structural restriction or where a traumatic experience is stored. It may be a signal that the baby feels that someone senses its discomfort, or it could be a defensive reaction: "No, I don't want this." Often the baby is crying because it must, because crying is how it expresses its need.

Crying and screaming are a means of expression and communication. Both usually express a particular need, and we can learn to recognize the different kinds of crying: sometimes it will be vigorous, demanding, energetic, or shrill; at others hesitant, muted, or weak.

If the baby does cry or scream almost incessantly during the treatment session, it is important for us as practitioners not to take a constantly hands-on approach. We should not apply excessive stimulation by our touch. If the child cries or screams for long periods, we should consider allowing everyone to pause for a while.

The mother or practitioner can use a clear and complete change in the situation to offer the child a fresh impulse from outside. This change might be a different position on the treatment table or for the mother to hold the child differently. The reason might be that the baby wants to be rocked, needs its mother to soothe it by singing, or needs her to give some other gentle acoustic stimulus. On the other hand, when the time is right to follow through a theme, and there is the strength drawn from resources to continue and conclude the process, we should continue with no interruption. In that case the change in situation is not required.

As craniosacral practitioners, we can strengthen bonding and help develop parents' understanding of their baby's new world. We can support and help parents recognize their own feelings during their baby's long crying sessions: for example, irritation, rejection, annoyance, anger, helplessness or inadequacy, the sense of being overwhelmed, and feelings of guilt for being a bad parent.

Some sources recommend establishing strict rules and structures to deal with a crying baby or a child who has difficulty sleeping. This can sometimes be effective, although it is more helpful to the parents than the child. Each child has its own rhythm, and parents should try to discover it and take account of it. The timing and need for sleep vary among individuals, but a bedtime routine (brush teeth, put on pajamas, sing, a bedtime story) gives a clear signal and can make matters easier.

FURTHER CONSIDERATIONS DURING THE CHILD'S DEVELOPMENT

20

20.1. Children Need Their Fathers Too

It can be a great challenge for working parents with a stressful daily schedule to combine work and family. Good interaction between the parents is one very important factor in good father-child relationships. Is a good father also a good husband, life partner, and breadwinner? Does he arrange for enough leisure-time activity for the family as a whole? To what extent does he fulfill his role as trusted family protector and guardian of each individual family member? What kind of effect does he exert on the family and on the child: is it protective or threatening?

The clear distinction between the roles of mothers and fathers is increasingly being eroded, and this varies among cultures. For this reason the father is an important point of reference for children. How much is he there for them? Children usually understand if their father simply needs a break and a rest, but they do not understand if he is permanently unwilling to give them any attention. In order to achieve a trusting relationship, fathers need to know what their children want and need. What does the child most like doing? What does the father know of what goes on in the child's life? Does the father have the empathy to understand and respect the child's development process instead of simply seeing it and understanding it intellectually?

Fathers become more important to their child as the child starts to move beyond dependence on its mother and explore the world. If it receives loving, patient attention, the child will turn increasingly to its father. Does the father have a sense of his child's feelings? Does he know which subjects the child enjoys or dislikes at school? Can he name the child's three favorite pastimes, two best friends, favorite sport, or hobbies? If he does not know these things, the way to catch

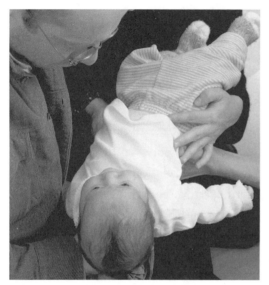

Figure 20.1. Valuable contact between father and child.

up is to spend time together, playing or talking, perhaps in surroundings chosen by the child. The father can help with the toilet routine, diaper cream, brushing teeth, or tidying the child's bedroom. They can find just as much pleasure being together with no set task, observing nature, splashing around in the water, or watching animals, for example.

The stages of a child's growth and development mark the progress of life and the passage of time. The first seven years of a child's life bring huge changes, and the next seven bring even more.

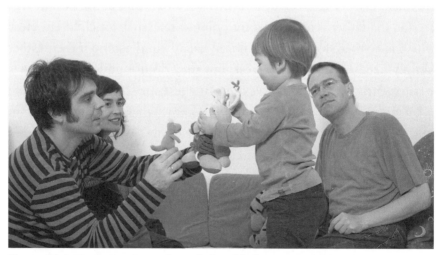

Figure 20.2. Exploring the caring relationship between child and parents.

20.2. Parenting Style and Family Environment

Looking at the parenting style, are the parents able to set boundaries as well as give the child a sense of caring support? Do "yes" and "no" mean what they say? Do the parents communicate in a constructive way with their child? How do they deal with fear, anger, hatred, sorrow, aggression, envy, and joy?

The family environment is also important. Is the family intact? Does the child live in a single-parent family, or an alternative type of family? If so, the child's relationship with its primary caregiver is still important.

For toddlers, there is the possibility of attending day care, a playgroup, or a mother-and-baby group. Playing together in a group promotes development and is easier for the child to relate to than putting it in front of a television or computer game too early.

Many of today's mothers go out to work and place their children in day care, where children can learn to achieve greater independence. They also learn more quickly to deal with emotional stress by themselves. On the other hand, they are not receiving constant emotional care, and therefore they should not normally remain at day care for periods longer than six hours. At kindergarten or once they are in school, the important factor is the relationship the child builds with the adult responsible for the group. If that relationship is inadequate, the child is thrown into an attachment desert every day, and this can have a disturbing effect on attachment and the child's ability to orient itself. The child may develop a emotional thick skin in self-defense and adapt as best it can so as not to attract attention or find itself excluded.

20.3. Early Training

Early childhood training is enjoying rapid widespread expansion. What this means in practice for the early encouragement of linguistic, musical, and scientific development is to some extent still the subject of controversy and discussion. It has been recognized that babies not only learn passively but can already think about cause and effect and try to place new experiences in abstract categories. By the end of the first year, babies are able to distinguish all one hundred phonemes that make up the world's languages. Until their fourth year, children can absorb foreign languages quite naturally and speak them without accent. For a child who is going to have a professional career in music, the best time to begin training is between the ages of two and ten. However, enforced early training is counterproductive, despite the good intentions. A child's primary need is for loving caregivers who respond to its needs and help it progress in its special interests.

When small children start to explore a particular interest, they need to be able to follow it through to a conclusion, when they know enough to satisfy themselves—even if all they are exploring is their own big toe. If someone intervenes while they are doing this and gives them well-intentioned learning tasks, this distracts them from their exploration and may cause permanent overload. It disturbs the child's own process of discovery, which is important for the child's personal development. Another unhelpful approach is to give the child a mass of toys and leave it to its own devices. Children faced with this situation constantly turn their attention to something new and never complete anything. On the other hand, parents, educators, and therapists can support children's natural curiosity and desire to find out by involving themselves in the child's play and gently offering space to learn more.

20.4. Bed-Wetting and Enuresis

The acquisition of bladder and bowel control is mainly determined by the development of the child's nervous system. It is a process of maturity that begins at around twenty-six months and is not fully complete until about age four. Later, incontinence is mainly associated with pressure and stress. Children who wet their pants may be doing so from stress or to attract attention if there is some unhappiness weighing on them. Such children do not need any additional pressure. Instead of compulsion, children in this situation need plenty of patience and to be lovingly guided and reminded. Parent and child can generally work together to establish a toilet routine that the child learns to carry out regularly on its own. The child should still work to achieve sphincter control, but this should be done without imposing any stress.

Treatment options for incontinence are outlined in section 30.5.

20.5. Disorders of Speech and Tongue Function

A child's ability to speak depends on complex well-coordinated inter-action of muscles. Speech involves a number of different muscles of the tongue, cheeks, and lips, the muscles of facial expression and mastication, and the muscles of the soft palate. Disturbance of just one muscle always affects the entire system of articulation. Disturbances can come about through paralysis of the facial nerve or the tongue. They can also be caused by the child's emotional state, for example if the child has faced either inadequate challenge, excessive demands, or is under too much pressure; these can have a paralyzing effect.

The organs needed for speech are the same as those we use to chew and swallow our food. Disturbances of mastication and swallowing do not necessarily lead to disturbances of speech, since the human body, as we know, has some capacity for compensation. Mastica-tory and swallowing disturbances may, for instance, be the result of a congenital problem such as a cleft lip, palate, or jaw; birth trauma; or inadequate sensory and motor stimulation of the region. Alternatively the cause may be peripheral, in the suboccipital region or restricted breathing through the nose. Dysfunctions of the tongue can lead to compensatory problems later on with the alignment of the teeth, jaw growth, or breathing.

When providing treatment, as craniosacral practitioners we concentrate particularly on the superior thoracic inlet, atlanto-occipital joint, jugular foramen, and hyoid, applying intraoral treatment as necessary. An increasing number of speech therapists and occupational therapists have taken additional craniosacral training over a number of years and have acquired considerable knowledge and experience. The rehabilitation exercises provided by these therapists and the balancing provided by Craniosacral Therapy to harmonize the musculoskeletal, nervous, and hormonal systems each potentiate the other, representing a source of valuable healing impulses.

Impaired speech, tongue, or swallowing functions can be treated at preschool age by craniosacral and speech therapy. Once the child is of school age, more active learning can be introduced to help the child to swallow or improve function. This involves using muscle exercises designed to develop awareness of muscle tone and the ability to regulate it. Improvement in function of the tongue has a positive effect on patterns of articulation and assists in producing sounds such as the sibilants *s, sh,* and *ch* and dental consonants such as *d, l, n,* and *t*.

The craniosacral practitioner should explore whether it is the form that has caused the functional disturbance or the other way around: has the functional disturbance led to the form? Examine the appearance of the regions surrounding the tongue and pharynx, cranium, shoulders, spinal column, and pelvis. Are there any signs of scoliosis, pelvic obliquity, or headache? To what extent are other factors also involved, for example too little stimulation or too much stress in the environment, nutrition, exercise, social interaction, or emotional states?

20.6. Nursery School, Kindergarten, and School Age

Early recognition of speech difficulties and social deficits is possible in the day-to-day activities of nursery school or kindergarten. For children, this stage is an important time of transition and preparation for school.

In school, children are expected to be able to sit still, work independently, and respond appropriately to all kinds of different people. Times of change always arouse strong emotions, so a degree of emotional tension is understandable at this time of mixed happiness, anxiety, and pride. Schoolchildren therefore need constant orientation and clear structures. They should be given encouragement and enough time to adapt to the many changes.

Parents can ease the pressure on themselves and the child by checking and adapting daily schedules. When planning the day, they should try to reduce unnecessary sources of stress and allow enough time both for homework and for play and exercise. It helps to involve the child in planning homework time. Some children like to do their homework immediately after they arrive home from school; others need a break first. Schoolchildren who are able to work out their own rhythm of learning and working succeed better in their learning and also discover a great deal about themselves. Homework should aid the learning process and help the development of self-reliance. The role of the parents is to ensure that the child has the right conditions. Taking a genuine interest in what the child is doing is highly motivating. Children are naturally curious, interested, and eager to learn. If they feel that they are taken seriously and supported at home, school also becomes easier. It is important to create a relationship of trust so that the children feel able to talk to their parents about anything, such as things that happen at school or on the way to school. The child has to be allowed to become independent, and the parents need to find out how best to support their child in this.

During this stage of childhood, the issues that become important are those of freedom and boundaries, tasks and responsibilities, and free time and friends. This is consequently a good time to encourage and assist children to develop their talents, perhaps in sport or learning to play a musical instrument. However, the many expectations on the part of parents and school often present children with difficult tasks.

The current situation in Switzerland, as an example, is that half of all children are assessed as needing therapy of some kind at least once. There is, of course, a difference between slightly delayed development and long-term problems. For those with long-term problems, Craniosacral Therapy is no substitute for speech and language therapy, training in psychomotor skills, remedial and special teaching, treatment for dyslexia and dyscalculia, special classes, and coaching. Craniosacral bodywork can, however, help these children as a form of additional assistance in a holistic way to promote their strengths and resources.

Helpful as it undoubtedly is for children to receive special therapy, support, and assistance, if there is too much of it or if it continues for too long, it can undermine their self-confidence. This can lead to a downward spiral. Years of special treatment demonstrates to children that there is something wrong with them, and this diminishes their sense of self-worth. Is the "problem" simply a harmless variation from the norm? Between the ages of four and six, natural developmental differences in speech, motor skills, attention, memory, and behavior can be considerable.

Increasing numbers of children have difficulties during their nursery and school years and suffer from headaches, backaches, and postural disturbances; extended periods of sadness; bad moods; and even depression. Even gifted children experience difficulties if they receive too little stimulation to develop their individuality and instead find themselves always required to fit in.

The need to remain sitting for so much of the school day, and then at home in front of the television or computer, is often harmful for children. It is a constant source of amazement to me to find out how much stress school-age children, at junior high and high school in particular, have in their bodies. Imbalance of tension in the locomotor and craniosacral systems can be resolved in a few treatment sessions, however, depending on the individual situation. The earlier this is done, the better.

Another issue that particularly affects schoolchildren is the orthodontic brace. Craniosacral Therapy can support children through this process. It is simpler, more effective, and more helpful to treat and release restrictions before puberty in order not to affect the next stage of development.

20.7. Therapy to Accompany Orthodontic Treatment

Problems that are appearing more often in children include not only allergies and learning difficulties but also more frequent disharmony affecting the teeth and jaw. These symptoms are often an expression of imbalance on the psychological and emotional-spiritual level. Abnormalities of the jaw and dental alignment can arise as a result of earlier dysfunctions of articulation or of the tongue in infancy. These problems in turn can be associated with restrictions of sucking, masticatory, and swallowing function in the newborn, which may have their origin in a difficult birth, as in a C-section where the aftereffects were not treated. Tensions caused in the body by malocclusion can place undue strain on the temporomandibular joint (TMJ) and its muscles and ligaments. The constant tension also affects the craniosacral system, especially the cranial base. This can sometimes lead to restrictions, specific learning disabilities, pain, and illness. Pediatric craniosacral treatment promotes the healthy development of the bones of the jaw and improves occlusion, for example. Holistic orthodontic treatment does more than simply stretch the jaw and correct the alignment of the teeth; it primarily helps restore sound basic function, for example in breathing, swallowing, digestion, and speech. It is important that this treatment not make excessive demands on the child, so not too much should be attempted at once. All too often, too much treatment tends to be done simultaneously.

Eurythmy therapy and other accompanying therapies that the child likes can be used to support the process of jaw development. Great progress can be made in a short time if children are allowed to form their own plan and choose the right time for treatments.

Orthodontic misalignment is often caused by dental or skeletal problems. Problems of dental origin are crowding, loss of space for the permanent teeth, distal bite or mandibular prognathism, supraocclusion or infraocclusion of individual teeth, and rotation or displacement of the midline of the maxilla. Skeletal causes include tension or posture of the rest of the body. The position of the upper and lower jaw and the interaction between them determine masticatory function, and they are influenced by muscular and skeletal factors. The more balanced body tension produced by Craniosacral Therapy and the organizing impulses of the Breath of Life improve the child's basic regulation. This has an effect on such things as digestion and posture and thus helps to improve occlusion. Improved occlusion can also help posture and digestion.

I apply Craniosacral Therapy before, during, and after orthodontic correction. When a problem in the way the jaw and facial bones are tending to develop has been recognized early and the need for correction is not urgent, dental impressions can be compared: the earlier or first impression is compared with one taken after nine to eighteen sessions of craniosacral treatment. This shows how the jaw and teeth have developed with the aid of regular craniosacral treatment. My experience has shown that sometimes no further correction is needed at this stage, or that the correction needed has been much less. If the child still needs orthodontic help, such as a dental brace, it is still helpful to have a freer craniosacral system, which can better compensate the correction or the restriction of the craniosacral system in the mouth region than a system that is already sluggish and beset with dysfunctions. The benefit is that there is sometimes a reduction in headaches or back problems, the body needs less strength to function, and children become less tired. Following orthodontic correction, we can evaluate the craniosacral rhythm in the structures that had been restricted and seek to improve its qualities, and then support the improvement of mobility and motility in the whole of the cranium and the whole of the craniosacral system, including the sacrum.

When providing craniosacral treatment for problems of the teeth and jaw, I work extensively for a while in the neighboring regions and those directly affected: the cranial base as a whole; the viscerocranium and, if possible, also regularly working intraorally; the mandible; the hyoid; and the sternum. At the same time, in each session I examine and treat the entire craniosacral system. I include the level of the organs and entire locomotor system, and also consider the extent of mobility or restriction of structures such as the pelvis, hips, knees, and ankle joints. It is well known that restrictions in the lower limbs, for example a previous Achilles tendon tear, or pelvis, for example due to a difference in leg length and pelvic obliquity, can be transmitted to the superior thoracic aperture, cranial base, and TMJ or can exert a compensatory effect on these regions.

See section 30.30 for an example of possible treatment for problems of the teeth and jaw.

20.8. Disturbances of Attention and Ability to Learn

See chapter 30 for a discussion of selected indications with pointers for Craniosacral Therapy.

Symptoms can sometimes arise as a result of stress, shock, or trauma that can even date back to events in the prenatal stage of human development, birth, or early childhood. These early effects alter the anatomy and physiology of the developing child, especially the brain and the nervous, hormonal, and immune systems, which finds expression in reduced capacity to deal with the demands of everyday life, for example in learning and speech disorders such as dyslexia or dyscalculia, disturbances of perception, or difficult social behavior.

When talking with the parents of children with restless behavior, possible questions to ask include: When did the attention disturbances begin? At what times of day is the behavior most marked or acute? What foods does the child eat, and do these include candy and foods containing artificial colors and preservatives? Is there anything happening in the child's life at the moment that could account for the disturbance or play some part in it, such as a divorce, change of teachers, difficulties at school, or a death, for example? Are the parents providing challenges without putting excessive demands on the child?

No child should watch too much television or spend great lengths of time in front of a computer. This is even more important for children with attention problems. Children learn to focus and concentrate, sustain their efforts, and endure through the support they receive from their parents, whose help can extend to managing homework and other tasks as well as family meals and games. Parents should make sure that this does not place unremitting fresh demands on their child. Craniosacral practitioners should ensure the same during our treatment sessions.

It is important to note that not every instance of difficulty in learning and concentration is necessarily a sign of attention deficit/hyperactivity disorder, described below. There are times in the development of a child, adolescent, or adult when they are especially full of energy and exuberance. It may simply be this that makes them less able to concentrate.

20.9. ADHD, ADD, HKD, MCD, MBD, POS, or Indigo Child?

The percentage of children with functional neurobiological disorders appears to be rising. The trend is increasing all over the world; recent figures show the percentage of children affected ranges five to fifteen percent. Boys appear to be affected three to six times more often than girls. A similar difference is seen for stammering and autism. Although the details differ from one study to another, the trend is nevertheless clear. Various different terms have been used over the years to describe the diagnosis, including minimal brain dysfunction syndrome (MBD) or minimal cerebral dysfunction (MCD), psycho-organic syndrome (POS), and hyperkinetic disorder (HKD). The best-known is the term agreed on in 1987 by the American Psychiatric Association, attention deficit/hyperactivity disorder (ADHD), formerly called attention deficit disorder (ADD).

20.9.1. Possible Signs

Attention deficit disorder, with or without hyperactivity, is not yet clearly defined internationally. The recognized descriptions of the disorder are those given by the World Health Organization's International Statistical Classification of Diseases and Related Health Problems (ICD-10), which is used in Europe, and the American Psychiatric Association's *Diagnostic and Statistical Manual of Mental Disorders* (DSM-IV), used in North America. The criteria are essentially similar, and the World Health Organization has been working to establish an agreed harmonized definition. The main signs of the disorder can be summarized as:

- inattention
  - inability to sustain attention and concentration
  - problems of perception
  - forgetfulness
  - inability to engage fully in work or play activities
- impulsivity
  - impulsive precipitate behavior
  - generally immature problem-solving behavior
  - inability to defer needs even for short periods
- hyperactivity
  - persistent pattern of excessive motor activity
  - often "on the go" or acts as if "motor-driven"
  - often talks excessively

20.9.2. ADHD

The term *ADHD*, which has now become the preferred term, emphasizes the fact that it is the degree of activity that is excessive. When all three types of behavior are present, children appear restless and find it difficult to sit still. ADHD manifests as hyperactivity, disturbances of motor activity, dreaminess, and inattentiveness. This can sometimes even be dangerous for the child and those around. These children exhibit an urge to keep moving, an inability to concentrate or to maintain effort during play and other activities, difficulty in following instructions, and a lack of attention in class.

Children with ADHD experience a whirling confusion of different thoughts, sensory impressions, and feelings stemming from all different levels. This makes it difficult for them to identify their own emotions or even distinguish them in the first place. In their constant state of unrest, they lack a sense of time, and everything seems the same. They experience either powerful feelings or lack of emotion and take an all-or-nothing approach. These children are creative, chaotic, and finders of new solutions; they want and need constant fresh stimulation and can sometimes achieve great successes in creative or physical fields. They sometimes give me the impression of unrecognized genius: more inventive and intelligent than adults, but children nevertheless.

Other features almost always found in these children are a reduced tolerance of stress along with disturbances of coarse and fine motor function. Memory is sometimes extremely good, and at other times nearly absent. Inattentiveness and poor memory can lead to learning difficulties and specific learning disabilities. Children who increasingly cut themselves off over time because of these difficulties can show behaviors not unlike those of autism.

The circadian rhythm is sometimes affected. The child has difficulty falling asleep and waking up. There are often disturbances to regular eating behavior—so much so that there are ADHD drugs available that are effective even if the child eats no breakfast, for example.

The child's sense of hunger and thirst can vary widely, with ravenous hunger alternating with lack of appetite. There is also a noticeable desire to eat too much sugar. The children concerned are unable to help this and should not be considered less intelligent because of it. Schoolwork is a struggle because of the lack of ability to concentrate. Problems of perception make it hard for these children to achieve their full potential. Homework time is inevitably a stressful time for the parents. Vigorous activities give these children a chance to compensate for their lack of fine motor skills: they may be daring cyclists, adore action and adventure, and be among the first to join a fight, which accounts for their higher injury rate.

In some children the symptoms may be similar but do not include hyperactivity. This is now seen as a subtype of ADHD, formerly called ADD, and the term is sometimes still used. These children experience everyday life as a constant flood of stimuli. They find themselves having to take in too much, unfiltered, at once. They are easily distracted, appear not to listen, are forgetful, and show little ability to sustain effort. They are often impulsive and act without stopping to think. They are unable to wait their turn, often interrupt, and in class they disturb others—when they're not daydreaming and appearing lazy. They have a low frustration threshold and tend to react immoderately. When faced with resistance, they respond with displays of temper. Children with this disorder sense that they are different, that their achievements are inadequate, and that they provoke irritation. As a result they are often aggressive or moody. They are inclined to boast, show off, and tell lies. The effect is to produce still greater rejection as they appear insolent and badly behaved. These children are like a whirlwind, sometimes increasingly defiant, ignorant, and fidgety, with a tendency to violent temper or even mad rage. This is not a form of stupidity; these children are, above all, helpless.

20.9.3. Society and Social Issues

Are the ADHD phenomenon, and problems of perception generally, a reflection of increasing problems in society or in schools? Is the apparent tendency to react by automatically prescribing drugs a feature of a society that thinks there is a medicine for everything and that there is no need to address the effects of growing social and communication problems? The disorder we now call ADHD has always existed but has increased enormously over the course of the industrial revolution and along with changes in society. The family and social environment play a part, as does the fact that the world around reacts more and more unsympathetically to symptoms of attention deficit and hyperactivity.

In the industrial and machine era, it became important to react at the press of a button. Recent decades have seen huge changes in the conditions we live in. As a result, healthy characteristics have become a handicap: human qualities such as inward awareness of feelings, sensing rather than cerebral thought, listening to each other, and beautiful storytelling have all been neglected. Yet these are precisely the aspects that provide a counterbalance to a whirlwind of action, the hectic behavior of those with concentration and hyperactivity problems. In our consumerist and performance-driven society, people are already subjected to extra stress and to social structures that create loneliness; it is an enormous additional challenge for the individual and for the human brain to find appropriate ways of meeting the many demands of the information age.

The situation calls for a response: as a society, we need to discuss the implications and perform a rethink. Our responsibility for our children's future is at stake. We need to ask ourselves where we are heading in our development as human beings, and whether we really want millions of children and adults to be taking drugs as the only way to adapt.

20.9.4. Individuality and Indigo Children

There is really no such thing as a typical ADHD child; these children, like any other, are individuals. Anyone who has experience with them knows how easy they are to inspire and what brilliant and creative ideas they produce and want to put into practice.

Their constitution, their whole being, and their path in life do not belong on any preset treadmill. In fact, their very nature makes this almost impossible. It makes them unruly; they spontaneously resist and rebel against the alien path marked out for them in an environment they find completely strange. They live in their child's world, and the ADHD label seems to signal that they will have difficulty assimilating in everyday school and work life.

It may be that this "abnormal" or conspicuous behavior contains a healthier potential than has been recognized—the potential of individuality and perhaps creativity that seeks to be fostered. Such children's resistance to social conditioning could also be seen as a healthy sign of responsible human beings with self-determination. Genius is, after all, sometimes close to madness. These children's brains and nervous systems were not made for school stress and the constant influx of stimuli. They need an environment that concerns itself more with them as individuals. To put forward a provocative argument, ADHD and all the names it goes under could also be seen as an interruption of conformity that challenges what is considered the appropriate behavior of people today.

The view is spreading, primarily in spiritual circles in the United States but increasingly elsewhere, that many children being born today are "indigo children" or "children of the light." They differ from previous generations in that they have a highly developed capacity for perception, are sensitive, and have potential clairvoyant ability. There are four types of indigo child: humanist, artist, conceptual, and interdimensional. Indigo children exhibit characteristics that are new and unusual and represent a challenge to their parents and to school life.

20.10. What Causes ADHD?

The question as to how children come to lack concentration, fidget, and behave in a way that suggests disturbances of perception is much discussed in psychological, educational, medical, and neurobiological circles, and it arouses much controversy. Various possible causes have been proposed.

Some point to genetic factors, for example if the father and mother have problems with their own dopamine metabolism or have mild ADHD. If genetic factors are responsible, ADHD symptoms can occur at any age.

Feelings can escalate very quickly. One of the factors that lead to this is restricted function of the dopaminergic system, important for the sorting and suppression of emotions, sensory impressions, and actions. Imbalance of the dopaminergic system appears to be of central importance. Dopamine is a biochemical precursor of norepinephrine and epinephrine, and along with serotonin is viewed as a happiness hormone, although it has other functions, including an effect on motor function. Dopaminergic neurons are found in the CNS, especially in the midbrain. Dopaminergic systems are also involved in regulating hormone balance; dopamine from neurons lying along the third ventricle operates via the pituitary to inhibit the release of prolactin. Dopamine also regulates the perfusion of the abdominal organs and is involved in governing renal function.

It is also possible for a mother who is hyperactive, overwhelmed, or under psychological stress to overload her fetus with stress hormones from her own hormonal system during pregnancy, which can have a decisive effect.

The school of thought that refers to this disorder as MCD or POS sees it as an organic dysfunction, believed to be observable on an EEG. According to this line of thinking, individual brain structures mature more slowly than average, believed to be caused by minimal brain damage occurring in utero or during birth. The frontal lobe region is thought to be smaller than average. There appears to be decreased glucose metabolism in the forebrain, which can affect brain function. Could this explain these children's extreme desire for sugar?

One hypothesis related to the frontal part of the brain runs that the symptoms resemble those of a frontal-lobe injury. The reduced regulatory capacity in POS or ADHD children could also be caused by a lack of sufficient clear information moving from deeper-lying regions of the brainstem to the forebrain, so that the brain is constantly seeking fresh information.

An earlier model suggested the opposite: the cause was thought to be inadequate filtering in the brainstem, thalamus, and hypothalamus, so that the brain was confused by too many stimuli.

A dysfunction of the frontal lobe, striatum, and nucleus accumbens can be involved in disturbances of perception. These structures of the brain communicate with each other by means of the neurotransmitter dopamine. However, it has not yet been possible to clearly demonstrate a dopamine deficit in the brains of children with attention problems. Other contradictory reasons are also being discussed. The neuroscientist Gerald Hüther believes that hyperactivity in children is not due to too little but rather too much dopamine production.[1] He argues that methylphenidate (as in Ritalin® and other medication) stops the brain being flooded with dopamine but at the same time hinders optimum brain development. If the drug prevents the growth of the nerve tree for dopamine-producing cells, we could soon find that older patients who had received methylphenidate in the past develop Parkinson's-like symptoms. Hüther also speculates that ADHD, or excessive dopamine production as the cause of the ADHD, could also be an effect of previous faulty development in the maturing brains of children who have been subjected to influences that include excessive or inadequate psychosocial stresses.

Other triggers that have been proposed for some years are allergic reactions to phosphates, artificial colors, and sugar. A study by the University of Southampton in Great Britain found that certain artificial coloring additives used in candy, snacks, and fizzy drinks, namely azo dyes such as tartrazine and the preservative sodium benzoate, cause concentration difficulties, sleeping problems, and aggressive behavior in many children.[2] The extent of the problem was recognized when the British Consumers' Association found these additives to be present in over one-third of foods. The British Food Standards Agency (FSA) advised all parents of hyperactive children to avoid giving their children foods containing them. These additives appear to be involved with marked frequency in how much ADHD symptoms are expressed. They can produce changes in brain metabolism and alter behavior. The FSA requested manufacturers to remove the "Southampton six" additives voluntarily pending legislation. In the meantime, many manufacturers are replacing them with natural alternatives, and warning labeling has become compulsory in Great Britain.

The number-one drug for many children is sugar. From the neuro-biological point of view, the effect is similar to that of heroin, although less drastic: consuming addictive substances activates the reward centers of the brain that create dependency. One of the effects of sugar is to activate these same reward centers.

20.10.1. Diagnosis

It is remarkable, in view of these different causes and effects and the range of symptoms, that it has proved possible to reduce them all to just one clinical syndrome. Some parents and professionals welcome a diagnosis because at last it provides them with certainty that the problem is indeed a syndrome or disorder. It means that they do not need to torment themselves with the thought that they are part of the cause. It reduces the need to question and change their own behavior. There are no standardized diagnostic tests, however. Not all family doctors and pediatricians who diagnose ADHD have sufficient training and experience, even if they have attended a crash course in the "correct" drug dosage. Extensive discussion with the child, parents, and teachers is necessary, together with tests and assessment of the child's emotional competence, social behavior, and performance at school. In many cases, those affected—the child and its parents and teachers, who are all under pressure—and their doctors do not take the time needed to do this; more and more they immediately turn to the traditional approach of medication.

The usual treatment is methylphenidate, sometimes with the support of additional behavioral therapy. This is astonishing; although this approach may temporarily alleviate the pressure on the children, parents, teachers, and educators involved, it does not solve the error in the system. In so many cases, instead of addressing the individual needs of the child, psychotropic drugs are used to treat learning and behavioral problems. Physicians are quick to prescribe them for children who are restless or do not conform to the usual norms—even for dreamy children, with the professed aim of helping them to concentrate better.

Concerned remedial and special-needs teachers are worried not only by the increase in the number of children and adolescents with learning and behavioral difficulties but also by the tendency to pathologize these problems and class them together. On closer examination these children differ considerably, and not every behavioral difficulty is necessarily ADHD.

20.10.2. Methylphenidate and Its Prescription

Methylphenidate, most commonly known in the United States as Ritalin®, was first synthesized by the chemist Leandro Panizzon in 1944. The first proprietary drug with this active ingredient was introduced in Switzerland and Germany in 1954. With the expiry of patent protection, a number of products have entered the rewarding psychotonic market.

As an example of the increasing trend, the estimated sales figures for methylphenidate in Switzerland, a country with a population of 7.4

million, amounted to 648 pounds in 2010.[3] In 2006 the amount was 375 pounds, and in 1999 just 84 pounds. According to the German newsmagazine *Der Spiegel,* in 1999 in Germany the pharmaceutical industry sold six times as much of an ADHD drug as it did in 1995.[4] Around the turn of the millennium, the number of children receiving regular treatment with methylphenidate was estimated to be half a million in Germany alone. The German newspaper *Frankfurter Allge-meine* reported sales of drugs with this active ingredient from German pharmacies as 2,692 pounds in 2006; the amount sold in 1996 was 194 pounds.[5] This represents an increase in its use of thirteen times over ten years. The figures for the United States are the highest in the world. For years the prescription and use of methylphenidate have been extremely high, and the drug is even taken by adolescents and adults as a performance enhancer. *Frankfurter Allgemeine* reported worldwide sales for 2006 of products containing methylphenidate to be worth around 1.2 billion dollars.

20.10.3. Side Effects

Characterizing such a large proportion of the population as medically or psychologically abnormal should cause us to stop and think. Methylphenidate is a psychotropic substance. It stimulates blood circulation, and in the United States has been reported to have led to complications in individuals with existing cardiac conditions; manufacturers now issue warnings. The side effects are well known and can be considerable: depression, sleep disturbances, loss of appetite, tics, and disturbances of brain and body growth. Some children taking drugs to combat hyperactivity not only had cardiovascular problems but variously suffered from hallucinations, heard voices, saw horrific images, or had panic attacks.

To what extent can drug treatment of difficult child behavior really be helpful for the child? Some parents report an improvement in the symptoms; others say that their child underwent marked personality changes. Some children became apathetic and conformed to the point of being puppetlike, exhibited loss of appetite, and had difficulty going to sleep. These signs are also seen in cocaine and ecstasy (MDMA) use. Methylphenidate belongs to the amphetamine class of drugs. It is a synthetic psychoactive substance that enables a child to sit and concentrate for several hours and improves learning, especially in school. At the same time, however, it can suppress emotions, curiosity, creativity, humor, and joy, which tends to reduce the number of experiences involving these human qualities for these children.

Drug treatment of ADHD is controversial among physicians and psychiatrists because it can play a part in delaying a long-term solution to behavioral difficulties: although the problems may initially appear to be lessened, medication seldom provides a complete solution. No drug can achieve a lasting effect in resolving severe problems within the family, at school, with peers, or in childhood development. Some physicians therefore urge better care in place of medication for these children, to enable them to adapt naturally rather than artificially to their environment.

My concern in discussing medication is not to call it into question in general. I neither advocate nor advise against its use. There are children for whom these drugs are helpful: they are enabled to learn better and keep up with others in the class. Some craniosacral practitioners only treat children who are not on medication. In my practice, I treat both those who do take methylphenidate, sometimes in combined preparations with other drugs from various manufacturers, and those who do not. My main concern is not to do anything to oppose drug treatment, but to help the child in whatever situation it finds itself at the time. In all cases, however, I do recommend that the child be under the care of an understanding child psychiatrist, remedial teacher, or school psychologist. This will help the child develop basic strategies to improve attention and social behavior.

20.10.4. Alternative or Complementary Therapies

Three studies, including a five-year study by a medical team from Inselspital, the university hospital of Bern, Switzerland, found scientifically demonstrable evidence that homeopathic treatments can help children with signs of ADHD.[6] The study showed clear improvement in over half the subjects. One important point to be kept in mind, however, is that successful homeopathic treatment takes time; children need comprehensive help.

Craniosacral Therapy offers interactive social and neurophysiological approaches that can be extremely helpful as additional treatment. The use of Craniosacral Therapy and homeopathy enables children to become more attentive and emotionally stable, and their social behavior improves—with no side effects. We can recall that Sutherland treated many hyperactive children and those with learning difficulties and psychosocial deficits. He found structural changes such as compression of the atlanto-occipital joint, a cranium that was hard and showed no sutural mobility, and meningeal tensions. Viola Frymann, whose work is discussed in chapter 4, found that in eighty percent of the children she encountered with learning difficulties, factors included a difficult birth, and neuromusculoskeletal deficits were present.[7] Children are in a critically susceptible phase until age two, and during that time strain patterns can contribute to learning difficulties. Even beyond age two, Craniosacral Therapy can assist the growth processes of the child, as the brain has enormous plasticity, or capacity to adapt.

It is possible to reduce pressure on many levels by assisting the child's own resources and through regular Craniosacral Therapy on the emotional level, on the level of the body, and in relation to themes of birth, self-attachment, and bonding behavior. This produces greater equilibrium. Sometimes the results of Craniosacral Therapy can mean that planned medication does not need to be considered any longer, that the dose can be reduced, that the medication only has to be taken on the rare occasions when it is necessary, or even that it can be stopped altogether.

Craniosacral treatment does not always lead to an observed improvement in performance at school. It does, however, help the child in terms of better orientation and adjustment to the situation and helps develop sound self-confidence. I am also concerned with supporting the child's individuality, personality, and strengths. This has a much more positive effect on development than concentrating entirely on problems and symptoms. One point that I have noticed over the sixteen years that I have been treating children with symptoms of ADHD is that during history-taking and treatment, it has emerged that around ninety percent of my young clients had a difficult birth, in many cases by C-section or with the umbilical cord around the neck. This leads me to think that a lack of oxygen during birth may be one of the causes contributing significantly to later ADHD symptoms. It is very probable that the extent to which ADHD symptoms are expressed is a result of the shock and the impression left by the shock, the inadequate supply of oxygen to the frontal and temporal lobes, and problems on other levels as discussed above, including postnatal bonding, the child's environment, allergies to food additives, and so on.

Treatment options for concentration and learning difficulties and ADHD are outlined in section 30.1.

20.10.5. What Parents Can Do

The earlier that signs of ADHD are recognized and holistic therapy is begun, the better the chances of overcoming problems. Affected children need clear boundaries. Consistent, caring guidance and a structured day are helpful. Of course, parents also have to stick to what they have agreed on with their child. Parents can help the child in the following ways: reducing the stimuli the child may be bombarded with, insisting on times of quiet, encouraging and demanding dependability, addressing careless mistakes, and involving the child more in general—enquiring, trying as far as possible to focus the child's attention on the matter in hand, and working together to look for creative solutions. Activity can aid in self-regulation because it helps bring order to confused thoughts. If the child becomes exhausted or takes a break, it can also be a sign that the brain is organizing impressions and that it requires time.

Several studies have shown that behavior improves in four out of five children if certain foods are consistently avoided. One-quarter of children were assessed as symptom-free when this was done: they were cured.[8] The affected children sleep better, for example. This is necessary for memory and the ability to concentrate as well as to enable balanced social behavior and movement.

Parents are also key players because of their adult ability to identify the essential and their role in creating the right environment to counter the action-filled qualities of everyday life. Parents can perhaps allow themselves times of respite during the day: oases of calm and of sensing and observing. In this way they could provide an example to their restless children. If they then establish a balance of alternating "action" with "no action," it helps children to alternate better between the two.

If children feel themselves to be a problem to their parents and their school, they find it difficult to deal with, and unconsciously, at least, they sense even greater pressure on them. They need the space and opportunity to work off excess energy, and on the other hand they need help to follow through a given theme in quieter moments. This calls for a great deal of encouragement and emotional closeness.

20.10.6. Concluding Thoughts

What is ultimately needed is for the various specialists concerned in education, psychology, medicine, and complementary therapy to bring together their expert knowledge and work together in an interdisciplinary approach to find comprehensive solutions for children and parents. These solutions are by their nature holistic.

Various structures of the brain continue to mature considerably through puberty, which means that in adulthood, the tendency to ADHD is minimal—as long as the children affected receive enough acceptance, care, expert help, clear boundaries, and patience. As long as conditions are favorable, our brains remain adaptable and able to produce new cells and create new networks even into advanced age.

20.11. Adults, Adolescents, and ADHD

Many adults and adolescents today are hyperactive. They are in constant need of stimulus and action. Even during meals or when using a mobile device, they tap their feet, and while sitting at the computer they drum with their fingers. They can be roused to great enthusiasm, become deeply involved and even totally absorbed in a particular concern, and are skilled in multitasking.

Increasingly, drugs designed for children with attention and hyperactivity disorders are also being taken by adults. An estimated four percent of the adult population is thought to be affected by ADHD. These people are often restless and may be workaholics. They have difficulty relaxing, are impulsive in their behavior, and find it hard to plan and organize. Each new officially recognized syndrome affecting adults creates a new set of patients and a fresh marketing opportunity. Other designer medications have entered this promising market, and even more will continue to do so. Used to enable individuals to adapt, readapt, or enhance performance, they affect and alter the neurotransmitter balance of the brain. A number of drugs to combat depression raise levels of the happiness hormone serotonin, for example. This changes regulatory processes so that a drug can have the side effects of anxiety, nightmares, and hallucinations and can in addition cause restlessness of movement. This in turn increases the likelihood of violent acts.

Another cause for concern is the fact that serotonin and dopamine act on regions of the brain that are involved in social and antisocial behavior: the limbic system, amygdalae, and inhibitory regions of the frontal lobe. Individuals who have damage to the limbic system usually lose the capacity to feel sympathy; they may, for example, be quick-tempered in their reactions and tend to lack a sense of fear. The frontal part of the brain above the eyes contains important centers for social coexistence. For example, these centers ensure that an emotional impulse, such as anger, does not immediately result in action, such as striking out. Individuals with damage or injury to this region often have a reduced planning capacity and poor sense of responsibility. They are often compulsive and moody. In 2006 a sixteen-year-old in Berlin who had taken methylphenidate randomly attacked and injured thirty-seven passersby with a penknife. He remembered nothing after the event.

20.12. Assisting the Development of Psychological Resistance and Resilience

Crises, with all their associated emotions, such as fear, sorrow, and anger, are part of life, simply the other side of the coin. In times of crisis, craniosacral practitioners can help build reassurance that difficult times, like any other, will come to an end. In stressful situations or periods of life, people are able to trust their own strength and know that coping with difficulties and obstacles builds up their capacities. Young clients are also encouraged to nurture solid, helpful contacts and friendships.

A person who has resilience, psychologically speaking, has the strength to stand firm in adverse circumstances and maintains a sound and healthy course of development despite the situation. Emmy Werner was among the first to apply and develop this concept in psychology. She visited seven hundred individuals on a Hawaiian island over a period of forty years. Around two hundred of them lived in difficult circumstances, including poverty, neglect, parental sickness or death, and violence, during childhood or adolescence. Werner wanted to find out whether it was possible for at-risk children to break out of the vicious circle of their family circumstances and live a trouble-free life later on, or whether they would inevitably become failures. To her surprise, one-third of the two hundred people investigated who had originally grown up in difficult circumstances suffered no ill effects: they were successful at school and at work and well integrated into social life, started families, and set themselves realistic goals. A further one-third had established stable personal and professional relationships by age thirty-five, and only one-third showed any abnormalities of behavior or unwillingness to integrate socially.[9]

The conclusion to be drawn from this is that even with a severely disrupted family background, for instance with an alcoholic father and depressive mother, it is still possible for people to care lovingly for their siblings and mature into stable and contented adults. The psychological resistance and resilience of children give them the power to deal with and overcome defeat and injury. They realize that although life may not be a picnic, they have the ability to cope.

The act of withstanding intolerable circumstances builds strength that can be reexperienced later and used as a resource. It is therefore important to pay attention to a person's powers of resistance and strengthen them. Resilience is strengthened by dealing with other children and by increased social interaction, quite distinct from the benefit that social contact has in opening the door to other worlds. Children always want to hear from their parents that they are valued and loved for themselves and not simply for their achievements or normal everyday occurrences. They should also be confronted with new challenges, learn through them, and gain in self-confidence, assurance, and resilience as they overcome them.

Success in confronting problems or setbacks teaches the young client to deal successfully with tasks and to prevail even when faced with difficult starting conditions. They will emerge stronger and more self-confident.

Supportive relationships, including those outside the original family, are an important protective factor that helps produce children who are resilient. These relationships may be with a teacher or neighbor, for example. Early challenges, assistance with progress, and accepting responsibility give the child a sense of achievement and can develop self-worth. A special hobby or talent that gains the child recognition has a positive effect. Resilient people are open, interested, and flexible. They do not simply collapse whenever fate causes a setback, and if they do collapse, they are quickly on their feet again, recovering as they have done before. The lesson is clear: overcoming difficult situations promotes resilience and is a resource.

20.13. Preadolescence and Puberty

Preadolescence is the stage between childhood and the onset of puberty and adolescence. Puberty occurs earlier now than it did a few generations ago: in girls it can begin around age nine and in boys around age eleven. At this stage children become moody and begin to argue for no apparent reason. They need something to push against and so may refuse to obey. Among the causes are hormonal changes. There is also a marked change and reordering of brain structures—especially in those regions that are responsible for motivation, concentration, discipline, and the capacity for judgment and empathy. They begin to explore their identity: who am I? What role do I want to fulfill in life? What is my role or function now? During this time it is important for parents to be people that the preadolescent can confide in, a stable support to lean on or occasionally perhaps to collide with.

Many adolescents in Western societies have deficits in the field of the emotions: problems with relationships or achievement, depression, and so on are all increasing. In Switzerland, for example, the suicide rate among children and young people is the second-highest in Europe.

Many children in Western cultures are lonely; their social connections often turn out to be unreliable or are nonexistent. Sometimes adolescents experience a lack of recognition and direction in their families and quite soon leave home. Aggressive children react defiantly from a young age. If the cause is not removed, this often continues through subsequent developmental phases in the form of excessive obstinacy. This is sometimes later expressed as hardened youth aggression and violence or as depression and suicide. Boys exposed to violence in childhood are more likely to become violent themselves as husbands or fathers. Their wives and children are then exposed to violence in their turn. Many adolescents have no role model to show them how to deal with tensions in a group, small or large, without resorting to violence. This later results in a situation where adults and even nations try to solve their problems with violence and cause yet more harm.

Adolescents want adults to take them seriously and accept them as they are. They want understanding and tolerance, even when things go wrong. They need to feel that adults believe in them, trust them, and have confidence in them.

The treatment of children with problems or symptoms is often simpler before the onset of puberty. Children of ages eight to ten may be more open to new learning opportunities than those going through puberty, when a new personality is taking shape and patterns of avoidance and aversion to the adult world begin to appear.

When school-age children are unable to relax during treatment, I ask them about their favorite subject at school, which enables them to talk about a resource. I may then ask them what subject they do not like so much. That opens up the question of emotional stressors or pressures. I then turn back to matters they enjoy. In this way, the child learns to alternate between the resource and the school stress, returning to the resource. This helps ease the agitation of the nervous system a little, in this case the agitation brought on by stress at school. I might then ask what they like to do in their free time. This question stabilizes or deepens the resource.

All of this strengthens the child's resilience and also helps develop the therapeutic rapport. While the child is talking, I observe such things as body posture and tone, or monitor the craniosacral rhythm during these various stages. I meanwhile continue treating, occasionally asking whether the touch is experienced as pleasant. I sometimes ask children older than age ten what job or profession they want when they are older. This usually inspires them and stimulates their creativity. It helps children develop a vision and perspective, and it often helps them learn better. Many children react with spontaneous pleasure to being asked what they would like to do in the future. The subject stimulates their imagination and inspires fascinating new ideas.

PART THREE

Elements, Assessments,
and Practice

THE MIRACLE OF SELF-HEALING

21

As pediatric craniosacral practitioners, our immediate experience of the polarities, rhythms, and cycles occurring in nature, in humankind, and within ourselves serves to stimulate our confident trust in the natural biodynamic processes of nature, humankind, and the cosmos. Everything is part of a rhythmic flowing process; everything is in motion to a greater or lesser extent as an integral part of the larger whole.

Self-regulating processes are a central theme in Craniosacral Therapy, one of the key objectives of which is to improve self-regulatory capacity on the physical level, especially in the nervous system, as well as on the emotional level, because all levels interact directly with each other. This objective is achieved primarily by balancing the craniosacral system, as reflected, for example, in improved metabolic processes and strengthening of the neuroendocrine-immune system. For instance, a stronger and more harmonious craniosacral rhythm supports the increased secretion of neurotransmitters in the brain, in the organs of the immune system, such as the spleen, and in the glands. The pituitary, which is located on the sella turcica, has a great deal of work to perform and must not overheat. A degree of cooling is achieved via the sphenoidal sinus due to the air that circulates through the paranasal sinus system. The self-regulatory capacity of the hormonal system is supported by the increased mobility of the bones that make up the viscerocranium and neurocranium.

It is a fundamental tenet of Craniosacral Therapy and Osteopathy that the body is a unity and that each individual person is a unity made up of body, mind, and spirit. The body is believed to have the capacity to regulate itself, heal itself, and maintain its state of health.

If too many restrictions are present, these forces of self-regulation and self-healing are diminished. Another fundamental principle is that all living things are in motion, that everything is continuously changing, and that a balancing process is always under way to improve equilibrium and homeostasis.

Craniosacral Therapy brings about changes that relieve tension, improve balance, and enhance the self-corrective processes; these changes are seen in the nervous system and in muscle and organ tonus, often immediately after a treatment session or over the ensuing hours and days. Sometimes it is good for the patient to sleep for one or two nights so that the brain can also process these changes and anchor the new improved state of balance. At the level of the bones, for example, changes produced by Craniosacral Therapy can reveal themselves relatively swiftly, depending on the age of the child, but sometimes it can take several days, weeks, or months before they become evident. Even where spontaneous healing has taken place, the person's body needs an individually variable period of time to anchor this newly gained equilibrium and to express it on all levels.

The pathway to an improved self-corrective process and hence to self-healing may also proceed via symptom intensification—a phenomenon known as initial deterioration, or in other words, a healing crisis. This may possibly be a healthy response that is indicative of deep cleansing from chemical substances or a reorientation in the organism as a whole. Organic comprehensive self-healing is a process that does not take place either at the touch of a button or in a linear manner.

Healing always occurs in the here and now, not in the past, and not in the future. Healing is the continuous process of change toward greater wholeness. By contrast, disease denotes a breakdown in the interplay between the various parts of the whole, a fragmentation that can no longer be satisfactorily compensated for. Even disease is an attempt to compensate for progressive fragmentation rather than having to discontinue basic functions. The craniosacral practitioner can best support the process leading to improved self-regulation, greater harmony, and wholeness by being present in the heart and in the moment.

In the model proposed by Wilhelm Reich, what does supporting the development of self-regulation look like, and what are the repercussions of it? The child is helped to pulsate in its own rhythm and, at its own individual tempo, to turn both inward as well as outward to the surrounding world. If practitioners and parents basically support and affirm the line of development that the child specifically wants to take, its pattern of living will unfold in a natural way. The various characteristics of a child with a well-developed capacity for self-regulation include: a generous and giving nature, actively seeking social contact, coordinated movements, litheness, grace, relaxed and supple shoulders, and mobile pelvis and legs. The characteristic features of a child with a pulsation disturbance are: hostility, avoidance of eye contact, stiff and uncoordinated movements, shoulders held high, fists chronically clenched, pelvis "locked in place," and legs extended stiffly. Where the organism is in a free and balanced state, in contrast to a blocked, contracted, or hypotonic state, the vital energies will be able to flow freely.

The body's ability to compensate for any imbalance is important as it seeks to restore balance. However, this activity uses up a certain amount of energy that is consequently not available for fundamental regulation, thus weakening the immune system, for example. If this state is then compounded by further imbalance, the body again has to compensate for this, which consumes even more energy and ultimately leads to disease.

Our organism strives to achieve local balance within its individual systems, such as the locomotor apparatus, internal organs, hormonal system, and nervous system, and within its segments, which are the different bodily regions, such as the pelvis, abdomen, thorax, throat, mouth, and eyes. At the same time it also strives to ensure balance among all the various systems so that the body as a whole can function as a unity. Regarded holistically, human beings, with our body-mind-spirit components, are anything but static; instead we are constantly in motion as a multiplicity of functions. From our subsystems right through to our totality, we are constantly seeking to maintain the best possible balance. In the broader context the organism also strives for balance with its immediate surroundings and with the cosmos.

21.1. The Holistic Matrix and Cell Memory

With regard to self-regulation, particular importance is assigned to the myofascial chains that link all parts of the body and the holistic matrix—the connective tissue as a whole—that links all structures right down to the cellular level, including the fluids they contain.

The biomechanics of the body demand robustness and strength, on the one hand, coupled with sufficient elasticity, on the other, to be able to adapt to asymmetric tensions. Stability and mobility are facilitated by tension networks known as tensegrity structures. *Tensegrity* is a portmanteau word that combines the concepts of tension and integrity. Tensegrity structures transmit tensions from tensile and compressive forces and commonly take the form of three-dimensional triangular or hexagonal structures, such as tetrahedrons, that are stable in themselves. Similar structures are found in honeycomb and even as far as down the molecular and cellular level.

The pelvis, for example, is a unified tensile field that in turn forms part of a wider tensegrity construction. Each tensegrity structure is able to organize itself and is simultaneously in contact with other structures. This model clearly illustrates how, for example, the position and mobility of the sacrum has repercussions for the entire pelvic structure and how it influences the balance of forces acting on the body as a whole via the straight and crossed fascia, ligaments, and myofascial chains. Tissue, cell, and cell nucleus structures are also built on the tensegrity model.

Connective tissue acts as a type of whole-body matrix and possesses a high degree of intelligence. This "living matrix" forms an energetic and biomechanical communication system that comprises, organizes, and energizes the body as a whole. In 1975 Alfred Pischinger originally published his book about the system of ground regulation in the body that, in his view, consists of capillary vessels, connective tissue, ground substance, terminal fibers of the ANS, and extracellular fluid.[1] Albert Szent-Györgyi, the scientist who discovered vitamin C, was convinced that molecules do not even have to touch each other in order to interact, and that energy can flow through electromagnetic fields. Together with intracellular and extracellular water, this forms the ground substance, the matrix of life. As reported in detail by James Oschman, among others, the tissue tensegrity-matrix system was first described in 1991 by Pienta and Coffey.[2] This system enables vibrational information not only to travel from the cell membrane to the nucleus but also for it to be transferred via the cell and the extracellular matrix throughout the entire body. Thus all cells are interactively in contact with one another via the tissue tensegrity-matrix system.

In Craniosacral Therapy it is held that traumatic experiences may have repercussions extending down as far as the cellular level. Our cells have memory. Among other things, Craniosacral Therapy also improves the mechanics of the forces at work in the body as a whole, bringing balance to the connective tissue and tensegrity structures, and thus exerting a harmonizing effect down to the cellular level. In other words, noninvasive Craniosacral Therapy may resolve traumas that have been stored at the cellular level.

21.2. Salutogenesis and the Origin of Health

Salutogenesis is a concept that was developed in the 1970s by the medical sociologist Aaron Antonovsky.[3] Instead of dealing exclusively with pathogenesis, which is the development and treatment of disease, and the strict dichotomy between health and disease, salutogenesis views the two as being at opposite ends of a continuum. The question is therefore not whether someone is healthy or unhealthy, but how close to or distant from the endpoints of health and disease that person is. Among other things, it depends on the individual's underlying attitude toward the world and their own existence. The basis for this is the individual's enthusiasm for life and sense of coherence, meaning how much the individual feels part of or at one with the flow of vital energy.

Health is not something static but rather an ideal target objective, a dynamic process that leads via holistic experience to health and wholeness. By contrast, disease is a process that leads to fragmentation, separation, and isolation. Every natural development is a biodynamic process of being and becoming, of change and transformation.

Starting from the basic premise that we as craniosacral practitioners see ourselves and the child as a whole entity, and that we then support the child in its healthy elements, meaning its resources and its sense of coherence, the focus is clearly on strengthening the capacity for self-healing. Orientation toward wholeness potentiates the healing effect. The sense of coherence, the fundamental ability to see the world as holding together and having meaning, is determined by several factors: the feeling of *I can understand it, I can manage this and cope with it*, and *This is important and it makes sense*. A strong sense of coherence enables the individual to react flexibly to demands and to cope better with physical, biochemical, and psychosocial stressors. It has a direct effect on the individual's state of health. Health is not the absence of disease but is a dynamic state of physical, mental, and spiritual balance.

21.3. The Polyvagal Theory and Social Engagement

Stephen W. Porges of the University of Illinois in Chicago has defined the concepts of the polyvagal model and the social nervous system, both of which have extended our understanding of the neurobiology of self-regulation.[4] Our ANS is neuroceptive, which means that our nervous system is subconsciously receiving signals continually from the world around us, and it immediately assesses whether we are safe or in danger. Neuroception occurs instinctively in all human beings and mammals to ensure an instantaneous fight-or-flight response in dangerous situations. If we cannot do either, then the nervous system switches to a self-protective reflex reaction of "playing possum," in effect a dissociative detachment from the here and now. When we feel safe, the parts of the vagus nerve that are most active are those that emerge from the nucleus ambiguous, located ventrally in the medulla oblongata. These vagus components cause our heartbeat to slow, our lungs to be better perfused, and our voice to sound warm and relaxed.

The vagus fibers emerging ventrally are myelinated, which permits lightning-fast reactions. They start to form in the fetus from about week thirty or thirty-two onward. In children and adults they are involved in such matters as expressing love, making contact with others, and the search for a partner.

When we feel threatened, the sympathetic part of our ANS becomes activated so that we can immediately defend ourselves or carry ourselves to safety: the fight-or-flight reflex kicks in, which increases the volume of blood reaching the extremities. If fight or flight in a given situation is futile and agitation is too great, the nervous system reacts by freezing or "playing possum." This type of emergency circuit comes into operation when the vagus nerve components emerging from the dorsal nuclei become activated to a high degree, immediately causing all bodily functions to shut down to the minimum level necessary for survival. This novel threefold view of the ANS explains how our reactions are adapted to our environment:

1. Calmness, relaxation, oneness with our surroundings, and social contact = mostly vagus nerve components from the ventral nucleus

2. Fight-or-flight situations characterized by relatively pronounced agitation or activation = mainly sympathetic involvement
3. Freezing and dissociation = mostly vagus nerve components from the dorsal nucleus

The social nervous system is made up of cranial nerves V, VII, IX, X, and XI, which are important in forging social contact and engagement with others. The child uses neuroception to scan and assess its surroundings: what does this facial expression mean? What is the tone of voice of its mother or of other caregivers? Are they turning toward the child or away from it? Cranial nerve VII also controls the stapedius muscle in the middle ear, which differentiates hearing to the extent that a mother can single out her crying baby, or the baby can distinguish the voice of its mother, from a chaotic jumble of background noise.

People who feel immediately threatened by some external stimulus often have "faulty" neuroception: without any obvious cause, yet conditioned by past experiences, the situation is classed as threatening and the nervous system reports danger, which leads to fear and stress and increases sympathetic activation.

The craniosacral practitioner can encourage the child's capacity for self-regulation by offering praise, strengthening its resources, and acting in unison with the child to determine the course of the treatment session. In this way the social nervous system and hence also the ventral vagus components are reinforced, and relaxation can become more profound. The craniosacral practitioner can also strengthen the social nervous system by specifically treating the five cranial nerves involved: the anatomical features associated with the course of cranial nerves V, VII, IX, X, and XI yield plentiful clues as to how the function of these nerves can be supported in practice. A list of the cranial nerves is provided in the Appendix; details of the pathways of these nerves can be found in standard anatomy textbooks.

21.4. The Second Brain: The Enteric Nervous System

The vagus nerve has an enormous number—approximately thirty-one thousand—ascending afferent nerve fibers leading to the brain. In his book *The Second Brain* the neurobiologist Michael D. Gershon points out some interesting associations.[5] Our "second brain" is located in the gut; it possesses a similar number of nerves as the brain in our head and also exchanges information with the brain via the vagus nerve. Moreover, the second brain, in particular the intestinal wall, produces endogenous substances such as dopamine and serotonin. The enteric nervous system constitutes a large association of peripheral ganglia that function like small organizing satellite brains governed by other autonomic nerves; these operate to switch the enteric nervous system on and off.

Relaxation of the transverse connective tissue layers, especially of the body segments as defined by Wilhelm Reich, coupled with visceral treatment affords enormous support to the second brain. Peristalsis provides direct feedback that points to the increased activity of the parasympathetic system, which is active in relaxation and release and is indicative of increased metabolic processes that imply improved self-regulation overall.

21.5. Mirror Neurons and Interpersonal Relationships

In its earliest forays into communicative behavior, a baby will imitatively seek to mirror the sound of its mother's voice and her facial expressions. With the discovery of mirror neurons, Giacomo Rizzolatti and his team at the University of Parma, Italy, have shown that our brains possess special neural networks that recognize and reflect the actions and signals of other people, which are then mapped into our own neural pathways in such a way that we, as observers, experience empathy and are also better able to mimic these actions and signals.[6] Rizzolatti has thus discovered a neurobiological basis for the fact that human experience and learning are made possible, in particular, on the basis of interpersonal relationships. Soon after birth, the baby begins to imitate the signals it receives and reflects them back with looks, facial expressions, touch, and sounds that together are formative in early mother-baby communication.

There is a close connection here with the social nervous system mentioned earlier. Additionally, the cingulate gyrus assumes an important role: according to Antonio Damasio, signals arriving from the body, from "inside," and from the mother, from "outside," come together in the neural networks of the cingulate gyrus.[7] This part of the limbic system appears to be active primarily in establishing empathy or in identifying with the feelings of others because it is here that neural network firing occurs. When the cingulate gyrus is at work, emotional core moods and a certain sense of self are activated: *I feel, therefore I am.* Neurons in this brain structure are activated in us when we observe joy or pain in other people, and a physical reaction is produced. It is therefore suspected that the cingulate gyrus mediates the qualities of empathy and of emotional understanding.

Neuroscientists have discovered that the behavior of the mother toward her child determines which genes in its brain are switched on and off. The notion of genetic determinism has been scientifically refuted by Michael Meaney and Bruce Lipton, among others.[8] Character traits—for example, whether the child is shy and fearful, well-adjusted, bold, or neurotic—are determined in large measure by the behavior of the mother and other immediate caregivers. Neuroscience has even made new discoveries with regard to adults, and the dogmatic assertion that the fully mature adult brain no longer forms new neurons is no longer unassailable. Not only the brains of children and adolescents but also the brains of adults possess a high degree of plasticity. This is determined primarily by lifestyle. The new neurons that are formed in the cerebral ventricles and that can also be found in the hippocampal formation are more easily excitable, form new synapses more readily, and link up to build new circuits.[9]

The topics of bonding, the social nervous system, and mirror neurons are addressed in this book because they all make a major contribution to self-regulatory capacity and thus to health. As you come to understand their impact and importance more clearly, you will be able to make use of these aspects as a craniosacral practitioner, even before you are hands-on. In light of this understanding, you will know that you can accompany and support children and their parents on these levels too—even though the actual hands-on treatment sessions may vary widely.

PRINCIPLES OF NONINVASIVE CRANIOSACRAL THERAPY FOR CHILDREN

22

This chapter contains a great many hints and tips that, in my understanding, rank alongside anatomical and specialist craniosacral knowledge in forming the basis of holistic Craniosacral Therapy for children. See chapter 30 for a discussion of selected indications, with pointers for Craniosacral Therapy.

22.1. The Role and Function of the Pediatric Craniosacral Practitioner

Pediatric Craniosacral Therapy demands the ability to empathize with and understand the world of the child, coupled with a high degree of creativity, flexibility, and spontaneity on the part of the practitioner. Healing is not merely the result of a specialist technical method but also of health-bringing laughter, compassion, and love. For example, as the emotional level regulates itself instead of remaining stuck, the body, mind, and spirit will also experience release. The whole person is then able to return increasingly to the vital energy flow.

If you are a practitioner intending to treat infants and children, you must first and foremost have good and balanced contact with yourself. Self-reflection helps to ensure awareness of your own physical and emotional state and especially of your own possible concerns. It also helps in sensing your own limits, for example the limits of your own ability to cope with stress—something that is generally vital when supporting other people. As well as your own personal state of mind, it is also helpful to become aware of the therapeutic intention before a session with the child: *Why do I want to treat this child? Is there perhaps some hidden motive that might better remain suppressed or that needs to be compensated for in this way?* Motivation and intention affect the course of the session because Craniosacral Therapy is also an interactive process in which both the child and the practitioner have a direct part to play.

KEY POINT

If you intend to treat babies or young children, you must have good contact with yourself and be capable of a certain degree of self-reflection. You will have developed the skill set needed to empathize with the child's world, to gauge and sense its needs, and to respond to them physically as well as emotionally and verbally.

Ultimately, it is the child who will determine the timing and the permitted intimacy of contact with the practitioner. Babies communicate primarily through body language, looks, and sounds, meaning voice and intonation. Beyond this, there is also uninterrupted two-way contact via instinctive factors, the social nervous system, and mirror neurons. Young children are not only aware of the facial expressions, voice, gestures, and touch of their practitioner counterpart, they also have all their senses set to "receive."

Where at all possible, a caregiver should also be present during pediatric craniosacral work, at least at the start of the first few sessions, so that the child is not left alone with a stranger and feeling vulnerable—factors that would probably unsettle it and potentially trigger stress.

As a pediatric craniosacral practitioner you will have built up years of previous experience of the powerful effectiveness of Craniosacral Therapy, both for you personally and having treated a great many adults and adolescents, and you will understand that as a facilitator you can support this natural process. You will possess a wide range of social and professional skills and will understand that you personally are not doing the healing but that you are acting primarily as a type of catalyst for the emerging process of self-regulation. As this happens, you function as a free fulcrum for the child, who—in a respectful and safe therapeutic space in the practice—benefits from a variety of learning opportunities and is thus enabled to experience and integrate new things. Physical, emotional, and mental-spiritual difficulties, symptoms, diseases, and conflicts are not necessarily negative. As long as they are not suppressed or rationalized but are instead approached in a solution-oriented way as a challenge, they carry the potential for change and growth for all parties involved. In the face of difficulties, it is possible for new perspectives, learning processes, and changes to emerge that later turn out to be steps in the right direction or even to be transformative in their own right. It is precisely through the difficult phases of life that we learn and grow.

Carefree areas of life are a joy and therefore a resource for the child. In contrast, difficult or burdensome areas, especially if they stretch back over a lengthy period, may trigger or intensify psychosomatic stress and be the reason that prompted the parents to bring their child to your craniosacral practice. I also take account of the child's psychological frame of mind and respect the child's wishes. The voluntary participation of everyone involved is important to me; anything else would merely generate extra stress.

As craniosacral practitioners, we learn from the children and their families. We support the life force within each child and each family member. The child is the main protagonist in the craniosacral sessions. With its inner rhythm, its impulses, and its individual tempo, it also determines which specific issues need to be addressed. As practitioners who are supporting the child, we can occasionally tell the parents what we are observing at any given moment, how we are accompanying the process, when we are gently applying a specific technique, and how the child is responding. In this way the parents become involved in the treatment. They develop an understanding for the natural principles of self-regulation and self-healing, and they learn to appreciate the potential of pediatric Craniosacral Therapy and how it operates. However, I only involve the parents fully in the session if they represent a genuine source of support for the child, meaning whether they are a positive resource. Otherwise I prefer to work separately with the parents and to support them individually.

KEY POINT

Craniosacral practicalities and your perceptual field:

- Impartially observe what comes to light in the session, whether from the child or from the parents.
- Be open to whatever awakens your interest and comes into your perceptual field, but without desiring anything specific, and without intention.
- Note how the child and the parents behave together.
- Note how congruent and resilient the parents and child are together and what inner and external resources are available.
- Support the child and the parents with craniosacral evaluation and treatment.

Many children have a hugely sensitive presence, as if vast numbers of fine antennae are operating subconsciously and consciously, instinctively, and with every sense engaged to perceive and assess the world around them. If they have no major disability or serious trauma, many children are able to size up the craniosacral practitioner quite spontaneously in terms of appearance, movements, expression, and personality as a whole. With children it is often not just the content of your words that is effective in widening or narrowing the field for the therapeutic process but also your vocal inflection, your presence, your intention, and your heart's coherence—the line that provides contact or connection with the child.

If you give the child the impression—verbally and especially on the emotional level—that you are open to it, the resultant security and trust generated will enable the child to relax mentally to the point where it allows itself to receive your touch. The child will also have a greater tendency to relax physically as a result. This is an important foundational aspect, alongside anatomical and practical knowledge and the cranial touch.

At each session the fresh challenge for you as the practitioner is to reattune yourself relatively quickly to the child and the parents, to be present in the moment, and to meet with each individual party precisely where they are. It is important that you use a linguistic register and vocabulary that children and parents can understand, and aside from your professional expertise, that you also offer your openness, clarity, integrity, and full support. Expanding boundaries and setting boundaries are also important issues for everyone involved; above all this should not be perceived as negative and limiting but rather as something that fosters safety and trust. This also means that agreements reached are adhered to by both parties in terms of both content and timing.

The dialogue—and this applies in fact to all interactions between

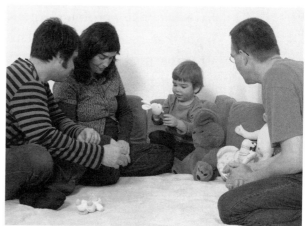

Figure 22.1. Identifying the concerns and wishes of the parents and the child.

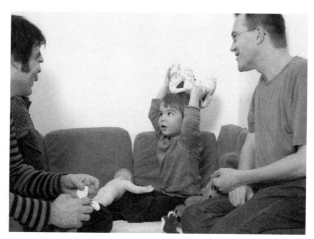

Figure 22.2. Getting to know the child in the therapeutic setting.

parents and child or practitioner and child—will follow an individual rhythm of its own. This rhythmicity can already be noted around the time of birth, even in preterm babies. The periodic ebb and flow of attention and interaction is evidently a natural phenomenon in learning processes. Therefore, before touching the child, I attune myself to its subtle messages in any form.

Anyone carrying out pediatric Craniosacral Therapy should first have acquired a profound knowledge of the structure and function of the craniosacral system and have gained extensive experience with Craniosacral Therapy in adults. Further training that covers the prenatal and perinatal periods is also helpful. Attending several pediatric craniosacral courses will also facilitate entry into the field of treating children. It is possible that such courses will impart anatomical knowledge, structural techniques, and a noninvasive core attitude that will enable participants to use these expanded perceptual and treatment options to support both children and parents in a comprehensive way.

22.2. Healing the Emotions of Child, Parents, and Practitioner

Permanently blocking off emotions has huge implications on the physical level. It becomes noticeable, for example, as marked tension in the locomotor apparatus, including the joints; shallow breathing, or drawn-up shoulders. The internal organs—especially the gastrointestinal tract, the "second brain"—also then commonly tend to be hypertonic, and the nervous system is mostly operating at full speed.

Emotions that have been suppressed can be reexperienced in a safe and protected setting and perhaps even expressed, regardless of whether the emotions are difficult or good. Release and subsequent autonomic and organic balancing are important for body, heart, and spirit. In the past the suppression of difficult emotions was believed to afford protection against excessive or prolonged pain. It is currently recognized that if they have not been resolved, suppressed emotions generally continue to operate at a subconscious level by avoidance, fending off, and rationalization. The suppression of emotions not only consumes energy but also prevents us from experiencing a broad spectrum of different emotions, and thus from shaping our lives in a vibrant and fulfilled way. To some extent the protective strategies of the past can impose considerable limitations on the adult's scope for action.

In the ideal scenario, practitioners will have free access to their own emotions. This enables them to better recognize the current emotional state of the child and of any accompanying adults. Practitioners themselves will have learned to move back and forth between their own difficult and pleasant emotions. This ability is highly valuable and most important for practitioners in the context of Craniosacral Therapy. It enables them to influence the therapeutic process considerably, because their own mood and their ability to handle critical situations will also affect the atmosphere in the room and the course of the session. When practitioners are able to move deliberately between difficult and pleasant emotions, sensing and utilizing their own resources during the session, they act as a firm anchor on a subconscious, instinctive, autonomic, energetic, and symbolic level. They also become a companion on the pathway through obstacles and emotions such as fear, anger, and emotional pain that previously seemed to be insurmountable.

The goal of pediatric Craniosacral Therapy is not to bring the child into a particular emotional or health-related state. Life is in flux, and therefore health is also not static but a process (see also section 21.2).

One goal of Craniosacral Therapy in children is to improve self-regulation and self-healing at the physical level, something that is also influenced by the emotional level and emotional balance. As we know, joy and fear produce entirely different biochemical reactions in the body, for example in our nervous and hormonal systems. However, the intention in pediatric therapy is not that the child should have only pleasant emotions or should always do as it is told. Children have a right to all their emotions and want to enjoy the freedom of being. There is no such thing as wrong emotions, but there can be wrong interpretations of these emotions. It is perfectly acceptable for children, and their parents, to be in a bad mood for a while. It is not therefore a question of having only good emotions, nor is it proper to deny all difficulties by claiming that there is no problem. By the same token it is important not to keep on finding new problems with the child; parents and practitioners alike should refrain from constantly searching for things that might be amiss and need treating.

During a craniosacral session it is permissible to sense and experience many old and new emotions without getting bogged down in particular emotions for long periods. With the practitioner's support, the child can increasingly develop the ability to move between difficult and pleasant emotions. This ability for emotional shuttling back and forth encourages self-regulation because it has a balancing effect on the person as a whole, especially on the nervous system and all autonomic processes.

22.3. Children as Mirrors for Adults

Children mirror to adults many emotions and existential qualities that adults may perhaps have forgotten or suppressed. By their very manner—with their innocent child's eyes, open heart, and vitality—children challenge those around them to open up to and embrace the moment. This enables children and adults to learn from each other. In this way children become a mirror for their parents and the practitioner, prompting them, for example, to become increasingly aware of their own inner child and to make space for it in their lives.

22.4. The Practitioner's Core Attitude

Through self-reflection, as when you continually reassess your own potential, capacity, and limitations, you will also learn a great deal with every session. At the same time, self-reflection during the session will help you to take stock so that you are not completely swept along by events and do not find yourself in uncharted territory but instead are able to guarantee a safe framework.

Personal resources are important for practitioners. They help you to establish a link with your personal strength and to remain in the here and now. This is important, for example, in the event of prolonged helpless crying, tensions in the room, or powerful therapeutic processes so that you retain your ability to guide the session with confidence—and to prevent you from becoming overwhelmed or even traumatized by the sometimes intense processes at work. A present and attentive practitioner operates on an instinctive level as protection for the child.

22.5. The Initial Session and Subsequent Sessions

22.5.1. Arranging the First Appointment

Wherever possible, during the first telephone call or when setting up the appointment, I provide certain preliminary explanations: I answer and ask questions and let the enquiring parents know how my pediatric craniosacral treatment sessions unfold. The more points that are clarified before the first session, the better able the parents are to form some ideas and to decide whether or not it will meet their expectations. Depending on the child's age, appropriate information can also be provided to the child. In cases where the parents intend to travel a long distance to come to me, I frequently recommend that they seek out a craniosacral practitioner closer to home because it is not ideal to travel for several hours to attend a one-hour treatment session.

Preliminary explanations may cover, for example, the following areas:

• Have any conventional allopathic medical investigations been performed and diagnoses made—for example, neurological tests, imaging techniques, and so on?

- What treatments have already been given, and what was the outcome?
- Is the child taking any medicines, homeopathy, or Bach flower remedies?
- Is there a treatment request or a prescription from a pediatrician or other physician?
- What are the parents' concerns and possible expectations?
- Where did the parents hear about Craniosacral Therapy or about me?
- Have the parents themselves already undergone Craniosacral Therapy sessions? If so, what was their experience?
- Depending on the child's age: has the child been asked whether it wants to receive Craniosacral Therapy? Has the child been informed about it, and if so, what was the child told? Was the child persuaded or invited to take part by bribing it with promises of a reward?
- Is it perhaps important for the child to be able to choose whether it would prefer to be treated by a man or a woman?

I inform the parents about the potential and the limitations of therapy. My preliminary explanations, perhaps over the telephone, are designed to promote clarity and to create an atmosphere of trust. When arranging the first appointment, I already make an effort, together with the parents, to find a time that will disrupt the child's normal daily routine as little as possible. This is so the child does not become a "special case" but can continue to attend school, play soccer, and so on. The mother and father are invited to be present for their child's craniosacral session. Depending on the child's age and desires, it will also be permitted to bring a favorite doll, book, or CD along to the session.

In each case I inform the parents that the initial session is designed first and foremost as an exercise in familiarization and building trust, to allow me to gain a first impression—not all parents understand the concept of evaluating the overall situation—and that I will touch the child only if it allows me to. If more is possible, then it is welcome, but the voluntary nature of participation in all areas is paramount. I mention the fact that as well as Craniosacral Therapy, I will use play-based elements to support the child—or if the parents want, I may perhaps start the session by briefly treating the mother or father; it often happens that parental release also has a positive effect on the child so that afterward it too wants to be touched and treated. I also provide information about the approximate length of the session (in my practice about fifty to sixty minutes) and about costs and methods of payment.

I suggest that after the initial session, or some days later, we discuss what will happen next, and depending on the child's age, I request that the child be involved in the decision-making process. I also point out to the parents that improvement or cure is an entirely individual process, and that although a body of empirical data has been accumulated, it is not possible to offer a prognosis in any specific case. The total duration of treatment is highly individual, as is the number of sessions required and the interval between them. I explain that I will be in a better position to estimate this after I have had some experience with the young client, because I will then be able to form a clearer picture of the overall situation and know how the child has reacted after two or three craniosacral sessions. Another source of variation is whether symptoms disappear for only a brief time or resolve completely. This is further dependent on severity and on any previous falls or surgical procedures that may perhaps already have been forgotten. If parents ask how long it will take to eliminate the problem or symptom, I might ask them what they believe to be the cause of the problem, thus actively involving them in finding a solution.

22.5.2. Duration of a Pediatric Craniosacral Session

The duration and intensity of a session should not be excessive, and the child should not be overstimulated. One of the golden rules, particularly with children, is: minimal stimulation, maximal integration.

It is not uncommon for children with pronounced agitation, stress, or unusual behaviors to already have a high degree of ANS activation. First of all in such circumstances the child's resources should be built up or strengthened. The child is strengthened and calmed as it is supported in its self-attachment, its bonding with the mother, and its individual tempo. Only then is it possible to work increasingly with more major difficulties or pronounced symptoms in a way that does not agitate or retraumatize the child even more.

The question as to the appropriate session duration is reassessed on each occasion on an individual basis, in line with the child's inner state, and depending on the situation, meaning the child's resources and the therapeutic process. It is consequently difficult to make any standard pronouncements or forecasts. It makes good sense to schedule about fifty to sixty minutes for the whole session, defined as lasting from the moment of welcome to the time of departure.

The session format can be structured as follows:

1. The initial dialogue with history-taking
2. The treatment section itself, in which predominantly hands-on treatment is given using play-based elements and Craniosacral Therapy
3. The follow-up dialogue

The treatment section—the actual hands-on part—can be subdivided into three phases:

1. Tuning in (synchronization), assessment and treatment both globally and locally, overall as well as specific
2. Targeted or specific treatment, possibly also local at affected sites or zones
3. Rounding off and integrating treatment, mainly global

The ratio among these phases may be altered during the session on an individual basis. The purely hands-on treatment time, for example, may be fifteen to twenty minutes in infants and twenty to forty minutes in school-age children. Hands-on treatment time is dependent on the intensity of the session and on when and how the therapeutic process can be rounded off and integrated appropriately.

Craniosacral practitioners can foster the parents' understanding of the initial signs displayed by the child by occasionally informing them about the impressions gained during the session; for example, regarding the child's capacity for increased self-regulation, or the individual tempo or needs of the child.

During the follow-up dialogue it is your responsibility as the practitioner to summarize with sufficient clarity your evaluation of the overall impression created by the child at that moment. In this way you will impart to the parents a degree of clarity, direction, and security. Excessively vague comments made by the practitioner can unsettle the parents, particularly if they have not personally experienced Craniosacral Therapy. Often the parents will want to hear your personal assessment.

The follow-up dialogue can be structured more easily if you are used to reflecting during the session about which dynamics are emerging and how structure, function, and the craniosacral rhythm or midtide are fluctuating as the session progresses. It is helpful for you to form an opinion without it being written in stone. You can remain open to new impressions; indeed, such openness is always essential. During the relatively short follow-up dialogue you should provide information to the parents and the child in a form that contains no forecasts or prognoses whatsoever so as not to rigidly label the child. Remember too that the follow-up dialogue at the end of the session is a momentary evaluation of the situation, not a diagnosis, and it may change during the period leading up to the next session.

Time management: depending on the practitioner and individual working styles, the craniosacral session should not last longer than sixty to seventy-five minutes. Since your role as practitioner also includes time management, you will determine this aspect. For everyone involved it can often be quite demanding to maintain attention for a whole hour. In addition, mothers will want to get home again, children might want to play, and so on.

22.5.3. Self-Reflection and Keeping a Record of the Session

For those newly embarking on Craniosacral Therapy it may initially seem a tiresome exercise to take a little time at the end of the session to review it internally from start to finish. However, it is enormously helpful for the novice—and experienced craniosacral practitioners can always learn something from each session—provided that you allow yourself a few minutes for reflection and keep a record of the session. Make notes detailing your impression and evaluation at the outset, and then the therapeutic process; the general physical and emotional level; the specialist level, meaning the craniosacral system with the craniosacral rhythm, mid-tide, and Long Tide; and finally what has changed by the end of the session. You should distinguish the issues or dynamics that become apparent during the session, both in the child and in the parents, and make note of anything that may have been triggered in you personally.

You can also keep a record of your own reflections on the emotional level, for example how you were affected, any difficult and pleasant moments, but also on the purely specialist level. This self-reflection may yield instructive questions for you as well as ideas that may prove fruitful in a subsequent session. A treatment record template can be found in my earlier book *Craniosacral Rhythm*.[1] Record-keeping after a session is important for the craniosacral practitioner not only because of the usual need for patient documentation but also because it provides a specialist basis as you work your way into the issues of the child and it reflects the child's emotional state, which is important for your own psychological well-being.

22.5.4. Subsequent Sessions

At the beginning of my day in practice or before a session starts, I review my brief notes or my record from the previous session. This helps me in many ways because it enables me, for example, to tune into the upcoming session. In this process I often find that important sequences from the previous sessions are recalled. I usually remember these sequences as if they had only just happened. It may be that physical anatomy questions or associations come to the surface, or perhaps an idea, an inspiration, or a sign concerning trails or levels that need to be pursued further may even intuitively suggest themselves. This may relate to something that was not yet possible in earlier sessions, either because the child did not want it or because the right time had not yet arrived.

22.6. How Many Sessions?

The number of sessions will be guided by the treatment goal, how serious a symptom is, and how long it has already been present. Craniosacral Therapy may already be highly effective during the first session; alternatively, resonance may be achieved only after several sessions have been completed. In addition, considerate regard and cooperation from the child's social environment has a role to play in terms of the likelihood of healing because these factors depend predominantly on input from the adult world. As a rule, unless the child has been through traumatic experiences, fewer sessions are required for the treatment of young children than for adults.

Whether and how therapy is having an effect should become apparent after about three to six craniosacral sessions. Perhaps the child is suddenly sleeping more, as if it wants to make up for lost time; or it becomes hungrier for social contact, bounces around more joyfully, moves more confidently, and is generally far more open. If the child's condition does not improve after six to twelve sessions, this may be attributable to the choice of practitioner or to the treatment approach adopted. At the same time, despite their expectant attitude, parents need to remember that lasting changes take time, even in children. However, it is also possible that Craniosacral Therapy may not be the method of choice at the present time. In such cases other interventions, for example physiotherapy, may be indicated.

Craniosacral Therapy is not a general substitute for specific therapies such as speech therapy, psychomotor training, or occupational therapy. Frequently, however, it serves to improve the child's ability to link back to its origins and early developmental processes. At the physical level, the effect of neurophysiological therapies can be amplified by pediatric Craniosacral Therapy and the resultant improvement in connective tissue and muscle tonus.

22.7. What Is the Schedule for Subsequent Sessions?

The timing of the next session in the sequence is agreed on an individual basis. This can often be better judged after the initial familiarization session with the child and its parents than beforehand. With children over age four, I advise parents to involve, or at least listen to, their child in decisions regarding further craniosacral sessions.

If the child's restrictions or symptoms are released or resolved very simply and quickly, longer intervals between sessions are more advisable, for example every three to six weeks, because the ground regulation system in such cases is evidently working relatively well on its own. However, if the healing process is making only faltering progress or even becomes clearly retrograde for a while, the parents should notify the craniosacral practitioner accordingly. In such circumstances, shorter intervals between sessions, for example every seven to ten days, might be more beneficial.

If the child experiences pronounced side effects after a Craniosacral Therapy session, such as severe diarrhea, vomiting, or dizziness, that do not resolve after twenty-four to forty-eight hours, a follow-up session is worth recommending. This should not be excessive, either in terms of the time taken or the techniques used. The child's craniosacral system should be newly evaluated and then harmonized, calmed, and balanced—all with the intention of achieving maximal integration.

22.8. Follow-Up Sessions to Consolidate Improvement or Symptom Eradication

In cases where improvement is noted after a few Craniosacral Therapy sessions, it is vital that the parents do not decide prematurely to dispense with further sessions for their child. In particular, if the child's symptoms are alleviated or disappear completely after just one or two sessions, there can be a great temptation for the parents not to make any further appointments or to cancel future appointments because they no longer appear necessary. However, experience shows that in such cases it is helpful for the child if its improved state is further consolidated by a couple of follow-up sessions. Otherwise the child could lapse back into its old pattern, and the parents might then think that Craniosacral Therapy had also not been beneficial. However, the sustained effect of craniosacral sessions is generally only reinforced or ensured by a sufficient number of follow-up sessions.

22.9. Total Duration of Treatment: Short Course and Long Course

Craniosacral Therapy in children can produce major effects and changes even in the initial sessions. Depending on the child, objective, and context, a short course of therapy often comprises about four to nine sessions, with a maximum of twelve. However, Craniosacral Therapy may also extend over one or two years, for example, to provide support in cases where there are repercussions from severe illness, surgery, or disability, as in severe cerebral palsy. For such children a long course of Craniosacral Therapy brings improved quality of life. As a result the child becomes solution-oriented and is supported and accompanied step-by-step in the process. In the treatment of children with ADHD, it is possible over the course of four to twelve sessions to minimize the effects of hidden causes, such as a difficult birth, and to improve bonding issues, and it becomes easier for both the child and its parents to cope with ADHD. In order to address the deeper, multiple layers of ADHD in a sustained way, and to change them at the level of cerebral physiology, consideration should be given to regular sessions, approximately every three weeks, over an extended period of about one or two years.

In practice a difficulty that is frequently encountered is that sessions are canceled or postponed for a variety of reasons, and a regular pattern of sessions, which would be important for these children and their parents, fails to materialize.

In terms of study, I would welcome it if our professional associations were to become more active and initiate a program of long-term studies, similar to what has already been done in homeopathy, therapeutic touch, and others.

22.10. The Pattern of Therapy

It is entirely possible for the first session to prove quite difficult, with the child not allowing itself to be touched at all. Not uncommonly, the next session is easier, for example because the child is now already slightly familiar with and more trusting of the surroundings, the craniosacral practitioner, and the gentle approach being adopted. For example, if it was totally impossible or only briefly possible to touch the child's head during the first session, this may perhaps not be at all problematic in the second or third session. However, the opposite may also be true, with the first session running very smoothly and the second session difficult because the child is no longer cooperative.

For the course of a session in general, many of the aspects dealt with in this book can be incorporated as supportive measures and utilized for therapeutic purposes.

22.11. Surroundings and Equipment

It is useful if the equipment for therapy includes a soft massage table, a mattress on the floor, blankets and cushions, and a collection of toys and books for infants and children. For sessions with children, the massage table can be adjusted to a relatively low setting, provided that it is still comfortable for the practitioner to work at. Depending on the age of the child, it is then possible see over the whole surface of the table. Perhaps the mother can lie on the treatment table so that she can be seen, encouraging the child to clamber onto and off the table on its own.

I personally always have a mattress or thick soft mat in readiness close by or to one side of the table to perform treatment on the floor. Not all infants are happy about lying on a massage table that they are unfamiliar with; instead they feel more comfortable on the floor where they can move or let off steam without restrictions. I am happy to have both options available for children, and they can decide when they want to try something out.

Using a colored model of the cranium, I demonstrate to school-age children and their parents the different cranial bones and sutures. This very quickly serves to illustrate that Craniosacral Therapy works not purely as an energy technique but that it can be used, for example, even to release cranial sutures that have been compressed by a fall.

Disposable latex gloves and finger cots are used to release the masticatory muscles inside the mouth and to test the sucking reflex. They are also employed for the assessment and treatment of the facial bones, especially the maxilla, palatine bones, and zygomatic bones.

A flexible pelvic model with a suitable newborn-baby doll is used to demonstrate the birth phases. Depending on the child's age, I sometimes set out two or three models that show the size of the fetus, for example, in the fourth and sixth month of pregnancy; one of these models shows twins. Use of these models has provoked surprising spontaneous reactions from the children on several occasions—their interest is clearly stimulated.

While this equipment is not absolutely necessary for pediatric Craniosacral Therapy, it does expand and enrich the sessions with children in most cases. Having said this, there are certain situations in which this kind of equipment is generally not available. For example, as part of a team of craniosacral practitioners, I am committed to a not-for-profit project that operates in developing countries to provide treatment free of charge to babies and children of parents who have no financial resources. We also provide training for health care professionals such as midwives and pediatric nurses. Even without any equipment whatsoever, the sessions are nevertheless effective. The most important things are an open heart, compassion, and listening hands; anything more is a welcome bonus.

22.12. Importance and Choice of Treatment Room

The treatment room should provide a safe setting for the session and should therefore be located away from external influences such as other practitioners, clients, neighbors, and so on, or disruptive sources of noise such as the telephone. Loud or intrusive acoustic stimuli should be avoided, especially with infants and nervous children; the same applies with powerful aromas. An uncluttered safe setting is synonymous with security and relative freedom from stress for the child, thus improving its capacity for self-regulation.

22.13. Practitioner Closeness: Distance and Regulating Distance

As a craniosacral practitioner you are connected with your resources, continually slowing down and remaining in the here and now. At the same time you tune in carefully to your inner space and the external space. For example, as you increasingly draw back the focus of your attention, directing it inward, increased and new space can also arise externally.

Throughout the session, you are ideally conscious of your physical, emotional, and mental distance in relation to the parents and the child, and you modify it as necessary, depending on the situation. During the treatment session it is perfectly acceptable to ask whether you are too close or whether the child has enough space.

Here too it is the therapeutic process that indicates to the practitioner how much closeness and distance the child needs. There are phases in which the child needs a great deal of closeness or protection on the physical level while it needs a great deal of distance and freedom on the emotional level, or vice versa. The more the practitioner is attuned to the whole person—the more tuned in you are—the better you can sense from your resonance how much closeness and distance are needed on which level in order for it to be optimally supported. In the process you should also regulate these levels in yourself to a high degree, in just the same way as you have often already done in routine practice, while attending courses, and during treatment sessions with adults.

Perform the case history by referring to the list in section 23.1.1.

22.14. Evaluation

As soon as the parents bring the child into the practice, I start to evaluate the overall situation. For this I do not proceed according to any fixed pattern or principle but am simply receptive to all impressions that enter my perceptual field. Does the child exhibit defensive aggression, such as a healthy defense mechanism, self-defense, and occupying its own space, or does it display destructive traits? This may, but need not necessarily, correspond to the current situation or the biographic level, but it may also be tied up with birth experiences. During the first session and perhaps during subsequent ones the mother or the father can be treated first while the child looks on or plays. While this is happening I occasionally explain to the parents and the child what I am doing and sensing. The child may look on with amazement at what is happening on the treatment table. Often it will sense very quickly if the mother lets go and relaxes more deeply. After that I might invite the child to allow itself to be treated too. In this process I observe the child continuously, in particular noting its body language. For example, does it reveal sites that require attention? Does it repeatedly turn over on one side? Do many aspects revolve around a specific point that the child keeps tapping to indicate that it wants to be freed from something? Where is its breathing free, and where is it reduced or suppressed?

In holistic Craniosacral Therapy, assessment and treatment go hand in hand, rather like an inseparable couple: even hands-on assessment, which involves listening while observing, has a certain effect. Also during the session, when I am using a technique, I am listening to the changes, which means that I am assessing at the same time. During the craniosacral session I continue to evaluate the overall situation, and I begin with the craniosacral-specific assessment of the child whenever the opportunity arises (see sections 23.5 and 28.8). Of course, I do not compel the child to permit me to perform hands-on assessment and treatment right away.

Sometimes it may be the reflexes that initially force their way into my field of view, whereas later on or in other sessions they may no longer be so prominent. Instead the stage may then be dominated by other aspects such as the locomotor apparatus, body segments, internal organs, or emotional support.

KEY POINT

In the setting of the general assessment (see section 23.1.3), I gauge the situation at that moment and explore the following points: what is ready? What are the current issues in the child that need to be dealt with and need to undergo change? What are the possible stories concealed beneath them, the issues that are perhaps expressing themselves in the form of these symptoms?

Going with the flow: if the emotional level is too stressed, the craniosacral practitioner can carefully release the structural, physical level. If the child senses the physical release and is subsequently able to relax more, a better platform can be created via the intermediary of the body for release and reorientation in the emotional arena.

If the physical level is too stressed, the practitioner can support the emotional level, thus making resources available to the child and preparing the body for change without generating even more stress.

22.15. Play-Based Approaches

Supporting the child during treatment can take a very playful form. For example, I might suggest to the child that it tries something new. This approach should involve multiple choices, but the practitioner should take care not to offer too many to ensure that the child can master the challenge and then relax afterward. An overly serious approach is rarely helpful for the child. Naturally, play and pleasure may also be transformed at any time into feelings of sadness and suffering, and yet a mood characterized by lightness and optimism is generally more beneficial. In the ideal scenario the practitioner will operate in a way that has a therapeutic and healing effect but does not at first glance have the appearance of arduous therapy or work.

Birth games: play-based approaches may also segue into games that simulate the birth process: for example, crawling under the massage

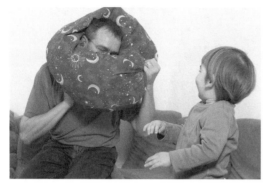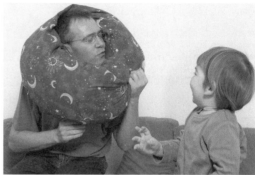

Figure 22.3. Play-based approaches.

table, making a nest in the blankets as in the womb, or offering resistance with the blankets and then letting the child use its own strength to push its head, shoulders, trunk, and pelvis through the tight blankets. Among other things, this activates and deactivates the nervous system and enables the child to regulate itself increasingly in a rich pattern of variations. For me and for the parents, it is often amazing, and touching, how children taking part in these symbolic birth games portray different phases and situations of their own birth without the link to the birth process having been made or even verbalized beforehand.

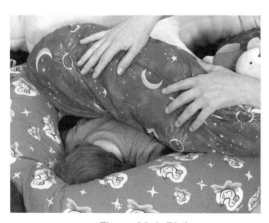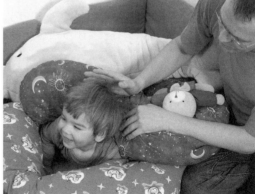

Figure 22.4. Birth games.

Pretending to be animals: the strength and joy that children derive from animals find expression not only in a wide diversity of sayings or customs; animals have been humankind's companions for millennia, and they are mentioned in various sacred texts. Nontechnological cultures have an especially close relationship with the animal world and refer, for example, to "power animals." It is no coincidence that animated films in which the main characters are animals are especially popular with children. Mammals in particular awaken more than just a caring and protective instinct in humans. They also symbolize other naturally inherent instincts such as motherly love, affection, interspecies connectedness, and aggression or fighting. Anyone who has

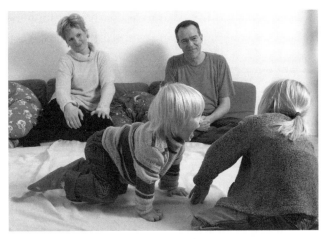

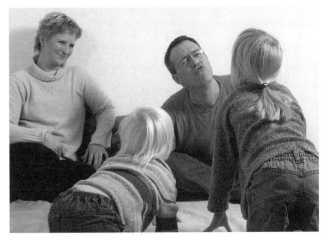

Figure 22.5. Pretending to be animals.

spent time watching puppies or kittens will realize how much they romp around as they chase each other and how they mix play with fighting. Through play the young animal gets to know its strength and its potential for aggression, fighting, and defending itself. All these are attributes that are also inherent in children and can be learned in play—for example, as they play with a stuffed toy or even imitate the animal, perhaps together with the practitioner. By slipping into the role of an animal, the child can explore and act out in play things that it perhaps might not dare to as a well-behaved human. Even the choice of animal can have a high symbolic value. Pretending to be an animal brings a great deal of pleasure, releases energy, and encourages self-expression.

Trampoline: would the child like to bounce on a trampoline? This movement can help simply to let off steam. On the other hand, I make sure that the child does not work itself up too much. As the child jumps up and lands back on the trampoline, I observe its movements, its general posture, whether it jumps tentatively, powerfully, too hastily, or even dangerously, whether its knees or other parts of the body are overextended, and so on. Sometimes I tell the parents what I have observed; in clearly positive situations, I praise the child for its skill, caution, strength, and good reactions.

Balancing games: another play-based approach involves balancing games on a tuning board or using other simple balancing aids. These allow the child to demonstrate its balancing skills, which may be impaired following falls, shock, or traumatic events such as accidents. Depending on the child and the particular situation, I offer the child an arm to hold on to from time to time if it wants to or if it is about

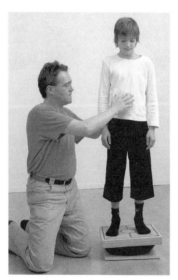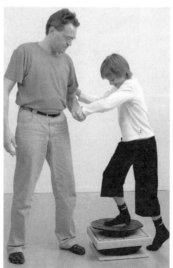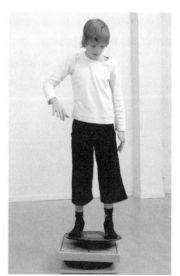

Figure 22.6. Using the tuning board to encourage balance and reactions.

to topple over. In these games I allow the child plenty of scope for experimenting and praise the child for its skills. At the same time I stay close at hand so that I can intervene instantly if the child starts to lose balance to ensure that no harm is done. If the child has already made good progress with its balance, I suggest as a new challenge that the child closes its eyes or stands with its weight on one leg.

The child is already familiar with the balance issue from its time in the womb, during and after birth, as it begins to crawl, learns to stand up and walk, and eventually learns ride a bicycle. The point of these balancing games is that the child gains or regains increasing confidence in a fun way and has the feeling that it can successfully overcome challenges; this strengthens its personality and development. Furthermore, these games serve to bring to light any uncertainties and fears as well as shortcomings in the child's sense of balance, which are almost invariably related to its past experiences and development. They offer a trail that the practitioner can trace back from the symptom to the previously hidden cause.

22.16. Resistance as a Strengthening Element in the Therapeutic Process

Occasionally the child wants to sense resistance as you apply your touch. It may be that the practitioner's appropriate contact and resistance help the child to sense itself better and to access its strength. In this case, offer light resistance—not so as to overwhelm the child in any way but so that it can push against you. Infants in particular sometimes like to feel definite resistance. The child then uses this, for example, to carry out its impulse to move away or to free itself from an unpleasant situation. In this process, however, the practitioner must be very careful and listen to establish whether the child introduces a break, waits, and senses itself. In these circumstances, do not offer any resistance but simply offer your supportive touch. You should also take care to ensure that the child really is taking a break. Under no circumstances should it enter into a violent process of struggle because the practitioner has offered resistance that is too prolonged or too strong. The child's strength may also stem from anger that might have had its origins in helplessness. For this reason I consider it extremely important, in a resource-oriented and solution-oriented sense, to deliver only minimal impulses and to provoke nothing, and afterward to focus primarily on maximal integration.

Here it is important to understand and to implement the bioenergetic principle: you should support the child in its natural sequence from buildup to release; in other words, any buildup or activation present is followed by release or deactivation. The energy set free by the release of tension helps the baby to establish better contact with the outside world and also to regain deeper inward contact with itself. In this way balance is also achieved at the level of instroke and outstroke. These terms were originally coined by Will Davis.[2] Instroke describes the gathering phase, the inwardly directed movement of biological energies from the periphery to the core. Outstroke is the outwardly directed flow of energy.

22.17. Rounding Off Incomplete Processes: Closing the Circle

The child's self-regulation can be encouraged very effectively if the practitioner identifies incomplete processes and supports the child as it takes up relevant impulses once again and rounds them off appropriately. The intention is to close the circle, meaning to support this natural sequence:

impulse/need → drive → activation/buildup → fulfillment and satisfaction of impulse/need → deactivation/discharge/release

The end result is physical and psychological balance. If the drive and the resultant sequence are rounded off in an apt manner, the child and the mother are content; if not, something is not complete.

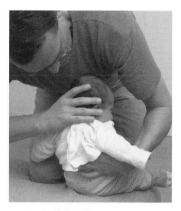
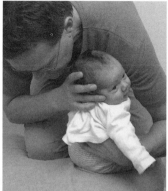
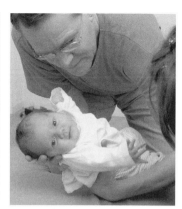

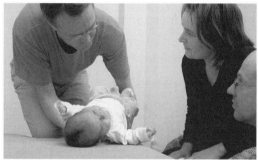
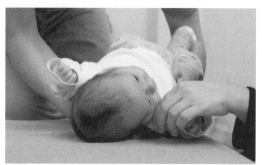

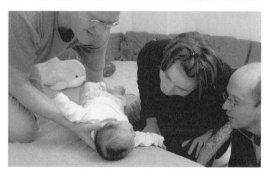

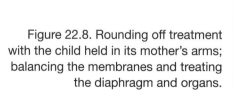

Figure 22.7. Careful assessment and treatment of the occipital bone, cervical spine, and torso, with the parents present.

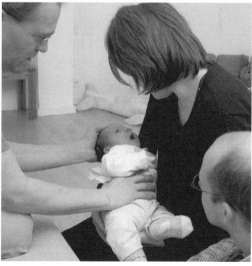

Figure 22.8. Rounding off treatment with the child held in its mother's arms; balancing the membranes and treating the diaphragm and organs.

If a drive is followed by an action that is interrupted instead of being properly rounded off, the outcome is not merely disappointment and frustration; the nervous system and the brain areas responsible for motor activity also become activated, but the incompleteness of the action has an irritating effect. In addition a certain amount of energy is mobilized in the body to execute a drive or to perform an action. If the action is interrupted, however, this energy is underutilized and not really released. It is self-evident that the child's every drive cannot always be fulfilled, and this is not a bad thing. However, if the child's needs and drives are frequently or permanently misunderstood and regularly interrupted, this will produce increasing physical and mental-psychological stress. This illustrates how the social environment also acts on the fine web of the body-mind-spirit unity. The higher the tension builds up, the greater the activation of the nervous system, especially the hormonal system, and the more important it is to round off the action or need, and to enjoy the resultant satisfaction so that sufficient release occurs. This insight into the process of self-regulation is extremely important.

Muscle hardening is frequently encountered in children who have a tendency to excessive tension buildup in the body. In such cases the nervous system very swiftly becomes activated or even overwhelmed in response to minimal or new impulses. Insufficient body tension, by contrast, may be a sign that the child has given up or become dissociated and that its nervous system, via the vagus nerve components from the dorsal nucleus, has shut down too far so that its capacity is being used primarily for those bodily functions that are important for survival (see section 21.3).

22.18. Attentive Presence Rather than Mere Techniques

Resource-oriented Craniosacral Therapy operates more using the principles of listening and assessing the body's own capacity for self-regulation, based on, for example, the craniosacral rhythm, the mid-tide, and the Long Tide (see also the introduction to chapter 21 and the introduction to chapter 24) rather than relying exclusively on techniques. Healing is therefore invited more by an attentive presence and through adherence to the fundamental Taoist precept of "doing by doing nothing." Techniques can be perfectly helpful, provided that they do not disrupt the therapeutic process but instead encourage it. Even Sutherland talked about treating "with thinking, feeling, knowing fingers" and of "allowing the fluids to do the work."[3] The fundamental principle of self-regulation is also encountered, for example, in the body therapies that borrow from the ideas of Reich. Among other things, they promote the organism's ability to balance the buildup and release of tension: entrapped life energies are set free and become available again for self-regulation, regeneration, and new growth.

At the start of therapy the practitioner will rarely approach and touch the child from its head end; if this does happen, it should on no account be done without advance verbal warning so that the child does not perceive the situation as threatening. However, once contact and trust have been sufficiently established, hard-and-fast rules are almost superfluous, and you may approach or touch the child from the head end without it being startled or fearful. Apply touch to the child in a respectful way, and during treatment, recognize nonverbal signals from the child as part of the therapeutic process and include these in the session.

During the session you may allow yourself short breaks, provided that this does not disrupt the process. You do not always need to be hands-on. The child can sense even without being touched, and you can consciously tune in to the "neutral" and do anything at all. It is also helpful to note your best standing and support positions at the treatment table because both can be important practitioner resources.

22.19. Practitioner Intention

Practitioner intention creates a field and a force that can affect the therapeutic process in a session. You should already have internalized your fundamental intention to support you before the start of the session: being present, regulating the physical and emotional distance, and having a deep fundamental trust in the forces of self-healing. The treatment room and the practitioner guarantee safe and trustworthy containment, and your fundamental intention prepares the ground for the therapeutic process of self-regulation and self-healing. It is helpful if you have been completely honest in tracking down your own conscious and unconscious intentions and if you have addressed them and reflected on them during your craniosacral training. For example: what is your task, your function, and your intention in general in treating the child? How do you directly support the process? To what extent do you, as practitioner, trust the therapeutic process? The more firsthand experience you have gained from sessions both received and given, the more self-evidently you will radiate a trusting core attitude that supports healing. Far from being simply a frame of mind, this attitude then becomes lived out and has the potential to become more deeply rooted with every session.

In contrast, the momentary intention serves as a therapeutic tool for a certain length of time during the session. It can be used specifically and in varied ways as the situation demands: for example, to support the therapeutic process. One of its main tasks is not simply to go with the therapeutic process but also to support it in a resource-oriented and solution-oriented way. In this setting, intention is a highly effective tool. Our intention influences energy. Intention or heightened attention can form a kind of focal point. A more prolonged intentional look, for example at the zone of a symptom or as we specifically alter the focus of perception, can also influence the therapeutic process. If the practitioner's or parents' eyes are directed to the place where things are happening, this intensification of attention can help something to be released. However, this heightened focus may also become too much and hence disagreeable.

22.20. Practice Nonidentification

The practitioner should be neutral and not identify either with the parents or with the child. As a practitioner I am loyal to the parents and the child. However, if there is a violent conflict during a session and I need to decide quickly in favor of one party, I would tend to take a position as the child's advocate, because support for children's rights in everyday life is generally less than optimal.

22.21. When Not to Involve the Parents in the Session

As discussed, parents are occasionally also involved in the session, especially in difficult situations for the child. However, you should do this only if the parents are a source of strength for the child, meaning that they have a good sense of themselves, are present, fairly calm, and not overwhelmed. If the mother, for example, is extremely nervous and the father is disinterested or feels out of place, they may not be a supportive resource for the child at that moment. It may happen that the parents are overwhelmed by their own situation so that their problems are being projected onto the child. Children are sensitive and able to pick up subtle impressions, and sometimes therefore end up carrying the sufferings of others. Where parent-child relationships are under pressure, it is therefore advisable to invite the parents to pay more attention to their own emotions. It may even be appropriate to recommend that they seek professional family counseling or psychological help.

The parents can be offered a chance to promote their own self-regulation if they allow themselves a time-out away from their child. While their child is being treated, they might go into the break room, for example, or take a stroll in a nearby park, listen to the birds, or admire the trees. In cases where the parents are clearly disrupting the therapeutic process, the practitioner needs to set some boundaries, perhaps in the follow-up dialogue or during the discussion before the next session.

22.22. Interacting with the Wisdom of the Body

While your hands are listening, it is useful to make discriminating use of the following therapeutic skills: nonverbal questions, intention, and the neutral. As a resonance to these three nonverbal tools, and if they are used appropriately, there often may be a spontaneous change, for example, in pulmonary breathing, craniosacral rhythm, or the fluid body; a stillpoint may become established; or something else may emerge more strongly into your perceptual field.

Nonverbal questions: at any time you can nonverbally—meaning inwardly—enquire of any structure, any function, any symptom, health itself, the child's inner healer, and so on as to what is really needed, what is most important now, or how the session should continue. As you do this you will be open to subtle and obvious signals because the wisdom of the body, the holistic matrix, and primary respiration know and will give a nonverbal answer. For example, at the start of the session, you may ask the child nonverbally—inwardly— which level is ready or particularly needs support at that moment, or you can address the child, its body, tissue, and cells in a nonverbal way. Sometimes you will receive an answer immediately, and sometimes soon afterward; perhaps this may come instinctively, intuitively from your resonance, energetically, or from the "knowing field."

I do not understand precisely which interactive levels facilitate this phenomenon. We are able to perceive things consciously even if we are unable to explain, understand, or classify them. Just because we cannot find a rational explanation for certain things does not mean that they do not exist. Many craniosacral practitioners have experienced this phenomenon and know that it works. I suspect that it is connected, among other things, with a simple transmitter-receiver principle, with the receptive tuning-in of the practitioner, with resonance, and with synchronicity—ideas that are familiar from the writings of Carl Jung. On a phenomenological level it is equally possible that the subconscious or the higher self of the practitioner and client communicate with each other. In resonance, and tuned in to the wholeness and perfection of the child, nonverbal communication is possible, as well as via mirror neurons and the practitioner's own body, which can briefly reflect the child's sensations and symptoms.

Internal questions of a fundamental nature in the treatment of children might include: what is blocking the child's system in such a way that it is unable to develop further in line with its potential and what is needed to resolve the issue? What is going on at the child's spirit or soul level? If we question the body nonverbally, it sometimes gives surprisingly clear answers that are consistent with what the child says later during the session or in the follow-up dialogue. On the basis of the practitioner's resonance with the child, these answers may arise from the subconscious, cell memory, the higher self, or the transpersonal level in a variety of ways, either through the child itself or as the practitioner experiences a clear picture, an emotion, or an internal scene like a short clip from a film, for example.

Intention: the practitioner's direct intention may serve to encourage or disrupt an effective field for a therapeutic process. Intention should therefore not be employed during the session automatically, following a particular set framework that suits the practitioner's personal predilections, as if it were a continuous mental program. Intention creates a specific field of attention and energy. It should be employed in a targeted way as an aid, for example, in guiding and supporting the process that is emerging at that particular moment in time.

Nonverbal questions and intention can also be used simultaneously. The practitioner's intention or nonverbal question can facilitate or hinder access to the neutral, a more balanced state. However, an intention or question is not the neutral. What is the system doing without my intention and without my nonverbal question? What is happening when both parties, practitioner and client, are no longer doing anything active and do not have any strategies, no longer even an intention, and nothing specific can be achieved?

Neutral: the neutral is located beyond questioning, intention, desire, will, and thought. If the neutral reveals itself during the therapeutic process, there is no further need for any possibly disruptive intention (see section 24.1).

22.23. Multiple Levels of Craniosacral Therapy

Craniosacral practitioners are aware of these multiple levels. Depending on the definitions used, we differentiate among the mental, physical, emotional, spiritual, and subtle energetic level or among the conscious level, the subconscious level with the collective archetypical subconscious, and the level of the higher self that is linked with cosmic consciousness. In healthy individuals these levels are all interlinked and accessible. Which level in the child is primarily being addressed by Craniosacral Therapy? Each individual person is a unity: we treat the whole person even though, with this type of Craniosacral Therapy, we are mainly working on the physical level. Consequently, gentle noninvasive Craniosacral Therapy and the resultant release address all levels. Depending on the child, practitioner, and treatment approach adopted, the treatment will have a differently marked effect on the various levels. Often the connection among these levels is severed by shock and trauma. This loss of wholeness results in fragmentation and impairs self-regulation and self-healing.

The whole is more than the sum of its individual component parts. As craniosacral practitioners, we perceive the child as a whole, as a body-mind-spirit unity. We assess which level in the child is currently more in the foreground and which level at that moment suggests itself as the most suitable area for change leading to greater wholeness. At the same time, throughout the session we are attentive and ready to meet with and support the child and the parents on the specific level that shows itself to be most clear, urgent, or ready. In the process we watch for reactions and changes on other levels too. As discussed, we evaluate whatever enters our perceptual field: the craniosacral system at the bone, membrane, and fluid level or the quality of the craniosacral rhythm, mid-tide, and Long Tide. In this way we gather additional essential information about the vital forces and about any impairment of the life force and self-healing power.

Our expanded simultaneous attentiveness allows us to perceive different levels at the same time and to invite changes with targeted therapeutic approaches. We recognize the directly emergent process and move among the various levels that are current in the child and parents. The levels that we primarily select depend on our own momentary assessment but also on our own life story, personality, social and professional competence, training, and personal preferences. These shape us as practitioners along with our individual therapeutic work. It can be justifiably claimed that there are as many types of Craniosacral Therapy as there are practitioners. It may therefore be entirely appropriate for us to organize our pediatric treatment session along totally different lines from those described in this book—and it may be just as effective. Our experience as practitioners and the trust that we place in the evolving process of self-regulation will help us during the session to relax at a level of being where the neutral and contact with the stillness or with the dynamic stillness can become deeper.

22.24. The Resource-Oriented and Solution-Oriented Treatment Approach

As a craniosacral practitioner, for many years I have used the resource-oriented approach. Resources are inner and external sources from which we draw strength, confidence, and pleasure. Each person's sources of strength are experienced and defined individually. We distinguish between inner and external resources. Inner resources may, for example, include a deep-seated trust in life, a firm faith, and calmness. Examples of external resources are nature, fulfilling relationships, pets, or a leisure-time activity. By establishing a link with our resources, we can sense changes in mood and how the body feels in response to that mood. Our resources have an immediate, sometimes involuntary effect on our thoughts and emotions—and ultimately on our bodily sensations.

The resource-oriented approach enables us to the see the glass as half full, not half empty. Even during the initial history-taking, during the dialogue with the parents and the child before the session starts, I look for positive characteristics. And during assessment and treatment I pay attention to which bodily structures are free and to the balance of the craniosacral rhythm or the mid-tide. In this way my focus is on movement, rhythm, and health, which are improved, rather than looking for what does not function so well. Of course, I am also aware of the restriction or dysfunction, ensuring that it has its place, but in principle more as an associated feature than as the main focus.

My dialogue is also resource-oriented. This has a much more constructive effect on the child, who is constantly used to hearing from parents, physicians, and practitioners what is wrong with it—a negative approach that often makes the situation worse and perhaps heaps up additional feelings of guilt. Questions about resources might include the following: What has recently given the mother/father and child particular pleasure? Recall a lovely experience during your last vacation: What comes to mind for the mother and father and child? The bodily region that feels most comfortable, expansive, or warm can be consciously sensed and experienced for a while. Examples of questions to ask the child might include: "What is your favorite fairy tale? What do you enjoy doing most? Which subject do you like best at school?"

The parents and child can be invited to take time now to sense their bodies and to feel the agreeable changes. I allow the parents and child sufficient time to experience these pleasant feelings more profoundly so that they become more deeply anchored emotionally, in the body and neurologically.

As discussed previously, as a craniosacral practitioner you should ideally be connected with your own resources before, during, and after the session and be resting in a relaxed manner in the holistic body-awareness. Even as you tune in to the session, you will already be connecting with your inner and external resources, rather than merely thinking about them; experience, sense, and feel the pleasant sensations as you do so. For example, you might recall a wonderful situation from your own childhood or last vacation, and then consciously perceive in your body the emotion that emerges. Sensing your own resources is important for the practitioner, for example, in a situation where a baby is crying long or loudly and is difficult to calm. Before this becomes too much for you, you should deliberately reconnect with your inner or external resources. The ability to consciously allow your own breathing to flow and to regulate your distance again will have an instantaneous resource-oriented effect during the session.

It is absolutely essential that parents and children with an unhappy history, shock, or trauma should learn to develop resources and to connect with them in the here and now. It is recommended that such individuals should be treated sitting rather than lying down, for the time being, and that treatment sessions should preferably be brief. Sensing resources while remaining present in the here and now will form a counterpole to the devastating trauma of the past (then and there), while well-established resources sensed in the body (here and now) will afford protection against retraumatization.

Shaping Craniosacral Therapy in a solution-oriented manner means that, as the practitioner, you must be creative both in proposing various solution pathways to the parents and child as well as in encouraging them to develop and try out their own possible solutions. While space is also granted to the trauma or suffering of the past, healing always takes place in the present. The problem is not lessened or resolved simply by complaining. If the present situation does not sufficiently promote healing, then it is important to find and implement approaches so as to create a suitable context for improved self-regulation and for healing.

For example, instead of allowing the mother to talk for too long about problems with the child, it would be body-oriented and solution-oriented to ask her to sense how she and her child are at this present moment. Having recognized the status quo of the mother, you can help to develop solution strategies by asking her, for example, "What could be helpful in this situation?," "What was helpful back then or previously?," "What has helped in the past, and what other possibilities might you explore?," "What would a good solution look like to you?" or "What would the best solution look like to you?," "What do you suspect are the causes of this symptom, and what are the various options to eliminate it?" It is not the job of the craniosacral practitioner to come up with solutions; instead, by your attitude and by your questioning, you stimulate the child and the mother themselves to contribute to improving the situation in a solution-oriented way.

22.25. Tempo, Tuning In, and Resonance

It is extremely useful for you as the practitioner to allow your own tempo to "run down" and become slower prior to the session. If you are very fast, very active, or want too much, it can often be a hindrance for the child, to the extent that it will not allow itself to be touched or treated, let alone lie down. As you decelerate yourself and rest in an alert relaxed state, not only is your own self-awareness expanded, but you additionally perceive your surroundings more clearly and sharply. This enables you to perceive what is happening at this moment, both now and from moment to moment. Your attentive presence acts in a healing way. As you slow down, your sense of time alters and may dissolve altogether if you remain attentively and calmly in the here and now. In this way you can shift increasingly into an underlying meditative frame of mind. Thus it becomes easier to tune in to the child and the mother and to proceed in empathic resonance with their moods and needs. After that you can use your touch to tune in to the child while remaining open to all sensations. Then proceed in resonance with the different rhythms of the child, for example, the respiratory rhythm, craniosacral rhythm, and mid-tide.

22.26. Expanded and Divided Perceptual Awareness

As a craniosacral practitioner, it is important for you to continuously expand your perceptual awareness and thereby train your divided attention. For example, by your relaxed seeing, listening, sensing, and observing, you can perceive the room as well as the child and its parents. Part of your perceptual awareness remains directed at you. You remain connected with your own resources and present with your heart. You are reflective, meaning that you are aware of your own feelings, possibilities, capacities, and limitations, and in this way you continuously train your own observer, your awareness. With constant practice you can steadily improve your attentiveness for events during the session, including subtle levels and changes.

The practitioner trusts the therapeutic process. You realize that pediatric Craniosacral Therapy is not something rigid and that nothing specific needs to happen, nor can it be forced; instead you help to shape and support the course of the session as a process characterized by myriad large and small healing moments.

Direct perception and observation on all sensory levels also reaches the nervous system's emotional level, the limbic system; self-reflection trains direct immediate understanding of the situation in the neocortex. Consciousness, perception, intuition, emotion, and intellect are not mutually exclusive but can contribute together to a comprehensive understanding in therapeutic work. Inasmuch as the intellect does not have sole command and does not restrict the senses, they can together promote alertness, clarity, and lightness in pediatric Craniosacral Therapy.

If you as a practitioner are open, sensitive, and simultaneously anchored in your self-awareness, your own system can react if a change occurs in the child, for example if a structure or an emotion demands special attention, or if there is a shift in levels. Your own body and your different perceptual levels are relatively balanced and function as a receiver for whatever the child wants to communicate, especially in a nonverbal way. The practitioner's resonance with the child is extremely important to support the therapeutic process. In this respect it is valuable if you have already received Craniosacral Therapy, are in a good frame of mind, and are continuously regulating your physical, emotional, and mental distance. All this will be hugely helpful for you as a practitioner and for the quality of the craniosacral sessions.

22.27. Contact and Dialogue with the Child and the Parents

22.27.1. Therapeutic Rapport

Any encounter involves nonverbal and verbal contact. This contact, the line connecting us to others, is also referred to as therapeutic rapport: therapeutic interaction, the practitioner's ability to empathize with the world of the child and its parents, to understand them, and to meet with each individual at that point where readiness is signaled. Therapeutic rapport therefore denotes the form of contact and exchange with the child and parents and should not be equated with the therapeutic process, explained in section 22.28, below.

Therapeutic rapport will be enhanced if the craniosacral practitioner speaks in a way that the parents and the child can understand. Adapting your linguistic style and register promotes rapport and helps to determine whether and how your clients feel understood, and consequently develop trust, during the session. If the child feels that it is recognized by you and trusts you, the healing process can be accelerated. Harmonious verbal support helps the child to continue with and round off its therapeutic process.

22.27.2. Dialogue and Communication

Communicating with the parents helps them to gain an increasing understanding of the holistic perspective and treatment method of the pediatric craniosacral practitioner. Once the parents develop a clearer understanding on a rational level of what had previously been obscure and hence nonexistent to them, they will be encouraged to engage more deeply on the level of emotion and understanding. This paves the way for them to experience and learn much about themselves and everyday relationships in the family. The pediatric craniosacral practitioner can therefore assist the parents toward helping themselves.

During the session, as the pediatric craniosacral practitioner, you can communicate your observations. You may emphasize the skills of the child and of the parents that are already present. An inestimably positive effect on everyone is achieved if verbal and joyful expression is given to aspects that are praiseworthy. You may speak with the child and the parents from time to time, and wherever possible and helpful, meaning when it is constructive for the child, verbally involve all parties in the session. In this way you will also help the parents to better understand the child's signals or situation.

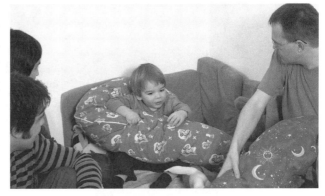

Figure 22.9. Establishing benevolent communication, contact, and trust; assessing the child; identifying emerging issues.

Through your benevolent communication and caring sympathetic approach, you can create, even without the application of touch, a space in which everyone present feels noticed and touched. Each one can be aware of their individual emotions and needs as you provide unobtrusive support through the session. Depending on the situation, however, you can take the lead by coaxing the child, mother and father, or both toward self-experience or interaction.

In the event of difficulties or even conflict, you have the possibility to mediate among those involved: invite them to talk about their feelings at that moment, or to express their needs. Your role is then to help bring about a situation that is more agreeable for all parties. Usually, this brings release, which in turn can be perceived and anchored. Insights gained from mediation, transactional analysis, Gestalt therapy, nonviolent communication, Somatic Experiencing®,[4] neurolinguistic programming,[5] voice dialogue,[6] or Rogers's client-

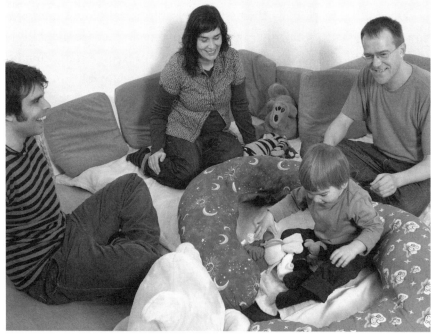

Figure 22.10. Contact and dialogue with the child and parents.

centered therapy can be extremely helpful here. Depending on the situation, however, attendance at a parent-child counseling center or psychotherapy assistance may be more appropriate than having the craniosacral practitioner act as a mediator. Ultimately, in most cases, Craniosacral Therapy for the child will take priority during the visit to your practice.

At the start of the session the craniosacral practitioner takes the case history and finds out what the parents know about the method and what the child has been told about the forthcoming craniosacral session. You can also explore the questions, concerns, and expectations of the parents and the child. Take care not to bring them from feeling into thinking. You should also avoid inundating them with so much information that it cannot be digested; this will merely serve to irritate all parties involved. Are the parents suffering excessively or feeling the need to succeed because, for example, there is a threat that the child may be moved to a special school? Are the parents placing you under pressure to succeed, or are you putting yourself under this pressure? Are you sensing a degree of coercion to answer the question "What is it that you actually do during the session?" (See also section 22.5.1.)

The intonation and pace of the dialogue of all parties involved will communicate at least as much as the content of the words used. During the dialogue with the mother or father and the child, be aware of your intonation and speed of delivery and ensure that these are appropriate to the situation. A pleasant and slow voice tends to have a calming effect, whereas a shrill or rapid delivery tends to achieve the opposite.

You should tune in to all the people in the room, especially the child with its needs and reactions. What is the issue at the start of the session for the individuals present? The main task will be Craniosacral Therapy for the child, but the mother and father are also central and pivotal. They may reflect interactions in the family system as a whole.

Using your notes from the previous session, you can briefly address the issues from that occasion in the forthcoming session and continue to hold them in your perceptual field. In the dialogue before the next session, you can ask about any effects achieved—for example, those felt immediately after the session, how the child felt in the days after the session, and how it feels now. This creates continuity from the previous session through to the start of the current session.

22.27.3. Open Questions

Almost invariably the pediatric craniosacral practitioner asks open questions such as what? How? Where? Where to? In what way? These are questions that cannot be answered with a simple yes or no but demand that the situation be described. Conditional questions such as "What would you do if . . . ?," "How would it be if . . . ?," and "How might it be if . . . ?" are also valuable for the therapeutic process.

22.28. Recognizing and Supporting the Therapeutic Process

The therapeutic process is something that is continually unfolding. Going with the therapeutic process has to do with development over time, and therefore relates to different segments and dynamics during a session. Not uncommonly, the therapeutic process will already be under way during your evaluation of the overall situation or during the craniosacral-specific assessment. The pediatric craniosacral practitioner recognizes and supports the therapeutic process as follows:

- Which issues, desires, or concerns are in the foreground at the start of, during, and after the session?
- What has priority for the parents? What has priority for the child?
- What is on the agenda? What wants to be seen?
- What is ready?
- What is revealing itself, and on what level is it revealing itself? Is the structural level or the emotional level more in the foreground?

- What is happening at the moment? What dynamics can you perceive in the room during the session?

While you, the practitioner, directly explore the actions and reactions of the child and negotiate your way, you are supporting and accompanying the therapeutic process. Equally important, however, is the ability to wait, so that the therapeutic process can be recognized more clearly and accompanied appropriately.

Using the child's resources, you should decide which of its impulses should receive increased attention. If no impulse is present, you might propose two options for the child to choose from. If the child does not respond either verbally or nonverbally to your proposals, the more active involvement of the mother or father in the session may support the therapeutic process. You can also tune in to the craniosacral rhythm or the mid-tide and support, for example, the three-step healing process (see section 28.7).

22.28.1. The Therapeutic Process Happens on Different Levels

In your capacity as a craniosacral practitioner, the more you are aware of the different levels (see section 22.23, above) and the better you are able to differentiate them in terms of their dynamics, the more healing your support will be. For example, it may be helpful for the therapeutic process during a session or a series of sessions to begin by working primarily with the emotional or the structural level and then later to take increasing account of the other. Through your heart and your empathy, you are continually in contact with the emotional state of the child. Through your hands and your perception, you are in contact with the physical structures, fluids, and primary respiration. Very often the child will unconsciously indicate the level that needs support and the timing of any change that occurs, or whether another level now seems to be more important. However, in line with the therapeutic process, you will also spontaneously codetermine where the treatment focus should lie—whether to prevent retraumatization or because the level you have selected is ready or because it urgently needs support.

With this open core attitude, with your faith in the therapeutic process to achieve greater self-regulation and self-healing, and on the basis of your experience, you are not occupied exclusively with one level; instead, several pathways are open.

22.28.2. Treatment Approaches and the Therapeutic Process

The deeper the child's trust and relaxation and the more the functional and biodynamic levels reveal themselves, the more fine and subtle the therapeutic process becomes. If you have experience as a craniosacral practitioner at these levels, this pathway is also open for the therapeutic process. In due course the competent craniosacral practitioner will take account of and support the physical level at least as much as the emotional, energetic, or biodynamic level. For many students there is a great temptation to neglect anatomy, physiology, pathology, or the differentiation of bodily structures, and hence also the three levels of the craniosacral system: bones, membranes, and cerebral tissue, including vessels and CSF, and indeed to disregard the entire basis of craniosacral work. This is because Craniosacral Therapy may also be effective without in-depth knowledge of these aspects. As a craniosacral practitioner, however, it does no harm also to listen for what can be sensed in the body and to identify the structure that require precise support. Almost invariably, due to the birth process, falls, accidents, or long-standing stress, children and adults have pronounced restrictions in their bodily structure that can often be resolved relatively quickly using the structural and functional approach to treatment.

The body remembers its developmental history. Past physical and emotional events are stored at the structural level and leave behind more or less clear traces, especially in the nervous system. In a space characterized by presence and stillness, listen with your hands both to the structure as well as to function or motion. Sometimes the structures begin to narrate stories because the craniosacral practitioner touches them carefully, listens, and allows time.

Craniosacral Therapy is not exclusively a spiritual or mind-based form of therapy; rather it is a body-mind (or "body-heart-spirit") therapy that touches all levels and supports primary respiration, the expression of the Breath of Life. In the same way the child is not exposed to nonstop techniques or to exclusively mental intentions. Instead Craniosacral Therapy involves the judicious use of all therapeutic tools in the directly unfolding therapeutic process and an understanding of the influence of primary respiration on the whole person. In the course of listening it may be that the three-step healing process reveals itself, the result of which—after a spontaneous stillpoint—will be greater balance of all bodily structures, for example.

A therapeutic process also takes place at the neurological level during pediatric Craniosacral Therapy; for example, the amygdalae store up fear-related emotions. With every Craniosacral Therapy session that enables the child to relax and eliminates the need for fear, the child's subconscious, and hence its ANS, is able to send the all-clear signal to the hypothalamus and the amygdalae, enabling any stored-up fearful agitation to be dismantled and released. This message is relayed onward to the brain stem, and neural networks become increasingly formed and strengthened, thus establishing calmness, joy, and new behavioral patterns.

As these ideas illustrate, the main point is to offer a safe and trust-filled setting in which changes can occur; this in turn promotes balance and strengthens the self-healing functions. Ultimately, the therapeutic process as such is difficult to define. It is something flowing and open that unfolds freely in the present moment. It is perceived not only with knowledge but also through tuning in to the world of the child through synchronicity and empathy.

This book outlines a great many principles and techniques that may be combined as appropriate to meet the needs of the individual child. As a general guide, see the example in section 28.1.1.

22.29. Relaxation or Therapy?

It is true that parents, midwives, pediatric nurses with sufficient firsthand experience in Craniosacral Therapy, and people undergoing training in craniosacral work may be able to help the child by using relaxing touch, for example, to calm it, to help it go to sleep, or to improve digestion, and so on. More energy is then made available to the child for self-healing.

However, it should be noted that when they are treated by a fully qualified craniosacral practitioner, existing structural restrictions generally resolve more rapidly and do not subsequently lead to further dysfunctions.

Dysfunctions caused by external factors such as emotional shock or a fall can be palpated in the structure and in terms of function and motion, such as the respiratory movement and the craniosacral rhythm. The intensity of the event is often traumatizing and is also stored in the body. The body remembers it through the phenomenon of cell memory. A multiple treatment effect is seen if we help to reduce or resolve the actual structural dysfunction directly, and if we also gently touch those zones where the repercussions and emotions of shock or trauma are particularly often stored: the diaphragm, solar plexus, neck, abdomen, kidneys, and bladder.

22.30. Should Symptoms Be Treated Directly or Only Indirectly?

How intense is the symptom for the child? Does the child possess sufficient resources? If so, how well are they anchored? It may be that the child should first be strengthened inwardly with a few craniosacral sessions. After that it is possible to treat the symptom without exaggerated aftereffects and without retraumatization. The craniosacral practitioner can move well away from the symptom or pain zone and listen and treat peripherally before shifting to a closer zone that is not so severely affected but is directly associated with the symptom, and then looking to see whether the symptom or pain zone itself can be touched. If the child's symptom has a clear physical location and the child finds that being touched there is agreeable or easily tolerated, treatment should not be exclusively peripheral. Moreover, with gentle and direct touch that has a receptive listening quality, the site of the symptom should be given the opportunity for release; this gentle touch will enable it to feel supported, to change, and to achieve a fundamentally new balance. It rarely makes sense to spend several sessions exclusively treating around the affected zone. In the words of Still: "Find it—fix it—leave it alone."[7]

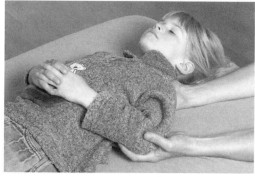

Figure 22.11. Peripheral release of the thorax and shoulder-neck region.

However, treating the symptom zone to the exclusion of all else is also not to be recommended. It is more beneficial to use craniosacral touch to briefly prepare the structures around the symptom. You can then ask the child verbally or nonverbally for permission to touch the symptom zone or pain zone directly. Proceed with treating this zone but make sure that the final one-quarter or so of the total treatment time is reserved for integration, so that the session can be rounded off in a stress-free and appropriate way. This approximate timetable when planning the session guarantees three things: first, there is sufficient time to support

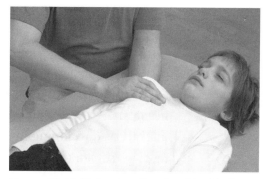

Figure 22.12. Releasing the shoulder blade and shoulder.

and round off an intensive therapeutic process; second, this period of integration serves to avoid any unwanted side-effects; and third, it helps to deepen the new body-awareness.

22.31. Respectful Attentive Touch

Before you apply your touch the child, you should ask the child for permission, or at least give some advance information of what you are about to do. Ahead of time you should tell the child that it can say "stop" or "enough" at any point, or can raise a hand to indicate that your touch is unpleasant or no longer agreeable, and that you will then stop at once. The child thus knows that it can decide for itself whether and for how long it is touched by the practitioner and that it will not simply be at the mercy of an adult. In my sessions with children it sometimes happens that the child tests me to see whether I will in fact disengage my touch when it says "stop"—which, of course, I do out of respect and to honor our agreement. This can turn into a game that is sometimes about assertion and sometimes also involves issues of power and powerlessness. In sessions with me the child must sense that it is respected in terms of its desires and needs, and must clearly understand that everything is done without coercion. This core attitude creates a sense of safety and enables the child to receive treatment in which no additional stress is generated by the practitioner.

As you negotiate your touch, proceed slowly and attentively so that the child does not interpret this as an assault but can clearly understand what is going on. As you apply your touch, do not exert any pressure whatsoever; your touch should be clear, gentle, and spacious at the same time. Afterward, keep listening for the reactions of the tissue and adjust the quality of your touch accordingly. In this way, instead of developing an instinctive defensive reflex, the child will display trust in the practitioner and in the treatment.

22.32. Therapeutic Intervention

If the child loses itself during the session in a lengthy or constantly recurring process that is no longer helpful but simply repeats an old pattern of total impasse, guide the child by dialoguing. If this is not possible, you must interrupt or prevent any retraumatization and energy-sapping tendency by using a clear therapeutic intervention. Examples of therapeutic intervention might include:

- Adjusting the tempo of the therapeutic process to match the situation, meaning to slow it down or speed it up, for example using breathing: ask the child to breathe more slowly or more deeply and frequently.
- Establishing and maintaining verbal contact; this helps the child to reorient itself.
- Speaking encouragingly, for example about resources and sources of strength.
- Addressing the child by name.
- Giving directive instructions, for example to open its eyes, sit up, orient itself again, perhaps by looking at mommy or teddy bear.
- Looking at each other by establishing eye contact.

During or after powerful processes, a definite change in the situation often helps the child to remain increasingly in the secure here and now and to reorient itself. The following are suitable options: gentle acoustic stimuli such as a child's rattle, walking around the treatment table once with your eyes open, offering something to drink, moving to another room, opening the window and together looking at the natural world outside, and so on. Treatment in the side-lying position or inducing a stillpoint may help to settle the child.

GENERAL AND CRANIOSACRAL-SPECIFIC ASSESSMENT

23

Comprehensive assessment of the overall situation and craniosacral-specific assessment together provide an overview of findings and are extremely valuable for subsequent Craniosacral Therapy. Diagnosis remains the preserve of conventional allopathic medicine.

KEY POINT

Your role as craniosacral practitioner is to assess and evaluate the situation. The more comprehensive the general assessment (your evaluation of the overall situation) and the craniosacral-specific assessment, the more complete the impression you gain will be. Your general and specialist assessment will determine the sequence within each session and the overall course of craniosacral treatment, enabling therapy to be more effective. Using visual assessment and palpatory listening with your hands, you will discover balanced body sites or zones as well as restricted sites or zones that are indicative of a compensatory pattern, a fall, or an injury. The more thorough your review, the greater the likelihood that you will locate any sites that may be the key to healing. The healing process would not really be supported if the child were merely to be calmed using gentle touch while at the same time there was a failure to identify and therefore resolve any restrictive structural imbalances.

However, this does not mean that you should spend a long time during the first session simply assessing: as your practical experience grows, assessment and treatment will increasingly happen concurrently, and the two will merge to become one. In this process you respect the needs and wishes of your young client. Rather than adhering to a rigid sequence of steps in your assessment, you might perhaps focus initially on building up interpersonal contact and thus on creating a trust-filled setting. With each touch that the child permits or even invites, the sensitive practitioner assesses and treats, and in this way increasingly receives an overall impression. All impressions gained during the process of assessment are like the smaller and larger pieces in a mosaic: during the craniosacral session these may be confirmed, move into the background, or fall away completely. After one or two sessions, you can usually form a comprehensive overall picture in this way and contribute increasingly targeted stimuli that will promote healing.

A balanced craniosacral rhythm has positive repercussions on the child's CNS and growth movements. Consequently, improvements may in reality occur on all levels. Many minute changes—greater lightness, improved orientation and motor activity, and many others—happen unnoticed and unconsciously. At the start of the session and during treatment you support the child, keeping watch for resources and occasionally addressing the child and parents. Mention aspects that elicit pleasure in the child and parents: subjects might include newly acquired characteristics or skills, the presence of a joyful or contented state, the child's warm and loving contact with the mother, a favorite animal, and so on. Give the child praise and recognition and reflect to the parents those things that occur to you. In this way the parents will possibly become more aware of what has changed over the course of one or several sessions. During the craniosacral session the practitioner serves as a fulcrum, coordinator, facilitator, and catalyst. After you have taken up verbal contact with the child and parents, a central element of this method will be available to you as you assess the craniosacral system, the craniosacral rhythm, or the mid-tide.

Remember that you will inevitably be encountering worried parents who have already received a great many unpleasant diagnoses and prognoses and may be quite fearful. Positive communication during or after the sessions is helpful and constructive in such circumstances.

23.1. Assessing the Overall Situation: General Impression, Dialogue with the Mother or Parents, Taking the Initial Case History

The following options for general assessment are particularly valuable for all craniosacral practitioners working with children. They are followed by an outline of the craniosacral-specific assessment.

During the initial dialogue and while taking the initial case history, the practitioner's attention is divided: you will be observing the child and its reactions even while you are in dialogue with the parents. As soon as possible after embarking on the initial dialogue, for example, ask the mother to recall some happy events, and then invite her to give herself time to clearly sense the pleasant emotions associated with those events, feeling them in her body too. If possible, it is important to begin by clearly voicing sufficient appreciation for those aspects that are good before moving on to discuss the difficulties that need to be dealt with.

The following list provides a suggested framework that can be varied from case to case. If the mother tends to be taciturn, introverted, or fearful, you might elicit just the key facts about pregnancy, childbirth, and the child. Alternatively, a minimalist solution might be to ask, "Is there anything about your pregnancy, childbirth, and the child's development that I should know?" After the session or in the dialogue before the next session, you may have the opportunity to address any important points.

23.1.1. Initial Interview with the Mother or Parents, Taking the Case History

- **Opening question:** "what is going well with your child?" You might then go on to ask about some detail, for example, "How is that seen in concrete terms?," so that the positive aspects can be reinforced and anchored.

- **Second or third question:** "what is going less well? What is the reason for seeking treatment?"
- **You might then go on to ask:** "do you have any expectations or fears, either regarding the child or regarding the treatment?"
- **Take a short family medical history:** ask about any illnesses suffered by the parents or grandparents, or in the parents' wider family.
- **Further suggested questions to ask:** how was the pregnancy? What went well? What went less well? How was the mother physically in terms of nausea, lower-back pain, and bleeding as well as emotionally and mentally-spiritually? What was her daily routine like: frantically busy, or lots of rest? Was she supported by her partner, parents, midwife, or someone else?
- How were the contractions in terms of their interval and duration? How did the birth go? Was it straightforward or difficult? Were there any complications? Were any medications used to encourage or inhibit the contractions or for pain relief? Did the mother receive epidural, spinal, or general anesthesia?
- How was the timing of the labor? Did it happen quickly, did it last too long, or was it just about right for the mother and the child? Protracted labor is exhausting for both the mother and the child. Very rapid labor can make the child feel as if it is being expelled. In either scenario the head and spine can become overstressed and compressed.
- How were the mother and the child immediately after delivery, and over the ensuing days and weeks?
- How is or was breast-feeding?

23.1.2. Overall Assessment of Mother and Parents

- How are the family members—the mother, father, and siblings— who have come to the appointment with the child? Are they inwardly balanced, stressed, or overwhelmed?
- How do they get along with the child?

- How good is the parents' physical self-awareness? You can gauge this by their breathing, for example.
- How great is the level of concern over issues relating to pregnancy, childbirth, and the health of the baby and the mother?
- Aside from their understandable concern, are the parents also able, at the same time, to sense and establish their own resources?
- How authentic is the impression made by the other family members?

23.1.3. Overall Assessment of the Child

- How is the child's self-attachment? How well is it connected with itself and with its inner self, and is it self-aware? Particularly during the initial months of life, this inwardly directed phase has a powerful self-regulatory and regenerative effect.
- How is the child's ability to orient itself outwardly, in the treatment room? Does it have contact with and interest in people, objects, or toys?
- How are the behavioral characteristics and skills of the newborn baby or child?
- The behavioral system of the baby or child can be described in terms of four levels, all of which tell us something about how the child is feeling and about its health at that moment:
  - **The autonomic system** regulates all fundamental physiological functions. It can be assessed in terms of skin color (pale or very flushed), breathing pattern (even or rapid, forced), digestion, saliva production, hiccups, twitching, and tremor.
  - **The motor system** regulates the child's movements. It can be assessed in terms of the type and tempo of movement (smooth movement sequences or disjointed, uncoordinated movements) as well as balanced, flaccid, or extremely tense muscle tonus.
  - **The sleeping-waking system** can be assessed in terms of alert or impaired attention, whining, screaming, or sleeping.
  - **The interactive system** regulates the child's readiness for direct

social interaction with other people. It can be assessed in terms of whether the child is open or closed to interpersonal contact, eye contact, facial expressions, voices, or gestures.

One system can be under stress while the others may be quite open. Instead of working primarily with the restricted system, you can use the levels under less stress as a resource, meaning as a source of strength in the session. The more you support what is going well, the less stress and the more pleasure and affirmation there is for the child. You can occasionally also subtly address the restricted system and issue an invitation to greater self-correction. If you sense improvements, you can communicate these in an appreciative way to the parents and child. In this way the parents become engaged in their child's process of self-regulation. You can briefly communicate your observations to the parents at once or during the follow-up dialogue. This enhances their understanding of the physical and emotional needs of the child so that they increasingly learn to tell whether the child now requires fresh stimulation or needs to take a break.

Clear signs of stress in the autonomic system are indicative that the stress is comprehensive and that stress activation is relatively high. In such cases the child's self-regulation and thus also its emotional state are impaired. This situation resembles the one described in section 22.5.2, in which care should be taken that the child is not activated even further by giving excessively long sessions or by offering too many stimuli during the session. Instead, a setting should be created in which the child can find a way back to greater self-regulation, flow and streaming, and readiness for contact. It may be that the child has a need for peace and quiet, or it would like to be held and sense some warmth and security.

If attention wanes during the course of the session and the child becomes tired, it will be unable to take much new input on board. This may also point to a nonrobust nervous system and to diminished self-regulation. In practice the child may express this, for example, by turning away from its mother or the practitioner (the interactive level), clenching its fists and pressing its lips together, moving jerkily or arching its torso (the motor level), accompanied by whining, crying, or screaming. The ANS may perhaps react with pronounced burping or irregular breathing.

The craniosacral practitioner can also observe the fine signals given by the child during the play-based phases of craniosacral sessions. The child's openness or stress in the autonomic, motor, and interactive systems will become apparent within a few seconds in its interaction with the mother. It is a major achievement if the child seeks to build up contact with a counterpart, to maintain it, and to remain inwardly balanced or become more balanced. And always remember that it takes a certain amount of effort to learn something: without resistance there is no growth. Signs of stress are not necessarily signs of poor interaction. The interactive system becomes disturbed and stressed only if the parents or the practitioner fail to understand or else ignore the child's own tempo, for example its momentary need for activity or for a break, or if they constantly place the child under too few or too many demands. In the case of infants, this disturbing stress on the interactive system very rapidly has repercussions on the ANS and the other regulatory systems. For example, it can cause the child to scream protractedly or to withdraw.

Use the following observations to assess the overall situation in the newborn:

- In its preverbal phase, what is the baby seeking to communicate or express through its body language, gestures, and the sounds it utters?
- How is its emotional state?
- What is its emotional expression like?
- What is its facial expression like?
- Does the child engage in eye contact, and for how long?
- Are its eyes clear, and is its gaze present?
- What are its eye movements like: coordinated or squinting?

- How is its hearing and its ability to listen?
- Is the child interested in social contact, in the people and things around it?
- Is the child capable of participating and taking up contact?
- Does the child deliberately seek to make contact?
- Is the child able to maintain its presence?
- How well does the child recognize objects and people again?
- Does it deliberately direct its attention from inside to outside, from outside to inside?
- How spontaneous, open, and interested is the child?
- How is the child's physical self-awareness? You can recognize and support this, for example, from the child's deeper breathing, especially in the abdominal region.
- What are the child's obvious resources, and which resources have so far tended to be hidden?
- How does the child communicate, and what sounds or gestures does it use?
- Does it like to experiment with movement and other forms of expression?

Assessment of the baby's or child's movement pattern:

- Do its extremities move smoothly and without jerky interruptions?
- Are the torso movements supple, even during deliberate stretching, extension, flexion, and rotation?
- How is its overall coordination?
- Is the baby able to raise its head and actively orient itself to both sides by turning its head?
- How is its muscle tonus, and is it balanced throughout the body?
- Are there any signs of tremor, twitching, or spasms?
- How are the child's nonverbal reactions to verbal, auditory, tactile, and kinesthetic stimuli? Which stimuli are the child able to identify and allocate?

- In response to stimuli, how is the automatic adaptability of the system? Do the child's breathing, pulse, and craniosacral rhythm react to an activity in a way that is commensurate with the demands placed on it?
- Is the child capable of reacting to changing sensory stimuli without losing its continuity of movement?
- How well can the child orient itself?
- Do body posture and movement interfere with the child's ability to orient itself?

Other aspects of the assessment include:

- What are the child's cycles of activity and rest like?
- Is a startle reaction evident only in situations of immediate and clear danger?
- What is the child's creative expression like? Does it play and explore creatively?
- What is the child's skin color like: vibrant, very pale, or highly flushed?
- How is its respiratory function? Is nasal breathing unhindered?
- How powerful is the sucking reflex or function?
- How harmonious are the functions of chewing and swallowing?
- How is the child's grip reflex, and is grip disengaged at the correct time?
- How good is the child's self-attachment now, at this moment?

In newborns and children who are traumatized, several of the aspects listed above will be abnormal, in the sense of being too weakly or strongly pronounced. Signs of shock or trauma in the baby or child may include:

- Feeble, shrill, inconsolable or frequent crying for no apparent reason.
- Glazed, distraught, or fixed gaze.

- Increased or reduced muscle tonus in general or limited to particular body segments.
- Constant restlessness, jerky movements, and involuntary tremor or twitching.
- Inability to stabilize its head unaided, possibly hypermobility in the neck or atlanto-occipital region.
- Limited or absent reflexes.
- Absent or extreme reaction to external stimuli, such as touch, light, or noise.
- Inability to connect with itself and remain connected while in contact with the external world.

23.2. Primary Personality and Secondary Personality

In the field of biodynamic body psychotherapy, Gerda Boyesen developed the concept that people predominantly live out elements of either their primary personality or their secondary personality.[1] The primary personality is characterized by a high level of self-attachment and pronounced body awareness; it is pulsating, streaming, sensual, appreciative, and powerfully expressive—the authentic child in us that senses and says what it wants. This personality seeks to realize its desires, pursues its own authentic needs and drives, and is simultaneously both autonomously freedom-loving and compassionately open to others. By contrast, the secondary personality is strongly conditioned and adapted. It senses authentic drives only rarely, if at all, and hardly ever pursues them; it is minimally assertive, gives up quickly, and identifies with its neurotic elements.

In pediatric Craniosacral Therapy I am always open to the signals given out by the child and the mother relating to elements of the primary or secondary personality. The primary personality is mostly able to self-regulate to a high degree. If it is out of balance, it requires relatively little therapeutic assistance. The secondary personality, on the other hand, tends to exhibit self-regulatory difficulties and requires more intensive therapeutic support in order to return to a state of balance.

23.3. The Dynamics of the Parent-Child Relationship

During the general assessment of the overall situation of the child and the parents, I sense the underlying mood in the room, the child, and the parents. I also try to sense the degree of concern or lack of it in the parents, especially relating to issues of pregnancy and birth and the child's state of health.

It is generally known that the cause of physical and psychological problems is not always to be found in the birth story or in the personal biography of disease and accidents; it may also be rooted in the structure of the family. During the initial session, therefore, I assess a variety of system levels, for example:

- How involved are the parents during the session? Are they inwardly and outwardly involved and reflective?
- Are the parents engaging? Too little, too much, or in a tactful way? Is their care for the child minimal, balanced, or somewhat exaggerated?
- Is the mother able to give time and attention to a need expressed by the child and to its individual tempo?
- How able are the parents to assess closeness: distance, their own boundaries, the child's boundaries? How able are they to adjust these according to the situation?
- Do the parents allow the child sufficient free scope while also setting boundaries?
- Is the child felt to be sufficiently capable for its developmental stage, or is too much being expected too soon?

- What individual resources does the mother possess, and how does she use them?
- Does the mother's time management tend to reduce stress or generate stress?
- Are the parents able to follow the ideas and structure of the session, experience what is happening, and allow it to take effect?
- Is the information communicated by the craniosacral practitioner understood? Or is it not heard, ignored, glossed over, or even dramatized?
- Is everything said by the craniosacral practitioner a confirmation of ideas to which the mother and father are obsessively attached, for example stemming from diagnoses or prognoses offered by practitioners of conventional allopathic or complementary medicine?
- Does the root cause of the parents' concern lie in feelings of guilt, shame, excessive demands, fears, or insufficient trust?

23.4. Cooperative or Controlling Interaction

Do the mother and child exhibit cooperative interaction that can be recognized from the mother's empathy and the child's cooperative understanding? Or is their interaction more that of a controlling mother and child that does what it is told? The mother-child interaction has a strong influence on the physical and mental-spiritual development of the child. In children who are born preterm, a controlling interaction pattern can have a considerable impact on the child's developmental state: they more often have behavioral problems and worse hearing and speech development than children who have a cooperative interaction with their mothers.

A positive effect on parent-child interaction can be achieved if the parents simply take their child lovingly into their arms and cuddle it for a while. As the craniosacral practitioner, if you are aware of the level of interaction, you can also heighten the parents' sensitivity to this, and the resultant improved interaction will make the parents themselves more attentive and understanding. Moreover, the child will be more joyful, more open, and more inquisitive as it explores new things. It will cry less and be empowered to develop secure emotional bonding.

The parents' capacity for bonding with and sensitivity toward the baby is influenced by parental temperament, their own physical, emotional, and mental-spiritual health, and any bonding issues with their own parents. Childhood experiences are relived through the birth of their own baby. In this way positive as well as negative tendencies are often replicated from one generation to the next. However, this does not mean that parents with negative childhood experiences automatically pass on negative relational patterns to their own child. The greater the willingness and ability of the parents to reflect the influence of their own childhood bonding experiences onto their current behavior and to improve it, the greater the likelihood that the baby will be spared from negative bonding patterns. Psychological or craniosacral support can be helpful in this context.

23.4.1. The Pacifier Issue

What do the parents think about this? How quickly do they resort to offering the child a pacifier? When and why do the parents offer a pacifier? Is it a help to the baby, or do the parents simply want to quiet the child with it? It may be that the baby just wants affection or physical contact, or it may be bored, discontented, or sad. For very tiny babies perhaps suffering from colic, a pacifier can effectively soothe them for a while. However, the pacifier should not be used as a long-term comforter. Infants can often manage without it, at least through the daytime. In the longer term a pacifier can interfere with the proper use of the speech muscles and adversely affect speech development. The child should be allowed sufficient time, without pressure, to stop using the pacifier.

23.5. The Craniosacral-Specific Assessment

Following is an outline of the options for the craniosacral-specific assessment as used primarily in the structural and functional treatment approach. Biodynamic craniosacral assessment is made using entirely different criteria because it does not take account of the physical structural level to the same degree. During the therapeutic process, after the craniosacral rhythm has been balanced, it may happen that slower rhythms—the mid-tide and Long Tide—can be perceived more clearly. For this reason, short examples of assessment and treatment using the biodynamic craniosacral approach are given in section 23.5.4, below, and section 24.2.

NOTE

Because assessment and treatment are rarely performed separately by experienced craniosacral practitioners, but rather merge fluidly with each other, proceeding hand-in-hand, further assessments are presented as an integral part of later sections.

23.5.1. Visual Findings

- Assess symmetry:
  - of the cranial vault
  - of the facial bones; during the birth process considerable compression is exerted on the facial bones, affecting the sphenoid, occipital bone, cervical spine, and the dural tube
  - from mastoid to mastoid, or the cranial base, for example in head tilt
  - from the root of the nose to the zygomatic bone
  - from the orbit to the mastoid
  - from the external occipital protuberance to the foramen magnum
  - of the torso: shoulders, clavicles, and pelvis

- of the throat and neck
- of the extremities; for example, how do the legs and feet lie?
- Skin and tissue: color and quality
- Segments: eyes, mouth, throat, thorax, abdomen, and pelvis
- Reflexes: especially the sucking, swallowing, and grip reflex as well as balance
- Contact level: visual, sensory, and auditory
- How are the balance of forces and the child's posture, as well as weight distribution while standing, sitting, and lying down?

23.5.2. Palpatory Findings

Most of the areas listed above can also be evaluated by palpation. Skin and tissue can be evaluated, for example, on the basis of warmth or coldness. External physical trauma, as in a difficult birth, a fall, or an accident, may affect the following anatomical structures, which we assess:

- thickness, firmness, and mobility of the scalp and cranium
- cranial bones: overlap, for example at the coronal, sagittal, squamous, or lambdoid sutures, or in the vicinity of suture junctions
- sutures that interrupt the force transmitted by a blow
- membranes and their tensions, in particular the dural tube and the intracranial membranes
- the entire cranial base
- the state of the ligaments, particularly in the pelvic and inguinal region and in the shoulder, thorax, and neck regions
- the mobility of the head at the top of the spinal column
- the atlanto-occipital region
- the TMJs and occlusion (the interrelationship of the maxilla and mandible)

What do you sense when palpating close to the structure or when touching it directly? How does your contact and touch feel?

23.5.3. Checking the Cranial Sutures

Examine the cranial sutures for signs of compression, frequently encountered at the lambdoid suture. How elastic are the structures of the cranial base and the cranial vault? This is an important prerequisite for muscle function, activated during breast-feeding, to contribute optimally to the development of the cranial structures. Compression of the viscerocranium (facial bones) during birth, for example, diminishes the craniosacral rhythm and may lead to the formation of pus in the paranasal sinuses.

During craniosacral assessment of the newborn, your attention should be alerted if the bones have a soft feel, for example, in the region of the parietal bones. Findings of this nature require ongoing monitoring by a conventional allopathic pediatrician, and such referrals must be made by the age of three months at the very latest. See also the discussion of ventouse and forceps delivery in section 15.1.

23.5.4. Evaluating the Craniosacral Rhythm, Craniosacral System, and Fulcrums; Sensing the Mid-tide, Potency, and Long Tide

Listen for and differentiate the following:

- The qualities of the craniosacral rhythm: strength, amplitude/range, symmetry/evenness, cycles per minute/rate.
- What are the features of the longitudinal and the lateral fluctuation?
- At this moment, which fulcrums in the body are most free? Are there any inertial fulcrums? Can you distinguish between primary and secondary inertial fulcrums?
- Is there any evidence pointing to traumatized body sites?
- How free or restricted are the three levels of the craniosacral system: the bone level; the membrane level of the dura mater and meninges surrounding the brain and spinal cord; and the fluid level, the brain including its vessels along with the CSF?

- How freely flowing are the blood, lymph, and CSF? How do they interact, and how are they flowing in the body overall? Do they form a unity?
- Is it possible to balance tissue tension using breathing, the craniosacral rhythm, or the mid-tide without actively applying any technique?
- Commonly a stillpoint will establish itself spontaneously. If this happens, is it a stillpoint in extension/internal rotation (CV4) or in flexion/external rotation (EV4)?
- What are the palpatory features of the craniosacral rhythm after the stillpoint compared with beforehand?
- How free is the flow of vital energies through the body?
- What is your sense of the physical level as a whole, as a unity?
- How is the mood in the room? Has it altered compared with before? Is it changing now?
- What is your sense of the energetic space between the midline and the limit of the biosphere or of the personal sphere of the child?
- How do you perceive the fluid body?
- Is the fluid field of uniform shape, without "bumps" or "dents," and does it have clear boundaries?
- Can you perceive the mid-tide?
- What are the features of the inhalation phase and the exhalation phase? How are the inhalation and exhalation phases in relation to each other?
- How strong is the potency or force in the fluid body?
- Is the mid-tide, the fluid body, changing?
- Is a stillpoint becoming established at this level? If so, is it during the inhalation phase or the exhalation phase?
- After the stillpoint, how do you perceive the mid-tide? How do you perceive the fluid body?
- To what extent does the potency coming from the inherent treatment plan have the ability to resolve inertial fulcrums and harmonize the different levels overall?

- How is the mood in the room now, and has it altered?
- Is the neutral becoming deeper?
- Are primary respiration and the potency transmitted by it working toward a holistic shift? What is happening during and after the holistic shift?
- Can you now perceive the Long Tide?
- Is the dynamic stillness becoming ever more present?

DIFFERING TREATMENT APPROACHES AND DIFFERENT RHYTHMS AS EXPRESSION OF THE BREATH OF LIFE

24

In his fifty years and more of research and practice in the field of Cranial Osteopathy, William Garner Sutherland continually made new discoveries. During what he termed his "bone phase" he developed the biomechanical cogwheel model that defines the axes of motion as well as the motion of the craniosacral rhythm of the cranial bones and sacrum in flexion/external rotation and extension/internal rotation.[1] From these insights he elaborated the biomechanical-structural treatment approach. With the passage of time he moved increasingly toward the membrane level, the meninges covering the brain and spinal cord. For example, he explored the function of the reciprocal tension membrane. The structural-functional treatment approach evolved over a period of decades.

The craniosacral rhythm refers to the motion of the CSF and the CNS at a rate of about six to twelve cycles per minute. The following qualities are distinguished: strength, amplitude or range, symmetry, and cycles per minute. Many authorities claim that the craniosacral rhythm in infants is slightly faster and more difficult to sense. Even though such claims are occasionally corroborated in practice, the statement does not necessarily apply in general. The practitioner should assess each child individually and without preconceived ideas.

Sutherland spent decades searching for the original spark that animated the primary respiratory mechanism that he had defined. In the final years of his life he carried out pioneering research into even more subtle levels of primary respiration, which he came to refer to as the Breath of Life. From that concept he developed what is today known as the biodynamic treatment approach.

In the biomechanical or structural approach, the practitioner works primarily to release restrictions using direct and indirect-direct techniques. Severe compression or restriction of the bone structures of the craniosacral system can be released in a relatively short time.

The structural functional approach does not involve any active testing and treatment of the motion restriction. The body and the craniosacral system are not confronted with the motion barrier; instead they are supported in the free motions of the respiratory rhythm as well as the craniosacral rhythm and mid-tide. Following the release of each restriction, the body rediscovers a new balance.

The biodynamic approach does not treat the physical level, the craniosacral system with its motion axes, nor does it harmonize the craniosacral rhythm with flexion or extension; instead the fluid body and the fluctuations of the mid-tide are supported. In this treatment model there is also a wide diversity of terminologies and perspectives. I owe my understanding of biodynamic Craniosacral Therapy principally to my teacher and mentor William M. Allen. As well as attending specialist courses devoted to this topic, I recommend the books by Charles Ridley and Michael Shea as well as the audio CDs by the osteopath James Jealous.[2]

The greater the balance of the craniosacral system, its rhythm, and the membrane tension, the more rapidly and clearly the neutral will deepen. The neutral is like a gateway, a threshold to the biodynamic treatment approach.

24.1. The Neutral

The neutral is a state that can be likened to neutral in a car's automatic transmission, and it illustrates the fact that the therapeutic process is now able to develop in different directions. The biodynamic approach to treatment becomes even more effective once the neutral has deepened. The neutral that we are speaking of here is located beyond intention, desire, will, and thought. This neutral is without intention and has a powerful connection with stillness—indeed, to a certain extent it is part of the stillness, which in turn has a powerful connection with the dynamic stillness. Client neutral is distinct from practitioner neutral—the two may be of differing depth.

The more the neutral emerges and deepens during the therapeutic process, the less appropriate are any intentions. In a state of neutral, the body-mind-spirit unity is in relative equilibrium, a state of balance. In this state not as much energy is needed to compensate for inertial patterns. Instead, the potency is available for the further therapeutic processes of self-regulation and self-healing. For example, the child being treated undergoes a holistic shift, after which the inherent treatment plan directs the session.

Intention can be used deliberately as a therapeutic stance, as a technique or for therapeutic intervention (see section 22.19). By contrast, in the neutral, as the biodynamic process deepens, the practitioner will usually not ask questions or have any intention but will instead act as a free external fulcrum. In this way the Breath of Life is empowered to take over the work, meaning the process of self-regulation, so that the life force—variously referred to as *od, prana, chi, mana,* orgone energy—can unfold in the individual. It is not the craniosacral practitioner but rather the inherent treatment plan that achieves the essential changes leading to healing.

24.2. Stages in Biodynamic Treatment

Access to the biodynamic field is a process that unfolds across various stages. There are some craniosacral practitioners working with the biodynamic approach who believe that as they connect with the stillness, the horizon, and the dynamic stillness, the biodynamic session can already begin. While practitioner neutral is certainly encouraged in this way, the child's neutral is also needed in order for the biodynamic process to be accessible.

In noninvasive Craniosacral Therapy, body structures—the locomotor apparatus, internal organs, and the craniosacral system—become more balanced both in terms of their tonus and with each other. The connective tissues as a whole are then in more balanced membranous tension locally, regionally, as well as globally, and the craniosacral rhythm is more harmonious in its qualities. The fulcrums are all in relative balance with each other, in a physical neutral in which the body requires far less energy for its functions. The neutral empowers the therapeutic process of self-regulation to continue developing in any direction.

If you are accustomed to palpating the craniosacral rhythm or connective tissue, you will find access to the mid-tide, for example, by using the three-step healing process to functionally support the balanced state of fascial and ligamentous tension. Rather than palpating the bodily structure (Zone A) in detail, use a random local body site to include the entire body together with the person's biosphere (Zone B) in your perceptual field. Your hands are permeable, transparent, and fluid and therefore do not constrict the fluid body.

Synchronize yourself with the stillness while simultaneously listening for a slower tide-like inhalation and exhalation motion. This manifestation of primary respiration is not just local but occurs globally in and around the body as a whole, sensed as a whole fluid body. The fluid body is "breathed" by the mid-tide at two to three cycles per minute. It reveals itself in Zone B, from the midline outward to the biosphere that extends one to two hand widths beyond the physical body. It is egg-shaped but is not identical to the aura. The aura belongs to the energetic body and its various chakras. The fluid body, on the other hand, is like a large single fluid drop that breathes as a whole in the inhalation and exhalation phases. The fluid body and the potency generate the structure. The potency is the energy in the fluid body, the fluid within a fluid. After the holistic shift, the potency enables comprehensive corrections to take place, and the inherent treatment plan is implemented automatically.

During the session, you can attune nonverbally to the child's wholeness, which has been present since the moment of conception and throughout the development of the embryo. The embryo is already a fully developed organism by week twelve of gestation. The original midline of the embryo, the notochord, also called the chorda dorsalis, can already recognize orientation and growth. It serves as an important fulcrum for the biodynamic process. This essence of the embryo, whole and complete in itself, provides a reference point, granting access to the original holistic matrix. It reveals the whole potential of the individual. The body, with its restrictions, injuries, or diseases, can now orient itself afresh using the original matrix.

Sometimes the child's life history from the very beginnings will come at you in waves, with its growth processes into a fully grown fetus, with its birth as the threshold and crossing point into this world, with its developmental processes as a newborn and child. The immense achievement embodied in development through to the present moment, the force of these formative and growth processes, serves in this context as a resource; so too does the momentary life force that expresses itself through the respiratory rhythm and primary respiration.

As the practitioner, maintain perceptual contact during the session with the health and wholeness of the child. These aspects will remain the principal element in your perceptual field while you are doing treatment and while you are accompanying the child, mainly nonverbally, through difficult memories or emotions. These processes are frequently accompanied by stillpoints and may occur very subtly in the stillness. Maintain contact both with the whole child and its resources as well as with the dysfunctions or inevitable events that have restricted or are still restricting the child's vital force and development. As you continue to hold the resources and the restriction nonjudgmentally in your perceptual field, the expression of primary respiration will ideally start to resolve the restriction—often without any mechanical technique being necessary to achieve this. The process of biodynamic therapy deepens firstly because of the more balanced state of the body, the craniosacral system, and the fluid body. Secondly, in the safe therapeutic setting, the child is enabled to relax ever more deeply, to let go of emotional pressures, and to identify less with thoughts or emotions; it comes to rest in itself. The child feels more and more carried, secure, and in harmony with itself, its surroundings, and the universe.

In addition, the fluid body may become balanced through fine impulses delivered by the practitioner, for example stillpoints at the outermost point of the inhalation phase or at the innermost point of the exhalation phase. However, for a long while you should do nothing other than remain connected with the stillness and go with the motions of the inhalation phase and exhalation phase. In the inhalation phase of the mid-tide, the fluid body widens, becomes freer, and opens up. Subtle transformations take place. The potency balances the fluid body. Afterward, in the exhalation phase, there is a sense of the fluid body emptying, narrowing, and receding. As the practitioner, synchronize yourself with primary respiration and go mainly with the inhalation phase, which is supported by this. If the fluid body is balanced at the level of the mid-tide, called balanced fluid tension, it will also be accompanied by stillpoints.

However, do not become obsessed with these subtle phenomena; instead widen your perceptual field to include also the treatment room (Zone C), the horizon, and beyond (Zone D). Connect with the dynamic stillness out of which creation, God, or the eternal source transmits the subtle energies with tidal motions of varying slowness— the Long Tide, the mid-tide, and the craniosacral rhythm—and provides the animating spark for the Breath of Life. Stay in contact with the stillness. In your connection with Zone D and the dynamic stillness, you will sense in the stillness of the fluid body "the sea around us," the Long Tide. The motion of the tidal body, the Long Tide with a cycle of about one hundred seconds, corresponds to a tidal rhythm of the macrocosm. The Long Tide "generates" the mid-tide. The tidal body is described by many as being more transparent than the fluid body, more like air or gas.

Terms such as *horizon, stillness,* and *dynamic stillness* are to be understood more in a metaphorical sense. You do not use them to influence the process, but they help you to come to a neutral, alert, expanded state of consciousness in which something greater happens. At this level, you sacrifice your ego. Rather than obstructing the process, you ensure a safe therapeutic setting in which the space-time continuum changes. In this way the expression of primary respiration and the potency are enabled to do the work.

24.3. Biodynamic Assessment and Treatment

In my view the biodynamic approach to treatment is suitable for advanced practitioners who are already intimately familiar with the structure and function of the craniosacral system with its craniosacral rhythm of six to twelve cycles per minute. As the foregoing account shows, assessment in the biodynamic field uses criteria that are different from those outlined in sections 23.5.1–3 and the first part of 23.5.4. Biodynamic treatment commences after the neutral, after still-points on the functional level, and after the holistic shift. The stages associated with these are described above. As you, the practitioner, observe the therapeutic processes in the biodynamic field, holding and containing them with as much space as needed, you support them with your perception. You are centered and relaxed, and you regulate the distance to the client. In this way you become a neutral fulcrum.

A brief overview of further assessments and options for biodynamic Craniosacral Therapy:

- Is the mid-tide balanced in the inhalation and exhalation phases? Are there complete in-breath and out-breath patterns with the appropriate physiological reciprocity, meaning can centrifugal and centripetal forces be sensed as full and relatively balanced?

- How is the fluid drive, and how powerful are its fluctuations?
- Are both the longitudinal and lateral fluctuations revealing themselves to be vital and balanced? Do they have the potency to release restrictions?
- Is the potency in the fluid body strong or weak? How efficiently does the potency build itself up?
- What shape is the fluid body? Is it balanced, or are there unbalanced zones, for example "bumps" or "dents"?
- Are free and inertial fulcrums present in the fluid body?
- Is the fluid body concentrated along the midline, and might it widen with a stillpoint in the inhalation phase? Or conversely, is the fluctuation along the midline weak, and should the midline be supported with a stillpoint in the exhalation phase?
- How does the ignition process reveal itself, and the individual ignition systems that are coupled with conception, birth, and compassion and love?

After the neutral in the fluid body, you can directly sense the stillness within it, and you are connected with Zone D and hence open for the Long Tide, the sea around us.

KEY POINT

When is it appropriate to use which treatment approach? With a holistic form of therapy it is impossible to give a general answer to this question. The choice of treatment approach, of session structure, and of techniques for the particular approach taken depend on the symptom, the age of the child, the setting in which it lives, as well as on your knowledge as craniosacral practitioner of the different therapies and treatment approaches. It is useful if you are able to clearly distinguish the different treatment approaches and know where you are.

In the majority of cases I personally begin with the functional approach and use the motions and rhythms that are present predominantly to support what is healthy. On the basis of the assessment using the functional approach and of the momentary attitude of the child, the functional, structural, or biodynamic approach will then reveal itself to be more advisable. If, for example, biodynamic Craniosacral Therapy has too little effect after several sessions, structural treatments are occasionally given.

With regard to the techniques mentioned in Section III, treatment in the majority of cases uses the structural and functional approach. I am of the opinion that it is not simply the choice of approach, position, or technique that is important but also the practitioner's attitude. The crucial consideration overriding all others is: what is it in the child that needs to be supported, and what is the child ready for? A structural treatment lasting twenty minutes can bring just as much relief or healing to the child as a sixty-minute biodynamic session, and vice versa. Transition from one treatment approach to another can be fluid. My current belief is that access to the biodynamic approach occurs via the functional level, in which the neutral deepens more and more. This is a process that can be encouraged by the practitioner's attitude but cannot be forced.

Ultimately, all rhythms are an expression of primary respiration. For me, *holistic* means not assessing which level is more likely to bring healing but rather supporting the particular level that reveals itself in the therapeutic process at that moment. I respect the child and do not interfere with self-regulation either by thoughtlessly performed techniques or by toying with the fluid body and tidal body by using subtle intentions. Some students of the biodynamic concept, in their passion for defining and assigning and their impatient desire to know and sense, firmly believe that they can sense everything relatively quickly. However, the fluid body and the tidal body and their slow tides are highly intelligent and cannot be duped.

Each treatment approach requires several years of practice in order to internalize it not merely as intellectual knowledge but also as experience. If you as the practitioner are not accustomed to treating in the deepened neutral, your mental conviction becomes active in the biodynamic field in the sense that it becomes transferred to the therapeutic process. It is then possible for treatment on this extremely subtle level to become invasive or interventional.

In terms of perception, if you are using the biodynamic approach, you no longer operate on the temporal level and are no longer busy. You do not actively desire to achieve anything; to do so would mean that you are not in the neutral that has deepened through several stages.

APPROACHES TO RELEASE FOLLOWING SHOCK AND TRAUMA

25

A situation is perceived to be traumatic if it is extremely painful, life-endangering, or hopeless. Trauma is often synonymous with high activation of the ANS; there is frequently a loss of defense capabilities, and boundaries are infringed. Afterward the child involved may possibly even freeze. In shock or trauma, more agitation for the ANS and the organism as a whole arises too quickly for the child to cope. In particular, the brain stem, hypothalamus, and amygdalae are placed on alert. However, all bodily functions are influenced via the ANS. Post–traumatic stress syndrome may develop at any age in the wake of overwhelming life events. However, an infant is more vulnerable than a school-age child or adolescent because older children are generally better able to muster some defense.

Some examples of events and situations that are potentially traumatizing: medical therapies, surgical procedures, accidents, family violence, abuse, chronic humiliation or neglect, separation from parents, natural catastrophes, physical injury with major blood loss, terrorism and war, or merely having to witness such things. Childhood trauma may also be caused by an apparently harmless fall, feeling lost in an unfamiliar environment, pediatric illnesses and high fever, sudden loss of a close family member, mere exposure to extreme temperatures, near-drowning in a swimming accident, and so on.

Abuse and violence toward children at home or at school are sometimes merely suspected, and sometimes really happen. Often the victims keep silent, tend to be rather defensive or withdrawn, and do not want to stand out; alternatively they compensate to the opposite extreme, later perhaps themselves becoming violent. Children in particular can be overwhelmed by traumatic events. Flashbacks may occur, or the child can be exaggeratedly fearful.

High global activation may arise during the birth process, especially where medical intervention was necessary during a difficult delivery.

After a fall, depending on the specific situation, the child's balance system may be affected, and this may subsequently be irritated, producing a need for a greater feeling of security. If there are further falls or if the child restricts its own mobility out of fear of further falls, it may later lead to motor disturbances, for example, or to psychological problems due to withdrawal.

How powerfully the child is traumatized by a physical or psychological shock will also depend on the situation immediately prior to the event and on how it was handled afterward. If the child or parents are already stressed, then the tragedy of a shocking event can often be more intense. If the child is comforted after a shock, it will find security, and if it is able to cry under the loving and watchful eye of understanding parents, it will be able to offload its agitation or feelings of powerlessness immediately after the event much more effectively than if it is defenseless and vulnerable or restricted in its spontaneous expression. Children often experience feelings of guilt or shame after shocking events. Sometimes they also feel guilty or partly responsible, even though they are not to blame for the incident.

Subsequently, children who have experienced shock or trauma commonly develop concentration problems, social and general apathy, and even dissociation, cutting themselves off from everyday life and entering a dream world. This distancing from themselves—for example, cutting themselves off from their own body so that they no longer have to feel physical or mental-emotional pain—can be a self-protective mechanism that is essential for them to survive, a kind of coping strategy (see also last part of section 23.1.3).

Craniosacral Therapy offers the child the opportunity increasingly to build up or reinforce its resources. Until these have become sufficiently anchored, craniosacral work should focus more on the issue of excessive demands rather than on the traumatic event itself.

For example, before or after a surgical procedure or illness, if the child perceives its own body as a threat, the body ceases to be a resource. In such circumstances, external resources can really assist orientation. If the child's environment is chaotic or if the risk of a renewed shock comes primarily from outside, it is more important to build up and utilize defensive and protective reactions and inner resources.

Signs of shock or trauma:

- on the physical level: fixed, empty, or cloudy gaze, superficial or rapid breathing, drawn-up shoulders, or autonomic dysregulation
- on the psychological and psychosocial level: lack of presence; diffuse communication, for example strange or inappropriate answers to clear questions; poor congruence, for example little or no agreement between body posture and what has just been said; difficulties in relationships and with boundaries; reduced spontaneity and creativity

We experience the emotions of the prenatal and perinatal period before we have learned to talk. These experiences leave behind at least traces of memory in our subconscious and in neurological networks. The amygdala, part of the limbic system, is close to the inferior horn of the lateral ventricle. It is where agitation is stored, and it enables us to recognize moments of danger instantly and to respond to them instinctively. The amygdala stores, and stores, and goes on storing—including feelings of constriction and congestion and memories of vertigo—and plays a part in the assessment of similar situations or dangers when we react with feelings of intimidation, fearfulness, patterns of violation and powerless, loss of orientation, or dissociation.

In situations of immediate danger, we react, for example, by the brain stem activating an extraordinary amount of energy, our heart rate increasing, blood flowing increasingly to the extremities, and muscle tonus contracting. Incredible forces can be unleashed within seconds. The defensive and protective fight reaction so essential for us and our kin or allies kicks in instinctively. The reptilian brain, a legacy that has taken millions of years to evolve, is located in the most primitive parts of our brains (see also section 18.6). When danger threatens, it reacts instinctively before it has had any time to reflect. Over the course of our phylogenetic development, our ANS has changed and adapted. This adaptation has taken place in the course of human evolution and reflects in particular our bonding-related interactions. We should also recall that during the gatherer period of human history, people performed quite different motor and neurological actions than those later required for hunting animals, or today at the computer or while changing lanes on the highway.

In the event of a major threat, if the high levels of excess energy, coupled with a variety of stress hormones, are not sufficiently reduced and released by successfully fending off the danger, this energy overload forms the potential for symptoms and syndromes to develop. Here too we encounter again the natural sequence of buildup, release or activation, and deactivation (see section 22.17). The effect of bioenergetic self-regulation is the improved pulsation and flow of vital energy, as described by Wilhelm Reich[1] and later by Gerda Boyesen[2] and other pioneers of body psychotherapy. Peter A. Levine has also incorporated into his trauma research his observations of wild animals and their reactions to trauma.[3] The nervous system can often be freed from the overwhelming effects of trauma in just a few sessions. However, the intellect, conditioning, and autonomic components often require further sessions in order to integrate this release on a permanent basis. For all parents, midwives, teachers, and body therapists interested in the subject of trauma, I recommend the book by Levine and Maggie Kline, *Trauma through a Child's Eyes*,[4] as well as firsthand experience in the form of a few treatment sessions.

Humor in therapy is health-bringing because it is the antithesis of the seriousness and tragedy embodied in past difficult situations.

Joy and humor produce something different in the hormonal system than sorrow, stress, or fear. This insight has brought about a rethink in some clinics and hospitals: hospital clowns and dream doctors, for example, help children to experience difficult times not only in a tragic way. The U.S. physician Patch Adams discovered as long ago as 1971 that patients regain their health more quickly if they laugh regularly, and he started medical clowning.[5] In a similar vein, back in the early 1960s, the science journalist Norman Cousins treated his own arthritic and spinal pain using a good dose of belly laughter.[6] When we laugh, the production of various neurotransmitters, such as serotonin, dopamine, norepinephrine, and endorphins, is increased while production of stress hormones such as epinephrine and cortisol is decreased.

Laughter brings strength, color gives energy, play enables us to forget pain and fear, happiness is contagious, and beautiful stories and music relax us. A kind word shatters loneliness, and even tiny positive moments and gestures can work miracles.

25.1. Pediatric Craniosacral Therapy and Trauma Healing

As a body-oriented therapy, craniosacral treatment for children is also suitable in the wake of accidents, shock, or trauma. It can be used in combination with other methods of trauma healing. For you as a craniosacral practitioner, a psychological and neurophysiological understanding of trauma is of tremendous benefit. Through a combination of expression and behavior, for example, the whole person reflects the robustness of the ANS. Even before you are hands-on, you can perceive the child in its wholeness and identify signs of trauma from its posture, speech and intonation, congruence, and so on. As you then gently touch the child's body during the session, you can additionally sense further subtle autonomic signs, for example balanced or unbalanced breathing, body tensions, the craniosacral rhythm, and the slower rhythms. These will provide you with information about the somatic-energetic-psychological state of the child.

Shock or trauma impairs neuronal, hormonal, and biochemical functions or structures such as the limbic system, specifically the amygdalae, the hippocampus, reticular formation, hypothalamus, and pituitary (see also sections 18.4 and 21.3). The individual no longer feels sufficiently secure because in the traumatized state the all-clear signal is no longer given. In response to just a trivial change in a given situation, faulty neuroception sends a danger message even though there is none evident.

This "no longer safe" feeling and the conscious or unconscious holding onto or avoidance of emotions has a direct effect on bodily structure. The throat-neck region, for example, is highly vulnerable and sensitive. When we sense fear or shock, we instinctively react by drawing in our neck—an important protective reaction. If a child or an adult remains in this physical-emotional protective posture for a prolonged time, however, the collagen fibers cause increased long-term thickening and hardening of connective tissue, and tension becomes chronic. On the other hand, if the individual is enabled to experience and release various emotions, it helps self-regulation. For example, the muscles and elastin fiber components of connective tissue relax in the region requiring protection.

During Craniosacral Therapy, the practitioner, in tandem with understanding warm-hearted parents, becomes a fulcrum to which the child can orient itself and which provides safety, hence serving as a resource.

The craniosacral practitioner with experience in trauma healing, as in Somatic Experiencing®, will begin by helping the child with shock or trauma to strengthen its resources. As a result, in the here and now, the child will gain a stable body-sensed counterpole to the past traumatic event, and retraumatization is more likely to be avoided. The child is present and able to express itself without the trauma being repeated. Afterward, as the practitioner, support the child as it rebuilds incomplete defensive and protective processes; for example, you can sense the instinctive, motor, and emotional drives that met with little success at the time of the traumatic event and "renegotiate" them. Of course, the trauma of the past cannot be undone; however, in a safe therapeutic setting in the here and now, it is possible to offer a choice.

Renegotiating trauma means that the child, supported by the practitioner, in the safety of the here and now, can explore different versions and can feel how the buildup of trauma energy can be reduced or resolved as a result. The vital energy that was bound up in the traumatic experience then becomes available again. The ANS is thus no longer in such a high state of alarm and begins to become increasingly balanced. A finely balanced ANS encourages "flow states"—feelings of lightness and joy, the sensation of flowing and pulsating—and improves self-regulation. The ANS is already functioning before birth and matures greatly up to the end of the first year of life. During the further development of the brain until the early twenties, other areas emerge that are responsible, for example, for regulating and balancing our ANS. The earlier infants and children are given the option for improved self-regulation, the better their ANS will also develop. This contributes to greater health and zest for life in adulthood as well.

The voluntary nature of Craniosacral Therapy sessions and the choices offered as well as a resource-oriented approach will enable the child in each session to unconsciously dismantle fears and anxieties that are also linked to traumatic events of the past. Traumatic memories stored in the body's structures down to the cellular level can be resolved through gentle and agreeable touch. The resource-oriented dialogue, perhaps combined with imaginative elements of trauma release, increasingly empower the child to improve its self-regulation.

Pediatric Craniosacral Therapy can be used, for example, before an elective surgical procedure. The body tissue affected and the surrounding areas then become more relaxed. The presence of fewer restrictions in the body means that only the more local regions will be impacted by surgery. After a surgical procedure Craniosacral Therapy helps to support the body tissue in its wound healing. The scar and the surrounding healthy tissue can be treated. If it is too early for this, the practitioner can work for the time being on the stress overload, the fear, or the high degree of activation shortly before the shock or trauma. Through the reduction in stress, the ANS achieves a balance that consequently supports the immune system and wound healing. It is also possible to reduce fears at the thought of surgery and the associated high activation or freezing of the nervous system. All this serves to achieve release in the child, and its autonomic processes can return to normal, which also strengthens its immune system.

See chapter 30 for a discussion of selected indications, with pointers for Craniosacral Therapy.

BASIC PRINCIPLES
AND PRACTICE TIPS

Structural treatments for pregnant women are described above in part II of this book. Helpful details relating to the treatment of children and mothers are presented in part II in the "Development" section, chapters 16 through 20. The material outlined in chapters 21 through 25 in part III provides a platform for practice. There, among other things, is coverage of issues such as history-taking, assessment, and the fundamentals of noninvasive Craniosacral Therapy for children. The theoretical aspects dealt with in parts I to III will help the practitioner during the craniosacral session to better identify the dynamics of pregnancy, childbirth, bonding, and development. These theoretical principles are important and valuable because they illustrate the many-layered nature of Craniosacral Therapy for children. Nevertheless, the practical implementation of Craniosacral Therapy itself should be straightforward. It ought to be imbued with a benevolent, constructive, and joyous core attitude and founded on trust not only in the immense power of the self-healing mechanism but also in intuition, love, and the practitioner's own hands.

A great many of the techniques mentioned in this book are explained in detail using photographs and text in my earlier book *Craniosacral Rhythm*,[1] and therefore are reiterated here only in exceptional cases. Pediatric Craniosacral Therapy is a special field of Craniosacral Therapy delivered mainly by fully qualified craniosacral practitioners who have acquired additional competency by undergoing further training. There are different ways of performing Craniosacral Therapy in children. Among other things, this is dependent on the craniosacral training of the practitioner as well as on personal background and professional experience. Even if a craniosacral practitioner performs treatment in children in an entirely different way and with different emphases than the approach outlined here, it may be just as suitable and effective.

26.1. Contraindications

Anything that is comprehensive in its effects may also have adverse consequences if it is used incorrectly. Without adequate experience of craniosacral courses and sufficient practice in adults, you should not use any CV4 techniques or atlanto-occipital release in children. In infants and young children, do not use pressure or compression when working on the head. Children with major difficulties or diseases should be sent for conventional allopathic medical diagnosis and should be treated only by craniosacral practitioners with many years of experience.

Note also the contraindications listed in sections 3.3.1 and 6.2.

26.2. How You Can Help the Child

Do not place yourself or the child under stress. Only treat children if you are in a calm mood and have already received many craniosacral treatments yourself.

Treating children demands a generous supply of openness, spontaneity, creativity, and tolerance, but it is also necessary to set boundaries. As a craniosacral practitioner, you should face with confident trust the unknown that wants to reveal itself, and you should welcome healing. To a certain degree you may go with the child and its drives, both when it is restless or extremely active, and in quieter phases or when it stays quite still.

Hands-on treatment is useful only for as long as it is agreeable to the child. It should not be overdone. About twenty minutes in infants,

and about forty to fifty minutes in school-age children, is often sufficient to encourage release and self-regulation.

Ask the child whether you may apply touch, or at least give
advance verbal warning that you are about to apply touch—even
in cases where the child may not yet understand the meaning of the
words. A "no" from the child or any defensive attitude should be
respected; otherwise touch and treatment become counterproductive
and would merely serve to increase the child's sense of indisposition or
crisis, thus increasing stress, which can never be the point of Craniosacral Therapy. It may be that the child would prefer to play, have a
baby massage, or explore the room.

When handling a newborn, as in when you lay it down on the
massage table or changing table, or when you pick it up, make sure
that you always pick the baby up and lay it down sideways—ideally
slowly and with a spiraling-rotating motion. Lightly support the neck
and back of the head as you do so because a newborn's neck muscles
are not yet able to support its head. To protect the cervical spine
and cranial base, the baby should never be picked up or put down
vertically or with a sudden jerk. Do not force a baby into a certain
position, for example on its back, but watch and note the position in
which it feels comfortable.

Presence and trust instead of pressure and will: things become difficult if you use deliberate intention to achieve something, for example
to sense the craniosacral rhythm or to quickly "treat away" the child's
symptom. Sensing different rhythms, such as the respiratory rhythm,
the slower craniosacral rhythm, or the mid-tide, is not possible using
your will or intellect. Instead, train yourself to sense these rhythms
using calm perception and trusting in your hands. A meditative core
attitude is helpful. For the most part, treatment should consist of
"doing by not doing."

As the practitioner, remain in contact with your own physical and
emotional sensations. During the session, pay attention to your own

relaxed body posture and allow your breathing to flow freely. This may perhaps sound banal or obvious, but the importance of putting this into practice cannot be overstated. How is the child to open up? How should it trust you? How should it respond positively to your touch if you are not really aware of yourself, are hardly breathing, lose contact with yourself, but at the same time want something from the child? Such subtle situations are already sufficient to unsettle the child, to stress and overwhelm it to the extent that, fearing danger, it loses contact with itself, freezes, or may go into a panic. As the practitioner, you will therefore do yourself and the child a major service if, before applying your touch, you become grounded and centered, breathe freely, expand your focus, and regulate the physical and emotional distance to the child. You can also expand your internal and external space by slowing down your own tempo and listening to the stillness. To begin with, wait to see what might develop out of this relaxed state and deliberately give the process of self-regulation and self-healing the opportunity to take effect.

Do not proceed in any sense in a manipulative way; instead grant the child sufficient time to sense and implement its own drives, and then gently accompany them. This releases the practitioner and the child—and the therapeutic process is given sufficient space and time to unfold.

For other health care professionals such as midwives, pediatric nurses, special-needs teachers, and craniosacral students, I recommend that you do not perform major techniques on the child. For the period of the session, simply offer a trust-filled safe space in which self-regulation, the pulsation and flow of the vital energies, can increasingly operate and become established. To support and accompany it *is* treatment, a key element of Craniosacral Therapy. A further component then comprises the many possible techniques with which the self-healing effect can be potentiated. You are already helping the child if you support it in its ability both to be with itself and to make contact with its surroundings, and in this way you reinforce its sense of self.

It is important not merely that the practitioner and the child should be in contact with each other, but also primarily how they are in contact. This is infinitely individualized and varied because both parties will have their personal style of communication. What you perceive, how you interpret it, and how you react to it as the practitioner will depend, among other things, on your own history. Contact with the child is also influenced by your own experience of early childhood communication, your own temperament, and how much you believe the child is capable of.

The more you recall and implement the core practitioner attitude described in chapter 22 and elsewhere, the more effective the treatment will be. As your experience grows, you will learn to pay attention both to your own attitude and to sensing the subtle motions and changes occurring in the child. For example, your hands will listen to the subtle motion of the respiratory rhythm. You will also listen for whether you can perceive the different slower rhythms. You will then decide whether to continue listening at the location you are touching, to use a technique, or to continue with listening and treatment at another body location. Craniosacral treatments that you have received, attendance at craniosacral courses, and the tuning-in exercise below will often facilitate and deepen the treatments that you give to others.

In a meditative core attitude, open yourself up increasingly to the level of your sensations. Drawing on the wise counsel of Sutherland, other trainer colleagues and I advise first that you trust your listening hands and then wait until your hands tell you what should be done. If your hands say "do nothing," then do nothing.

It is a key prerequisite to be receptive if resonance with the treated child and its subtle self-regulatory processes is to be at all possible. It is helpful to have no expectations or preconceived ideas as you remain open to everything that wants to reveal itself from moment to moment. Not only the child's spoken words but also its body language provide pointers to how it is feeling and to the issue that wants to be seen.

If you are a practitioner with little craniosacral experience, ensure that you round the session off at the right time; do not delay this phase if you notice that the treatment might become disagreeable for you or for the child.

EXERCISE: TUNING IN THROUGH SELF-AWARENESS BEFORE YOU BEGIN TO APPLY TOUCH

In a comfortable, relaxed posture, consciously ground and center yourself, let your breathing flow freely, and relax your lower jaw so that your mouth is slightly open. Sense your relaxed and supple body, and rest for a few moments as you perceive your body as a unity.

Without wanting to change or accomplish anything, direct your attention to your breathing. Now develop an awareness of where and how you are sensing the respiratory movements. You might also try this now while you are reading these lines.

Allow yourself to become slower, welcome the slowness, and as you do so, listen to your heart and the stillness within yourself. During this slowing down, you may initially also be aware of a certain excitement or of your heartbeat becoming stronger; after a short time this will regulate itself as you orient yourself to the stillness.

Now direct your attention simultaneously to your respiratory movements and your heart region. Allow yourself to sense your heart region and respiratory movements simultaneously for a few moments. Grant a few precious moments of time so that your self-awareness can deepen without the onus of having to change something.

Now direct your attention to both of your hands: in this process it is likely that they will autonomously become more present and more sensitive after a few moments.

Give yourself enough time to sense all these regions simultaneously over the next few minutes: your respiratory movements, your heart region, and both hands. This sensation may possibly be deepened if you close your eyes as you do this. When you open your eyes again later, remain connected with these sensations while you become aware of the room and outside space.

Give yourself permission not to have to accomplish anything during the ensuing craniosacral session.

Open yourself up to the unknown, to the momentarily emerging process of self-regulation that you will gently go with. Now and throughout the craniosacral session, while you remain attentive with all your senses, observe and note how you and the child are doing.

Which location on your body feels most pleasant at this moment? While you sense this location in yourself, this might be the first "question" to address to the child before you begin the treatment.

26.3. Treatment on the Massage Table, a Chair, or the Floor

You can work with the child on the floor, in its mother's arms, or on the massage table—it is best to keep all options open and see what is most suitable for the child, depending on its age and impulse. If you begin on the table, it is always possible to move down from it and change the level, perhaps to relive the birth process (see also fig. 22.4 and section 28.16).

26.4. Treatment with the Child in Its Mother's Arms

You can also treat the baby in its mother's arms. It may also be possible later to continue treatment on the massage table.

26.4.1. Method

Gently distinguish tissue density, for example, and the quality of the craniosacral rhythm or of the mid-tide. If you cannot sense the

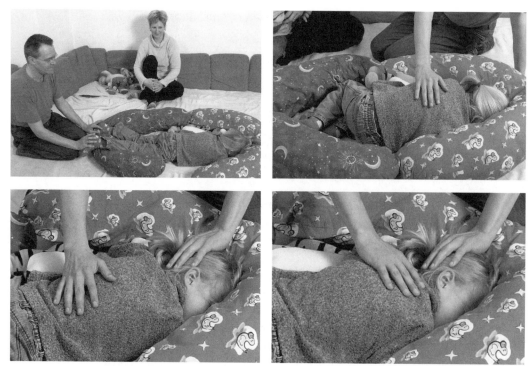

Figure 26.1. Treatment on the floor.

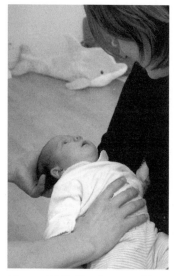

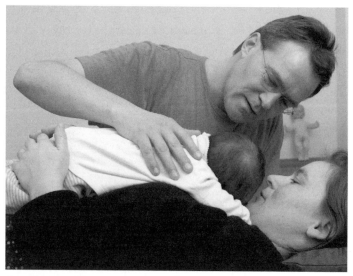

Figure 26.2. Treatment with the child in its mother's arms.

Figure 26.3. Treatment with the child lying on its mother.

craniosacral rhythm or the mid-tide, listen to establish whether and how the respiratory rhythm is perceptible. Afterward, listen to the slower rhythms.

26.5. Treatment with the Child Sitting

You can also treat the child sitting, for example, on a chair, or with legs dangling over the edge of the massage table, or on the massage table propped against a nursing pillow. Treatment with the child sitting is recommended as an initial familiarization stage if the child is not yet ready to be treated lying down or if treatment lying down is likely to result in crying, screaming, or loss of orientation. In the sitting position, the child is more likely to be connected with its everyday routine and familiar waking state. It is able to react more quickly to stimuli from outside and feels more secure than if it were lying down. In the lying position, the child is more in a resting state, more vulnerable, and more exposed than when sitting; on the other hand, letting go is more readily possible in the lying down position. The force of gravity means that the tonus of the body when sitting is different than when lying down.

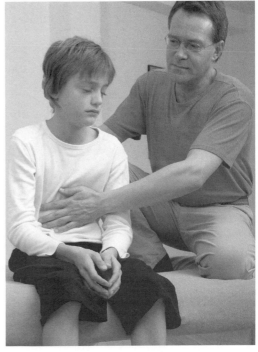

For the practitioner it is helpful if the child is sitting in an accessible position, for example, sideways on a deep chair, so that the entire back region and the front of the body can be touched without hindrance. If the child is sitting on the massage table, it should be in such a way that the practitioner can be positioned close enough to deliver treatment in a relaxed manner. Be careful that the

Figure 26.4. Treatment with the child sitting.

massage table does not become unstable from the one-sided distribution of weight.

Whether you are standing or sitting to deliver treatment, you have to frequently adjust and alter your feeling for the intensity of touch. At each moment you decide whether and for how long to apply your touch, whether you are attuned to the craniosacral rhythm or the mid-tide, or whether you will use specific release techniques such as the gentle ear pull, the frontal lift, or the parietal lift.

26.5.1. Method

You can also gently palpate the tissue and its density along the length of the child's spinal column. Alternatively, with your hand slightly off the child's back, you can scan relatively quickly along the spine to sense any "abnormal" sites. Tune in to any features such as unusual warmth or coldness, and then let your hand take the lead. Perhaps your hand will be "summoned" by the kidneys,

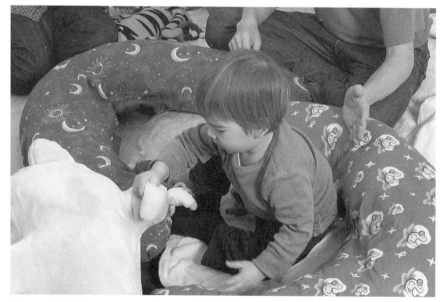

Figure 26.5. Treatment with the child sitting: assessing the back and spinal column.

or it may move intuitively to a particular location. With practice and a little patience, thermal assessment will become possible, in which pronounced warmth might point to inflamed tissue and marked coldness might indicate a withdrawn vital force and poorly perfused tissue. Sites that have undergone severe compression or have been the point of impact for a fall or blow can also be identified in this way and receive your healing touch.

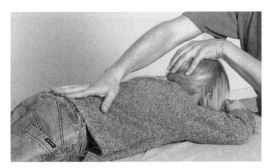

Figure 26.6. Treatment with the child lying on its front.

It does not necessarily have to be a "difficult" bodily zone that you are touching; a pleasantly reinforcing and warm hand supports the back and invites it to let go and lean inward. Instead of a hand at the back, the child might perhaps prefer to receive warm and supple contact on the front of its body, for example, in the abdominal region or against the ribs.

There is also the option of using both hands at the same time to touch the child's back and an area on the front of the body. The procedure is the same as described above.

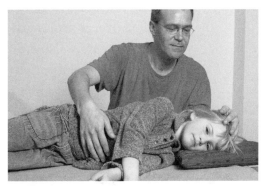

Figure 26.7. Treatment with the child lying on its side.

26.6. Treatment with the Child Lying Down

The child may be lying on its back, on its front, or on its side with a pillow under its head.

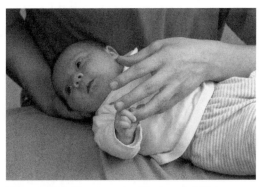

Figure 26.8. Treatment with the child lying on its back.

26.7. Where to Apply Your Touch

When embarking on a pediatric Craniosacral Therapy session, start by choosing a body location or region that feels pleasant, warm, or soft, or is least troubled by problems. This will serve at first to reinforce and anchor what is pleasant and positive, an approach that is more resource-oriented and solution-oriented than starting right away at a site where there is a problem.

26.8. Should You Apply Touch through Clothing or Directly to the Skin?

Touch automatically results in closeness. Because touch is often applied over a prolonged period in Craniosacral Therapy, a degree of intimacy may also emerge. However, the craniosacral rhythm can also be palpated through clothing, and the mid-tide can even be perceived in the sphere immediately around the body. Loose comfortable clothing is therefore not an obstacle in Craniosacral Therapy; quite the reverse: clothing may act as an important boundary, ensuring that your application of touch is not perceived by the child as being too intimate.

26.9. Touch

Sometimes subconscious agitation, insecurity, or wanting too much on the part of the practitioner can result in stress, causing energy and blood to withdraw from your extremities. Again, take time to regulate your emotional, energetic, and mental distance and apply touch to yourself in a relaxed way until your hands become warmer. Loosening and shaking out your hands will help ensure that the blood gets to your hands and fingers again (but avoid shaking your hands out in the immediate vicinity of the child). Feeling and massaging your forearms, wrists, and hands can also be helpful. If your hands are cold, apply your touch to a clothed part of the body rather than to the child's head. If you often have cool or sweaty hands, you might benefit from some Craniosacral Therapy sessions yourself.

Before starting to touch the child, you should verbally or nonverbally ask for permission to do so, or else at least give some verbal notice in advance of your impending touch. For example, I might ask, "can I touch you on your feet?" Alternatively I might say to the child, "now I'm about to touch you on your torso. You can say if you don't want me to do that." If there are no verbal or nonverbal signs to the contrary, I apply my touch slowly, clearly, and gently, and I listen with my hands.

As you apply your touch, continually fine-tune its quality, both to the tissue beneath your hands as well as to the emotional situation and the reaction of the ANS. You can also allow the child to experience different qualities of touch and then ask which it prefers. Perhaps it will prefer touch at the skin level or a clearer touch at the muscle or bone level. Remember that frequently modifying your touch as well as repeatedly changing your position sends out fresh sensory stimuli and may have a disruptive effect.

When you listen with your hands, you are sensing whether or not the tissue accepts your touch. If it is accepted, the tissue offers no resistance and becomes softer or warmer after a short time. If your touch is rejected, the tissue reacts with resistance, spontaneous withdrawal, and contraction; the child's breathing becomes hesitant; and its body assumes a defensive posture. In visual terms you can learn a great deal from the child's facial expression and gestures. Almost always the child will respond to your initial touch with a spontaneous reaction, for example with a change in breathing; by drawing its legs up; by becoming tense, rigid, or restless—or else it may relax.

Depending on the child's age or how much it has grown, adapt your touch accordingly. In infants it is frequently sufficient if you touch them lightly using only two or three fingers, and in school-age children it is usually appropriate for touch to involve the broader contact of your whole hand. The tissues will seek and find a new balance merely in response to your spacious touch.

TREATMENT OPTIONS FOR USE BY MIDWIVES, PEDIATRIC NURSES, SPECIAL-NEEDS TEACHERS, AND OTHER HEALTH CARE PROFESSIONALS

27

Treatments for couples experiencing fertility issues and for women during pregnancy are described in part II of this book, along with some additional practice tips.

With every attentive, listening, and receptive touch and treatment, you are honing your palpatory skills with regard to structure and the subtle inherent motion of the slow rhythms. It takes considerable practical experience and detailed knowledge of anatomy to be able to recognize, assess, and distinguish the structures, their inherent motion, and any changes that occur. Touch and release techniques for the head are performed very precisely using a weight of 0.04 to 0.1 ounces. Attending some number of craniosacral courses will also facilitate your entry to the field of Craniosacral Therapy.

Your heartfelt benevolent concern as well as your safe and yet spacious contact will have a positive effect on the child, who will start to play and will express its needs. The space provided by you, coupled with your harmonious contact, will open up the field for trust and the therapeutic process to emerge. This atmosphere enables the child to have new learning experiences at its own tempo. It is the child, rather than you as the person delivering the treatment, who reveals any issues it may have, such as self-attachment, expression of needs, and so on.

In order for the therapeutic process to develop, it is essential during the sessions that you continuously regulate your distance and maintain your contact. If your distance is not appropriate, this may instinctively activate defense mechanisms in the child, causing stress or resignation. If your contact with your inner self is inadequate, or if your contact with the child is insufficiently well maintained, the child may well respond in kind.

27.1. Supporting the Thorax and Respiratory Function

The child may be lying on its back, front, or side, or may be sitting. This treatment can be used to encourage maturation of lung function in preterm babies. It can also be performed on the back region if the baby has belly-to-belly skin contact with its mother.

This treatment may be used on its own or in combination with other Craniosacral Therapy techniques. Even before you establish touch contact, it is helpful if you sense your own thorax, your free breathing, and the expansion of your own lungs. While performing this treatment, remain within your breathing flow. For a time you may also consciously sense the dorsal aspect of your own lungs; periodically breathe deliberately into that area. In this way you will be less intensively occupied with the child's thorax and instead you will be setting a good example of full, free breathing. Remain in this touch contact and listen to the stillness.

27.1.1. Method

1. While using your gentle and spacious touch, at the same time sense the tissue and its tonus laterally on the child's thorax. Is there a sense of space and widening developing between your hands?
2. How is the respiratory rhythm perceptible at the thorax?
3. Next listen to the space between your hands. How do you perceive this space? Is the child's breathing changing? Does the tissue react after a while by becoming warmer or by expanding?

4. Support the flexibility of the thorax and lungs by clearly establishing contact with the bone level of the thorax, and next go with the movements of in-breath and out-breath. Retain your clear contact with the ribs. During the child's in-breath in particular, take care not to constrict the thorax in its expansion; instead, invite expansion.

5. As you perform treatment, widen your focus to include the whole body and the child in its body-mind-spirit unity.

6. After touching the thorax laterally, next apply your touch either to the front or the back of the child's thorax. Listen as described above.

7. Touch both clavicles and go with their movements in the respiratory rhythm with the intention that they should become even more mobile and free. This can also encourage lymph flow.

8. Another position involves the child's shoulders: mold your hands to their shape as you apply slow and supple touch. Listen as described above.

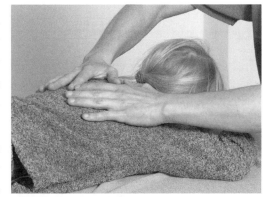

Figure 27.1. Supporting respiratory function and the lungs.

9. With the child lying on its back, slip your hands beneath the child's shoulder blades, taking care not to exert any compression via these structures onto the thorax. This can be additionally facilitated by the soft padding of the treatment table and by the position you adopt.

10. Via the bone level, make deliberate contact with both lungs in the thorax. Can you sense the left lung or the right lung more clearly during

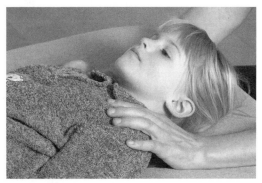

Figure 27.2. Listening to the respiratory and craniosacral rhythm, and perhaps sensing the mid-tide.

its in-breath and out-breath movement? Is the child's breathing changing? Is it becoming more even? Is it becoming deeper? Where does the greatest freedom and widening occur—in the upper, middle, or lower pulmonary regions? Invite the surfaces of the two lungs to expand on their own with each in-breath.

11. Next, invite the thousands of pulmonary alveoli to expand even more with each in-breath. This expansion of the thorax will also give the neighboring heart more space. Also include the blood vessels of the lungs in your perceptual field, then the heart, and both lungs—and subsequently these organs with their vessels and fluids as a whole.

12. The lungs themselves are relatively light. Can you sense their lightness and widening? What else is entering your perceptual field?

13. What is the mood in the room like? Has anything changed on or within the thorax? Has anything changed with you and the child overall? If so, how do you perceive this?

Disengage your touch slowly and gently. Allow yourself and the child sufficient time to enjoy the ongoing effects.

27.2. Touching and Releasing Body Sites, Supporting Organ Functions

The visceral therapy advocated and practiced by teachers of gentle Craniosacral Therapy is characterized by its noninvasive nature that acts primarily through perception. In no way does it involve robust, invasive visceral manipulation.

Purely as a precautionary measure, noninvasive visceral techniques should be used in problem pregnancies where there is a risk of miscarriage or pregnancy bleeds. Noninvasive visceral therapy is also indicated in preterm babies because their bodies are still very fragile.

Ideally, you should begin at less restricted sites or zones, which you will locate once you have gained some experience. Using touch that is both gentle and spacious, palpate the tissue and its tonus at various sites on the torso. Wait to establish whether a free location becomes even more relaxed. Then with your other hand, touch another body location that is perhaps restricted and needs support. Leaving one hand at the unrestricted site, place your other hand on a zone characterized by greater tissue hardness, a restriction, a previous injury, or on an organ such as the liver, kidneys, or bladder that you want to strengthen in function. Of course, as an alternative, it is possible after a while to use both hands to touch the zone requiring treatment.

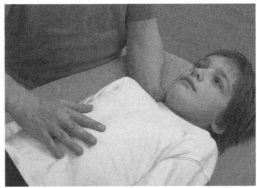

Figure 27.4. Releasing the liver and the apex of the lung (the right superior lobe).

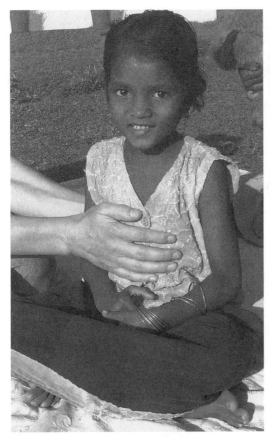

Figure 27.3. Releasing the diaphragm, esophagus, stomach, and kidneys.

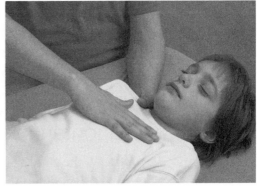

Figure 27.5. Releasing the pleura, pericardium, lungs, and the apex of the right lung.

27.2.1. Method

1. Once your contact and touch are right for the child (if necessary, ask), listen for a while to the tissue that you are touching with one hand, and then to the tissue that you are touching with the other hand. Are there any differences? Is one site less restricted than the other? If so, how do you sense this? Afterward, listen with both hands simultaneously. Are space and widening becoming apparent between your hands?

2. At the bone and connective tissue level, can you sense the movement of the respiratory rhythm with one hand or the other, or even with both hands?

3. Afterward, listen to the space between your hands. How do you sense this space? Is there any change in breathing? Does the tissue react after a while by becoming warmer or by expanding?

4. At the bone and connective tissue level, can you sense the movement of the respiratory rhythm or the motion of the slower craniosacral rhythm?

5. Expand your treatment focus to include the child's whole body and its body-mind-spirit unity. What is the mood in the room? Has anything changed in the tissue that you are touching? Has anything changed with you and the child overall? If so, how do you perceive it?

6. Ask the child whether you should remain at this location, apply touch to a different region, or stop the treatment. Disengage your touch gently and slowly.

27.3. Listening to the Craniosacral Rhythm and Spontaneous Stillpoints

As you touch the child's body tissue, sacrum, or head, listen occasionally to whether and how you are sensing the movement of the child's breathing at the site in question.

After a while you will be able to sense the even slower craniosacral rhythm. With increasing practice, you will learn to evaluate its qualities: how strongly can the craniosacral rhythm be palpated? What is its amplitude like, meaning the range of external and internal rotation or flexion and extension? What about its symmetry? Is the motion of the craniosacral rhythm equal or different on the left and right sides? What is the frequency of the rhythm beneath your hands? Is it closer to six cycles per minute or twelve cycles per minute? What is your overall impression of the craniosacral rhythm: is it relatively constant and balanced, or is it unsettled and changeable?

Is there a prolonged pause after a while, a spontaneous stillpoint? Does this last for about thirty seconds or two to three minutes? What are the sensed characteristics of the craniosacral rhythm after the stillpoint? To what extent have its qualities changed?

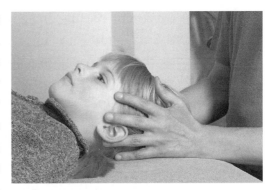

Figure 27.6. Cranial vault hold: listening to the craniosacral rhythm and spontaneous stillpoints.

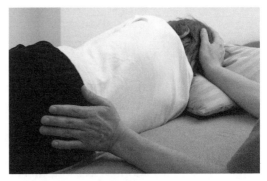

Figure 27.7. Hand position at the sacrum and occipital bone with child on its side.

27.4. Harmonizing the Craniosacral Rhythm at the Sacrum and Occipital Bone

Position the child comfortably on its side, back, or front. Encourage release of

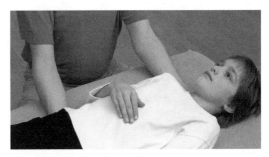

Figure 27.8. Hand position at the sacrum and occipital bone with child on its back.

tension by placing one hand on the child's sacrum and the other on the occipital bone. Listen to the slow motions of the craniosacral rhythm. Many children particularly enjoy this treatment. A description of the child's position on its side and the details of the method are as outlined for pregnant women in section 10.8.6.

27.5. Short Treatment Sequence

1. Touch the child's feet or knees with your supple hands. Listen for any fine micromovements that may emerge as a result of your agreeable touch. You may be able to sense in your hands the child's respiratory movements or craniosacral rhythm over the hips and legs.
2. Touch any paired bodily structure on either side—left and right—of the midline, such as the sides of the pelvis or the shoulders. Listen in a relaxed way.
3. Touch any site or region front and back in the vicinity of the midline, for example the pelvic or abdominal region in front and the lumbar region or shoulder-neck region, taking care not to compress the spinal column, in back. Listen with receptive hands.
4. Touch the middle of the child's torso with both hands on the sides or with one hand in the dorsal region and the other hand at the

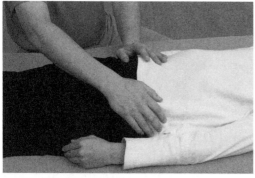

Figure 27.9. Releasing tissues at the sides of the pelvis; listening to the craniosacral rhythm.

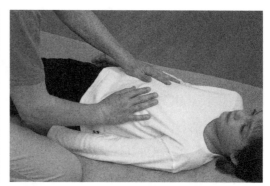

Figure 27.10. Releasing the mid-torso and diaphragm.

junction of the thorax and the abdomen. How can breathing be perceived here?

5. Sitting behind the child's head, place your arms on the table and rest the weight of your arms on the padded surface. In this way you will take the load off your own shoulder-neck region before you establish broad contact with the child's shoulders. Listen to the tissue, how the respiratory rhythm subtly moves the shoulders. Is the left or the right shoulder freer? Does one side come toward you sooner and farther than the other side? Go with the movements of the in-breath and the out-breath, and as the child breathes in, invite more space and more widening. Use this position to perceive the thorax as a whole. Does something change if you allow your hands to move on their own like corks floating on water?

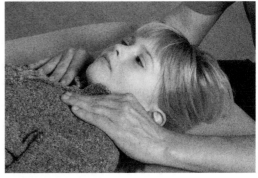

Figure 27.11. Supporting in-breath and out-breath at the shoulders.

6. Establish contact with the child's occipital bone using the cradle hold. The atlanto-occipital region is an important area in babies and children. Without using pressure you can ease the tension in

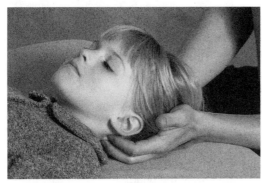

Figure 27.12. Massaging and lateral stroking of the muscles at the occipital ridge.

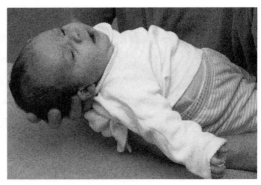

Figure 27.13. Hand position for cradle hold and upper back combined.

this region by positioning your soft finger pads directly on the occipital ridge, thus supporting the release of various neck muscle attachment points in that location.

7. Next listen to the craniosacral rhythm at the occipital bone.

8. Slowly and without pressure, gently apply touch to the child's head as a whole, invite space and widening, and listen with relaxed hands and fingers. Simply invite self-correction without performing any techniques. After a while, listen to whether the craniosacral rhythm makes itself felt in your flexible hands and fingers with its slow filling and widening motions or with a decrease in volume. Perhaps you can go with time-lapse slow-motion movements and then sense whether the craniosacral rhythm takes a break, meaning whether a spontaneous stillpoint is establishing itself.

9. Using supple and sensitive hands and fingers, listen at the child's head, as in the cradle hold, at the parietal bones, or at the frontal bone. Are you able to sense the craniosacral rhythm at the front, sides, or back of the head? If so, is it more pronounced in flexion/external rotation or in extension/internal rotation? Are the slow motions of the craniosacral rhythm relatively balanced and harmonious and flowing relatively continuously, or are they choppy and unbalanced?

10. To conclude, select a site on the child's torso, at the legs or feet, or a site that the child requests. Listen here with your hands and compare your impressions now with those at the start.

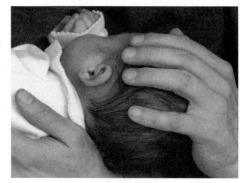

Figure 27.14. Palpating the craniosacral rhythm at the head.

27.6. Gentle Ear Pull Technique

The gentle ear pull eases tension in a number of cranial sutures and in the temporal bones, including the middle ear and labyrinth, and releases the TMJ and, indirectly, the superior hyoid muscles. It also helps the meninges, which are often taut or adherent, to become slightly stretched and more flexible. In the same way, tension patterns are released in the tentorium cerebelli, which is the horizontal component in the intracranial membrane system, and at its points of contact with the falx cerebri and falx cerebelli, the vertical components of the intracranial membrane system. It also has a positive effect on the drainage of blood from the brain and can reduce or resolve a sensation of pressure in the head and TMJ.

Via the connective tissues and the bony substance of the temporal bones, the auricle (external part of the ear) and the auditory canal are continuous with the dura mater and thus indirectly with the entire intracranial membrane system. The tentorium cerebelli covers the cerebellum like a tent and has attachments left and right to the petrous parts of the two temporal bones. Both consequently undergo easing of tension.

The gentle ear pull should not be used if it proves to be disagreeable to the child, or indeed to adults.

27.6.1. Method 1

Relax and deliberately ground yourself. With your hands relaxed, place them on the treatment table alongside the child's ears. Position each thumb in the bottom third of the external ear cartilage, not in the auditory canal. With your index and middle fingers, take hold of the back of the ear cartilage, without exerting pressure. Then, with both hands, slowly offer a very gentle suggestion of steady and continuous traction sideways, away from the child's head. It is important to calculate the intensity of pull extremely finely, taking care not to provoke the tissues. Instead, the mere suggestion of traction confers better contact with the temporal bone and its petrous part and with the tentorium cerebelli, which you invite to release its tension from the inside outward. At the same time, listen and simply be open to any possible direction of motion that you perceive in your left or right hand. Go with it in the direction of ease that is revealed. If you sense resistance, stop but maintain the steady gentle ear pull. Listen and do not define any direction. Go with it into the new free direction only if further release is evident. This is similar to unwinding, in which the direction of free motion is supported and any limit of motion is accepted.

27.6.2. Method 2

After you have supported the temporal bones, and indirectly through them the tentorium cerebelli, in their spontaneous free motion via the external ear, you may additionally define a clear direction in order to release these structures more specifically. Place very gentle traction on both external ears simultaneously along an approximately oblique posterolateral line that would roughly be an extension of the petrous part of the temporal bone, meaning slightly to the side and toward the child's occipital bone. Then release the gentle ear pull and let go of the external ear.

27.6.3. Method 3

Instead of easing the tension in the temporal bones and tentorium cerebelli as described above, in school-age children you can use the gentle ear pull during external rotation of the temporal bones, which is done in an anterocaudal direction. During internal rotation, maintain contact but without traction; then apply traction again during the external rotation phase.

Next listen to the craniosacral rhythm at the temporal bones and in the cranial vault hold (see figs. 27.15 to 27.17). Has anything changed,

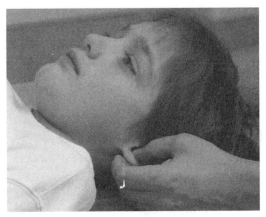

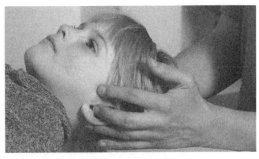

Figure 27.16. Listening to the craniosacral rhythm at the temporal bones.

Figure 27.15. Gentle ear pull: releasing the TMJs, temporal bones, and tentorium cerebelli.

and if so, what? Is the craniosacral rhythm more pronounced, more balanced?

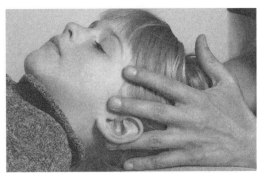

27.7. After Ventouse or Forceps Delivery

Figure 27.17. Listening to the craniosacral rhythm in the cranial vault hold.

This treatment is done as a supportive measure between sessions by a fully qualified craniosacral practitioner. With one hand, establish contact with the child's parietal bones together with the anterior and posterior fontanel. With your other hand, make contact with the child's sacrum, abdomen, or diaphragm region, for example. Do not apply any pressure with your hand on the parietal bones and fontanels; instead mold it to the child's cranial shape and establish a more levitating or lifting contact. Via the bones, this hand connects with the meninges and the falx cerebri as well as with the CSF. It is relaxed and goes with the slow motions of the craniosacral rhythm or the mid-tide. In the process you will often also sense spontaneous self-correction without these having been induced by your treatment. Assess the size of the fontanels before and after each session.

This individual treatment can be combined with other Craniosacral Therapy techniques, for example with the gentle ear pull or intracranial membrane release.

27.8. Nourishing the Soul and Encouraging Bonding via the Umbilical Cord Connection

The unborn child receives blood, oxygen, and many other substances from the mother and experiences its connection with her through the umbilical cord via the placenta over a prolonged period. Excretion processes also take place via the umbilical cord. Among other things, the umbilical cord symbolizes being nourished and our primal connectedness. Interestingly, the second chakra, known as the *hara* chakra in Japanese, is located in the abdominal region about two fingers' width below the navel; in Zen Buddhism and in Japanese martial arts it represents a person's inner center.

Deliberate contact and gentle touch in the umbilical region can bring nourishment for the soul and connectedness for the child. In this way the health care professional or the mother can simply support the child in its fundamental psychological needs. The prerequisite is that the person applying touch must be present, relaxed, and connected in the heart. The child will be able to sense whether the application of touch is nourishing to its soul or whether the person is inwardly absent. If the mother or father is connected in the heart and with the child, she or he can take a comfortable position to the side and place one or both hands over the umbilical region. The other hand may also be positioned over the back opposite the umbilical region. Alternatively, the other hand may also be placed over the child's heart. The important thing is the quality of presence in the contact and not so much the time factor or precise positioning. The health care professional may stand or sit behind the mother and touch her dorsal region to support her. In addition, the health care professional may tune in to the shared fluid field of mother and child, or to the mid-tide and Long Tide, the stillness, or dynamic stillness.

Prenatal or perinatal umbilical cord trauma may arise if the umbilical cord was involved in birth complications, if the cord was cut after delivery and before it had stopped pulsing, or if the baby's navel healed poorly or was painful. In such circumstances this form of treatment is particularly valuable. Every child can be supported in this way at a deep level. This application of touch simultaneously improves the perfusion of the abdominal organs, encouraging autonomic self-regulation.

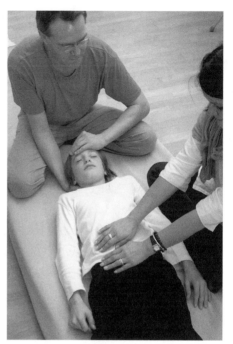

Figure 27.18. Strengthening the umbilical cord connection and the *hara* chakra.

27.9. Healing through Emotional Attachment and Its Expression on the Verbal and Nonverbal Level

The craniosacral practitioner may assist the parents and the child verbally, for example, by supporting the mother during the craniosacral session in sensing the emotions that she felt during pregnancy and childbirth. Today, at this moment, she has permission to experience these sensations and to give them spontaneous expression.

27.9.1. Telling the Story of Pregnancy and Childbirth

Even if the traumatic event, such as a difficult pregnancy or childbirth, was extremely intense, the mother and child have come through it. The mother should bring this to mind and consciously connect with her sources of strength. If the mother has feelings of guilt, she can let them go. She can exhale her tensions with a few deeper breaths and sense the relief, where possible, in her body too. She should allow herself sufficient time to be sad and to display other emotions. All this is helpful in making it easier for her to become calmer. Now she will increasingly sense her heart region. The emotions of the heart spread out via her arms to her hands and via her eyes. Then she can begin to make eye contact with her child. The mother continues to sense her breathing flow, which also reflects how she is feeling. Provided she is ready, the mother can now take the baby in her arms, or for infants, onto her lap.

After a time, once nonverbal contact with her child has deepened and the mother senses a heart-to-heart connection and feels the impulse to do it, she can begin to tell the child in simple words and sentences what happened. She may narrate the most important aspects from the time of her pregnancy. Then the mother tells the child the story of the birth, why there may have been difficult phases, and what the consequences were. If the child cries while this is happening, the mother should offer eye contact and tell the child in her own words that she understands that it was difficult and that all emotions are permissible. After the mother or parents and the child have sensed these emotions and have been able to communicate in their individual way, they should then consciously return to the present: the mother demonstrates to her child the pleasure she feels that it is here, holds it in her arms or in her lap, and continues to gaze at it. She can remain simply present and in heart-to-heart contact. Perhaps she will touch her child in the region of its heart, diaphragm, or navel. Now she is enjoying with her child the healing presence in the here and now, without distraction and without disturbing this newfound attachment through any overly hasty activity.

As the craniosacral practitioner, gently guide the mother in this process and allow her and the child sufficient time. You may occasionally support the mother by touch or verbally, particularly if she has little self-awareness or loses herself in violent emotions. Regulate your distance as appropriate for the situation, especially during the intimate interaction, so as not to disturb the profound process that is unfolding.

FOR FULLY QUALIFIED CRANIOSACRAL PRACTITIONERS

28

The treatment options for use by midwives and other health care professionals outlined in the previous chapter can also be employed by fully qualified craniosacral practitioners. In Switzerland, in contrast to the situation in many other countries, a craniosacral practitioner is someone who has completed a course of craniosacral training lasting several years and who has passed a final examination, rather than someone who has merely attended a few short courses.

Structural treatments to improve conception and for use during pregnancy are described in part II. A wide range of suggestions for the general assessment and the craniosacral-specific assessment are summarized in chapter 23.

The different treatment approaches employed in Craniosacral Therapy are described in chapter 24. Depending on the emphasis of the particular college or instructor, differing approaches and techniques will be taught. Biodynamic Craniosacral Therapy operates hardly at all with the craniosacral rhythm and the physical level but instead focuses on the slower rhythms of the mid-tide and the Long Tide. This approach requires entirely different skills that, in my view, are best suited to practitioners with many years of experience. The treatment options described in this chapter, predominantly in the gentle functional-structural field, have often brought relief for physical and emotional problems. I will allude only occasionally to biodynamic Craniosacral Therapy and would instead refer readers to specialist courses devoted to that topic.

Before you perform the procedures described in the following pages, I would recommend that you also attend some pediatric craniosacral courses once you have completed your specialist craniosacral training. Among other things, delegates attending such courses will learn how to treat children and their parents, and how to recognize and sense any changes that occur; this helps to minimize any fear of touching that you may have. Pediatric craniosacral courses will also enable you in your own sessions with children to develop a deeper knowledge and understanding of the various dynamics and to better distinguish the therapeutic process. In fact, during the practical demonstrations of treatment sessions with children, the collective group attending such courses, through the empathy and spacious support offered, has a potentiating effect on the therapeutic process. The group and the room form the containment, rather like the womb, and guarantee a safe setting.

Treatment of babies and infants—especially in the head and neck region—should be performed only after you have accumulated many years of experience in Craniosacral Therapy. Because they are central elements in the craniosacral-specific assessment and treatment, you will always tune in to the quality of the craniosacral rhythm and of the mid-tide and Long Tide, together with their inherent potency. See chapter 30 for a discussion of selected indications, with pointers for Craniosacral Therapy.

28.1. Treating Babies and Children

Craniosacral Therapy in newborns and infants can already take place after the initial prolonged bonding phase between mother and child, especially after a difficult birth; where organ function, for example pulmonary function, is poorly developed; or where the child is disabled. Even in healthy newborns, treatment during the first three to six months is helpful to ensure early release of bone displacement or joint compression and to bring about overall improvements in the tension state of the dura mater and intracranial membranes as well as in fluid exchange. The potency of primary respiration can then also perform its delicate growth-promoting work unhindered before any restrictions become more imprinted in the bodily structure.

KEY POINT

Correcting the position of a structure is not the main issue; rather, it is about encouraging its motility (inherent motion) and mobility (the motion of one structure in harmony with other structures).

To emphasize again: never apply pressure to the head when working with babies and infants. In general, up until about age six, compensatory restrictions are hardly ever encountered. For this reason you should use direct treatment for release techniques involving the head. In other words, instead of indirect-direct release techniques that involve compression-decompression, use direct release, meaning decompression. In contrast, in school-age children and young adults, who often already show compensatory head patterns, the indirect-direct techniques can also be used; gently go into the pattern of restriction (compression) and then follow with direct release (decompression). Naturally, you will need to adapt the following assessments to the age of the child.

In babies and infants it is not recommended to work exclusively at the bone level but that you also comprehensively assess and support the membrane and fluid level (see sections 23.5.4, 28.3, and 28.11).

Evaluate the entire craniosacral system and its rhythm in terms of its quality—strength, amplitude or spectrum, symmetry or evenness, and cycles per minute—and whether the mid-tide is perceptible. Are there any bodily structures that are affecting the craniosacral rhythm or the mid-tide? If so, to what extent? What are the free fulcrums? What are the inertial fulcrums in the head region and in the upper, middle, and lower torso regions?

28.1.1. Getting Underway in a Pediatric Craniosacral Session

In your capacity as the craniosacral practitioner, speak to the child: welcome it, introduce yourself, and as you do so, establish and maintain contact with the child. You may ask the child, "What can I do for you?" or "Where do you need my support?" The answer may come immediately in the form of a gesture, an emotion, or both at once. An infant at the preverbal stage of experience will not grasp the content of your words, but it will understand the inflection, the energy of the spoken word, and its accompanying intonation, and it will be able to respond using sounds, gestures, and body posture. Frequently the baby may indicate with a hand a particular body location that feels out of sorts or will touch the site more often, perhaps the face, forehead, occipital bone, ear, or the area around the stomach or liver. Using changes in facial expression, sounds, and pitch, it can offer a brief account using babbling baby talk or by crying out.

One of the responsibilities of the craniosacral practitioner during the session is to be continuously attentive and to guarantee the respectful, safe therapeutic setting. You should observe what is happening, the mother-child interaction, and the reactions to your specific therapeutic approaches from the start until the final minute of the session. At the same time you are aware of the emotional, physical, and energetic changes in the people in the room, and you accompany the directly emerging therapeutic process.

Observe and assess the child as follows:

- How does it express itself in terms of body posture?
- How does it control its coordinated movements, and is it mobile? Which positional changes does it like or dislike—lying on its front or on its back?
- Has it learned to hold itself erect against gravity?
- Does its posture betray an inability to hold itself erect, for example due to a restriction, weak muscle tonus, or visceral dysfunction?

- Does it react to a look by laughing, babbling, or displaying fear?
- Is the child's behavior defensive and introverted or open and extroverted?
- How well developed are the functions of breathing, phonation, articulation, and facial expression, and how can these be encouraged?

With one hand, apply gentle touch to the child's dorsal region while placing your other hand in the area of the costal arch, diaphragm, stomach, and solar plexus, or if this is disagreeable, slightly farther down in the lower abdomen. Always adapt your intensity of touch to the tissue tonus and the momentary situation. Note how your touch is received by the child: is it accepted? Does the child respond with relaxed breathing, softening of the tissue, or with defensiveness? Is the child at this moment more in the buildup-activation phase or in the release-deactivation phase? Are there any reactions or changes in response to your touch? How is the tonus in the area of the diaphragm and thorax? How free is the connective tissue under one hand, under the other hand, and between your hands? Is a fascial glide possible? If so, is it easy and smooth? How do you sense the breathing or the craniosacral rhythm? Are there any motor or sensory reactions in response to your touch? Which bodily regions, for example the thorax, the abdomen, or the dorsal region, are characterized by hypertonus or hypotonus?

If you change your position, always keep one hand in contact with the body if possible.

Assess and treat the following body levels:

- locomotor apparatus: connective tissue or fascia, muscles, bones, joints
- organs
- the craniosacral system, with its three levels:
  - bone level: sacrum, occipital bone, atlanto-occipital joint, and cranial bones, including the cranial base.

- membrane level: meninges covering the brain and spinal cord, important, among other things, for growth and development of the CNS.
- fluid level: CSF, and all fluids together. Use the fluctuation technique, for example to invite a stillpoint with CV4 or EV4.

Treatment can be performed using one or several approaches:

- Listen to the inherent motion, go with it, and observe any changes.
- Go with the inherent motion and amplify or exaggerate it.
- Ease tension or perform release using the direct technique or indirect-direct technique.
- Ease tension or perform release using "stacking."

Continue as in the general and craniosacral-specific assessment, outlined in chapter 30, and the further assessment and treatment options outlined in this section.

28.2. Assessing the Head and Dural Tube

In its birth position, the side of the baby that is conjunct with the mother's spine undergoes the greatest compression, displacement, or torsion during the birth process. In newborns and infants in particular it is important to gain an overall picture using the following assessment for the head and dural tube:

- How free and mobile are the individual cranial bones in relation to each other? Are the sutures free or compressed? Are the cranial bones floating on the dura mater, or do they appear to be fixed?
- How mobile are the individual cranial bones in themselves? For example, a baby's occipital bone may have a relatively pliable feel, and it may also undergo intraosseous compression or torsion in itself. Assess, for example, the frontal bone, with its two parts; the sphenoid, with its three parts; and the two temporal bones.

- Craniosacral rhythm: is there a more pronounced tendency to flexion/external rotation or extension/internal rotation? Are there other motion patterns of the SBS, such as torsion or side-bending, both with a compensatory effect, or lateral pull or vertical pull, both due to external physical trauma? Detailed theoretical and practical knowledge, comprehensively covered in many published sources, is essential for treating SBS patterns.

- How is the craniosacral rhythm perceived specifically at the individual cranial bones?

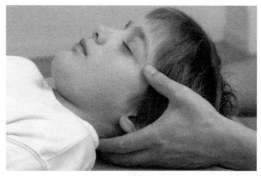

- How free are the spinal meninges in the suboccipital region, at the level of the thoracic vertebrae and the lumbar vertebrae? Is continuity freely accessible from the foramen magnum to the sacrum? Are there any abnormalities? Any differences?

Figure 28.1. Palpating and balancing the SBS via the sphenoid and occipital bone.

- How balanced is the tension state of the dura mater in the vicinity of the cranial vault, and how balanced is the tension state of the intracranial membranes?

- A restriction at the bone level or an imbalanced tension pattern at the membrane level always has repercussions on the other level. It is important to discover where the greatest restriction is located and to identify the primary inertial fulcrum.

- Can you perceive the inherent motion of the brain as a whole, embedded as it is within the protective bones and membranes and floating in the CSF, together with its vessels?

- What are the perceived characteristics of the tide-like motions of the CSF? Do they tend to be strong or weak, regular or irregular?

- Are stillpoints occurring spontaneously without being intentionally or actively induced? If a stillpoint has occurred, is it happening in extension/internal rotation (CV4) or in flexion/external rotation (EV4)?

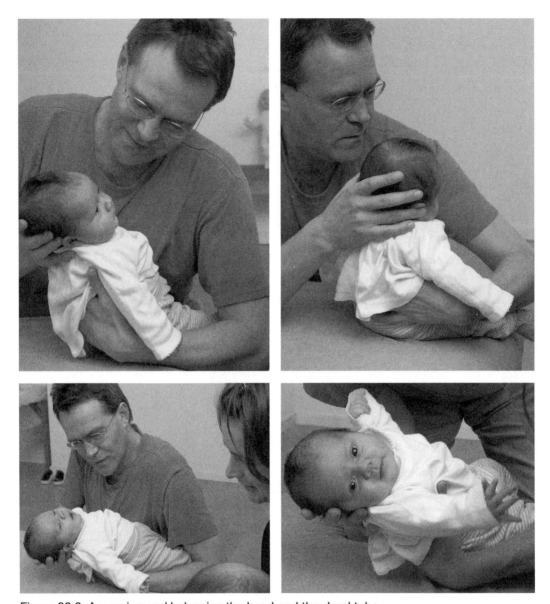

Figure 28.2. Assessing and balancing the head and the dural tube.

28.3. Balancing the Fontanels via the Bone and Membrane Level

28.3.1. Method

With one hand, touch a bodily zone such as the abdomen, back, or neck using pleasant, gentle contact. This hand serves as the anchor or support. Without using any technique, it supports the tissue as it seeks and finds a new balance point.

Using the loosened fingers of your other hand, gently palpate and touch the individual cranial bones around a fontanel and invite membrane balance. As you do so, remember not to exert any pressure at all; rather your hand should levitate slightly over or close to the suture junction, and the contact of your supple fingers will be simultaneously clear and light. Listen how your two or three fingers subtly move and, in time, display more balanced movements, possibly accompanied by a stillpoint.

Assess and treat the fontanel on the opposite side, and afterward evaluate using the cranial vault hold.

28.4. Balancing the Occipital Bone with Its Constituent Parts

Torsion of the occipital bone imparts incorrect growth impulses from above to the spinal column, in particular, a state of affairs that frequently results in lateral spinal curvature, called scoliosis, and other disorders. The occipital bone, originally consisting of four parts, fuses to form a single unit by age four to six. After that age, improvement of the given underlying pattern is still possible in most cases; because the bone grows, the method described below has a more beneficial effect on the overall development of the child than if the occipital bone were not treated. In hyperactive children there is often a tendency for the occipital condyles to be compressed. Compression of the foramen magnum is often detected in children with cerebral palsy.

Careful spreading can also be performed on its own without subsequent decompression.

28.4.1. Method

Slowly and gently position one or both hands beneath the child's occipital bone. Then listen:

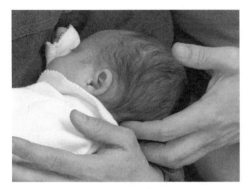

Figure 28.3. Start position for lateral spreading at the occipital ridge.

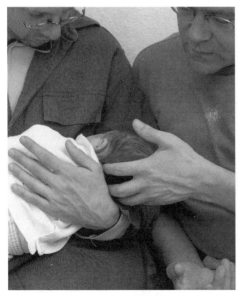

Figure 28.4. Continuing lateral spreading at the occipital ridge.

- What is the shape of the occipital bone?
- What is the position of the occipital bone?
- When you sense the craniosacral rhythm, what is it like? Ask it to reveal its motion pattern: Is there displacement, torsion or rotation, or an intraosseous pull of the occipital squama toward the SBS?
- There may be unwinding of the occipital squama. Allow space and time for this self-regulation.
- Next sense the occipital bone with all four of its parts (see fig. 18.2). Observe how these four constituent parts are positioned and whether the structures are evolving to a more homogeneous balance.
- Start position: with your supple finger pads at the occipital ridge, subtly palpate the muscle attachments there. Next broadly position your finger pads at the bony occipital ridge, or place your fingers beneath the occipital squama without compressing the lambdoid suture. With a newborn, position the baby's head on two or three of your fingers.
- Next listen without actively doing anything, and establish the connection with

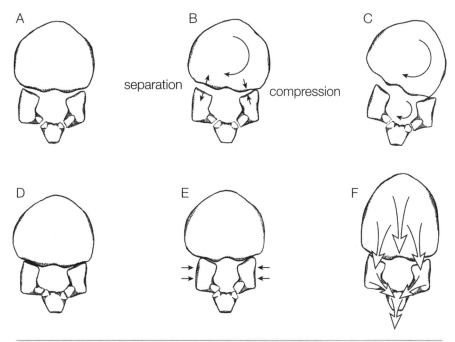

Figure 28.5. Common positional anomalies of the constituent parts of the occipital bone: *A*, occipital bone without positional anomaly; *B*, rotation of the occipital squama; *C*, rotation of the occipital squama with torsion of the lateral condyles; *D*, compression of the occipital squama with condylar and basilar parts; *E*, compression of both condylar parts medially; *F*, intraosseous elongation toward the SBS and cranial base.

the two lateral parts of the occipital bone to the left and right of the foramen magnum.

- How are the left and right condylar parts positioned—are they relatively horizontal, tilted, or compressed?
- Does anything change when you invite space and widening?
- Gentle spreading at the occipital ridge: Slowly spread apart your fingers (for newborns) or your hands (for bigger children) laterally; in this process your supple finger pads at the occipital ridge, or your fingers beneath the occipital squama, will slide slightly laterally and apart. This gentle lateral widening can be repeated because it eases the tension on the two lateral condylar parts and creates

space for the foramen magnum. The lateral condylar parts of the occipital bone may now also assume a more balanced position.

- After this lateral spreading, you may also release any compression on the occipital bone, including its constituent parts: from the start position described above, sense all four parts of the occipital bone. Begin by spreading the occipital bone and indirectly the two lateral parts, then deliver a mere hint of decompression on the basilar part away from the sphenoid and the two petrous parts of the temporal bones, and invite space and widening there. Then attune yourself to the articulation of the basilar part with the two lateral parts and release any compression, again delivering a mere hint of decompression. Perform these release techniques one immediately after the other without allowing the occipital bone to return to its compressed position.

- Direct or functional stacking is also an option. In direct stacking, each emerging pattern is held and stacked onto each new pattern to achieve release. In functional stacking, the occipital bone, membranes, and fluids are supported in the motions of the craniosacral rhythm in the free range so that they find a new balance point and so that dysfunctions are reduced or resolved.

- Listen to the reorganization of the four parts of the occipital bone.

- Listen to the craniosacral rhythm, whether a spontaneous stillpoint occurs, or whether and how the mid-tide can be perceived.

- If necessary, you can then assess and support the sacrum, SBS, temporal bones, parietal bones, intracranial membranes, or fluids.

28.5. Listening to the Craniosacral Rhythm and Inviting a Stillpoint

You can listen to the craniosacral rhythm and invite a stillpoint at paired body locations. You can also do this at the sacrum, occipital bone, frontal bone, or temporal bones. On the basis of your evaluation, you decide whether the craniosacral system can be better supported with a CV4, a stillpoint in internal rotation/extension that corresponds to compression of the fourth ventricle, or with an EV4, a stillpoint in external rotation/flexion that corresponds to expansion or opening of the fourth ventricle. The CV4 collects and centers, and it builds up potency in the center because it retains the freshly produced CSF for a while in the inner CSF spaces. In contrast, the EV4 widens and expands, enabling the CSF to flow immediately from the inner to the outer CSF spaces without first accumulating for several minutes. It is more likely to be used if the system has a tendency to be closed, is predominantly in internal rotation–extension, or is tight to the midline. CV4 and EV4 can be invited using intention, or they can be gently induced. For example, EV4 can be induced at the temporal bones, the occipital bone, or the sacrum.

The proportions of a tiny head can make it difficult to induce a CV4 stillpoint in a small child using the heel of the hand at the occipital bone. It is therefore advisable to position your index and middle fingers cranially, beneath the baby's head, and to invite a stillpoint in this way. It is recommended to attune predominantly to the membrane level and the fluid level of the CSF via the bone level and in this way to subtly invite the stillpoint.

A CV4 after delivery helps with the removal of medications that the child has received itself before or during the birth process; preterm babies, for example, receive medicines to further support pulmonary maturation, and medications that have been ingested via the placenta. Although CV4 has been questioned for some years now in certain colleges and by practitioners who claim that it is too invasive, it has immense potential for boosting the body's capacity for self-regulation (see sections 18.4 and 18.5). Techniques that have been used successfully for decades should not necessarily be ignored because of fashionable trends. We know that it is primarily the core attitude, coupled with the experience and the intention of the practitioner, that determines whether a technique is advisable in a particular client and how therapeutically valuable and effective it is. I am of the opinion that in general, no pressure should be applied in the head region in children under about age six, even for a CV4. In fact, pressure is mostly not necessary in older children and in many adults.

Stillpoints can be induced on the biomechanical-structural, functional, or biodynamic level. The procedure is different on each level. Inviting a stillpoint is more consistent with the functional approach, whereas gently inducing a stillpoint tallies more with the biomechanical-structural approach. In the biodynamic model, CV4 and EV4 are invited on an entirely different level.

28.6. Opening the Craniosacral System through Flexion/External Rotation

One of many possibilities in structural Craniosacral Therapy, after each local treatment, is to deliberately support or strengthen these individual components of the craniosacral system in their external rotation–flexion phase. This strategy is based on the fact that, during the birth process and development, the child often experienced compression. Due to compensatory dysfunctions or external physical trauma, its craniosacral system may have a greater tendency to remain in internal rotation–extension. The aim of supporting the child's craniosacral system more in flexion–external rotation after specific local balancing is to increasingly open the craniosacral system so that the vital force can spread outward or from the middle to the sides or periphery. This is not practiced if the craniosacral system is already clearly in a flexion pattern or if the midline is to be strengthened.

28.7. The Three-Step Healing Process

As an alternative to the previous technique, described here is a core attitude that is used predominantly in the functional and biodynamic approach. The practitioner can observe the process of the body's own self-regulation in terms of the three-step healing process, as defined by

Becker.[1] This process unfolds on various levels: in pulmonary breathing, in the regulation of tissue tension, on the level of the craniosacral rhythm, and in the mid-tide. The practitioner listens in a neutral to the three natural phases of self-regulation without intervening:

- **First step or phase:** listen to the motion of the tissues and fluids as they seek and find a new point of balance on this level.
- **Second step or phase:** has a new point of balance been reached? Is a holistic shift taking place, accompanied by stillness?
- **Third step or phase:** on this level the motions are now freer and more balanced. The holistic matrix, the craniosacral rhythm, and the fluid body find their way to a new state of balance. Make a note of any changes compared with your findings beforehand and assist their integration. This third phase in turn may itself transition into a new first phase.

28.8. Craniosacral Assessment and Treatment in Babies and Children

Chapter 23 details the general and craniosacral-specific assessments that you may opt to use in practice. The following list relating to assessment and treatment is extremely comprehensive. It is hardly ever fully implemented in every craniosacral session and may in fact stretch over several treatment sessions. I recommend that you assess and treat what the child can handle without stress.

When you are hands-on in your application of touch, the craniosacral-specific assessment and treatment merge into each other. To a certain extent the assessment already acts as treatment, and while you are performing a technique, you are simultaneously listening to the reaction—and therefore assessing once again.

Respect for the child is always foundational: treat the child in a way that it feels safe in the room and is able trust you, and so that it can also codetermine the tempo and the content of the assessment and treatment. In detail:

1. Slow down: decelerate your own tempo.
2. Allow the child time to orient itself, to arrive in the room.
3. Begin by looking for what is healthy in the child.
4. Visual findings: does anything stand out when you briefly inspect the child? For example, look at the eyes; does the child have a squint?
5. Speak directly to the child.
6. Ask for permission to be allowed to make touch contact.
7. Respect the answer if you receive one.
8. If possible, treat the child and the mother because they are very close to each other and spend a great deal of time together.
9. Bring your own hand close to the child, perhaps offering a finger first. Gently sound out together with the child the various qualities of touch and make a note of what the child likes and dislikes. Agreeable touch can become a resource.
10. Then look at the symmetry and tonus of the child's body, its reflexes, and the craniosacral rhythm, and use your hands to invite the fluids and the potency to release any restrictions.
11. Of these suggestions, use only those that the child finds agreeable.

If the child likes lying on its front or on its side, you can:

• Assess the sacrum, the spinal column, and the occipital bone.
• Support the spinal column more specifically: with one hand, establish contact with the child's sacrum or occipital bone. Using the thumb and index finger of your other hand carefully and subtly touch each vertebra. Without pressure, sense the position and inherent mobility, with the intentional objective that each vertebra should position itself in the most balanced way possible. Starting from the lowest lumbar vertebra, slowly touch each vertebra in this way up as far as the thoracic spine and the seventh cervical

vertebra, also called the vertebra prominens. Depending on the age of the child, you may also touch the spinous processes of the bottom three cervical vertebrae. Remain longer at any abnormal locations, but ensure that this particular treatment does not last for too long—about five to ten minutes, depending on the experience and the reaction. It can also be used as a change from the supine position or to round off a pediatric session.

With the child lying on its back with knees flexed, use soft, gentle, and lightly flowing rocking movements to assess:

- the mobility of the pelvis, sacrum, sacroiliac joints, and hips
- the mobility of the lumbar spine
- whether the pelvis is horizontal or tilted in leg length inequality
- the mobility of the abdomen
- the regions of the torso, for example below and above the diaphragm, for mobility and symmetry

With the child's legs extended, assess as follows:

- What are the visual and palpatory findings for the legs, feet, knees, and pelvic symmetry?
- How are the respiratory rhythm and craniosacral rhythm palpable at the feet, knees, or thighs?
- How free is the tissue in the pelvic region?
- Can the craniosacral rhythm be palpated simultaneously at the sacrum and the occipital bone? This can be done with the child lying on its back, front, or side.
- How free are the left and right hips?
- How free are the sacroiliac joints and sacrum?
- How free are the lumbosacral region and the thoracolumbar region?

Go with the craniosacral rhythm at the sacrum and sides of the pelvis and intentionally synchronize it gently.

Slightly raise the child's feet, and then assess the individual segments: using soft, gentle, and flowing rocking movements, first assess as far as the pelvis how free or restricted the pelvic segment is; how mobile are the joints and the surrounding ligaments and muscles? Then assess the abdominal segment, the thoracic segment, and the cervical segment: how free are they? Do not use this technique where hypermobility is present. Then move the child's legs flat again.

How free or fixed is the dural tube? This can be assessed with the child lying on its back, front, or side.

Afterward, the transverse layers of connective tissue or segment transitions can be released, or you can continue as follows:

- How free are the liver, kidneys, and other organs such as the gallbladder, stomach, spleen, and pelvic organs?
- Support digestion by placing one hand on the child's belly and slowly moving it in a clockwise direction over the stomach. This encourages peristalsis and relaxes the large intestine.
- How free and permeable is the diaphragm region, meaning the inferior thoracic aperture?
- Take hold of the child's thorax laterally and from behind, and test the mobility of each rib individually and of the thorax as a whole.
- With one hand, gently touch the solar plexus and stomach region, including the costal arch and diaphragm region, and listen; with your other hand, slowly and gently touch the neck region.
- Use two fingers of one hand or the thumb and index finger of both hands to test the position, structure and quality, and mobility of the clavicles.
- Assess the position and mobility of the shoulders, the arms, the entire superior thoracic aperture, and the thorax as a whole (peripheral release of the thorax and shoulder-neck region is depicted in fig. 22.11).
- How free is the cervical region, specifically the hyoid bone?
- Gently palpate: how free are the neck and throat region and the

cervical spine? Assess the position of the seventh cervical vertebra and the surrounding muscle tonus.

- What impression is gained with one hand listening in the neck-throat region and the other at the occipital bone? What can you perceive with one hand, with the other hand, and between your hands?

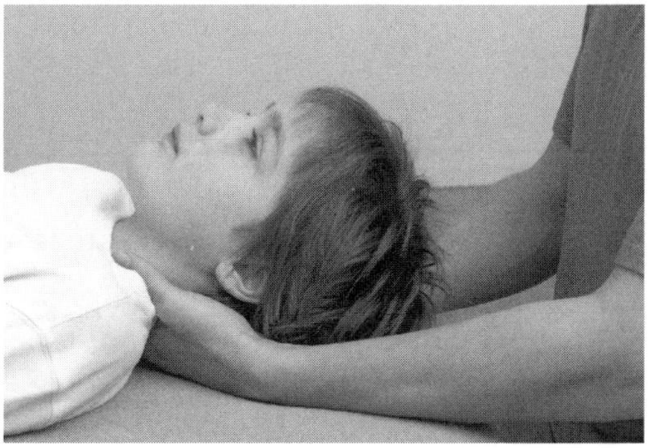

Figure 28.6. Releasing around the seventh cervical vertebra and the neck region.

- Ease the tension in the suboccipital region and the atlanto-occipital joint: position one supple hand transversely in the shoulder-neck region and the other longitudinally beneath the occipital bone and listen. Then, using your hand beneath the occipital bone, invite space and widening.

- How free is the atlanto-occipital joint? Is the second cervical vertebra, also called the axis, free? Is slight rotation in both directions smooth?

- With your hands on the occipital bone: What are the qualities of the craniosacral rhythm? How free is the cranial base?

- Is the occipital squama free? Is it "dancing?"

- How free is the occipital bone itself, and what is the interrelationship between its four constituent parts?

- Assess the position of the two lateral condylar parts around the foramen magnum.

- Next, via the occipital ridge, perform no more than a hint of subtle spreading of the lateral condylar parts, thus creating more space for the foramen magnum, the pons, and the medulla oblongata (for further treatment, see section 28.4, above).

- Using the cradle hold, listen at the occipital bone to the change in structure and motion; in an infant, place your thumbs on the frontal bone.

- Up to about eighteen months after birth, assess the six fontanels: how free and mobile are they?
- What is your overall impression of the head in the cranial vault hold? What is the quality of the motion of the craniosacral rhythm like at several cranial bones overall (see fig. 28.13)?
- What is your impression when you specifically assess and treat individual cranial bones, especially the SBS, the temporal bones, the parietal bones, the frontal bone, and the ethmoid?

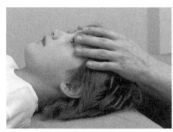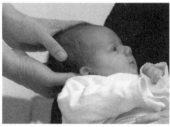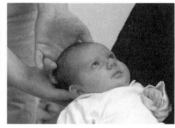

Figure 28.7. Listening to the craniosacral rhythm and releasing the parietal bones using light decompression.

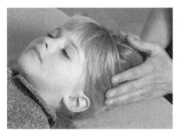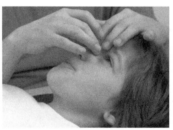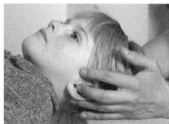

Figure 28.8. Listening to the craniosacral rhythm at the frontal bone and releasing with light decompression.

Figure 28.9. Releasing the frontonasal suture.

Figure 28.10. Evaluating and balancing the craniosacral rhythm at the temporal bones.

- Assess all the cranial bones plus the zygomatic bones. Acting as a kind of shock absorber, the zygomatic bones protect the maxilla, temporal bones, sphenoid, and frontal bone but may also compress these bones.

- Precise, minimal decompression is possible in the area around restrictions and compressions; for example, light decompression of the SBS can be performed via the sphenoid and occipital bone.
- Offer just a suggestion of the gentle ear pull in a posterolateral direction.
- How free are the foramina in terms of blood flow?
- Perform jugular foramen release (see section 28.10, below).
- Is there any compression of the sutures or suture junctions, for example at the asterion or pterion?
- Are there any other abnormalities that require treatment?
- Are the sutures free or fused? Are any sutures compressed? Pay special attention to the occipitomastoid sutures, the lines of junction of the occipital bone with the temporal bone on each side.
- Assess for the presence of intraosseous compression or torsion.
- Assess the dura mater, and treat its tension patterns.
- Palpate the occipital bone and frontal bone together, and listen for any change in structure and motion.

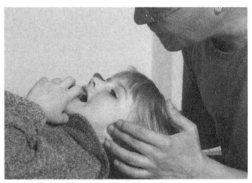

Figure 28.11. Stroking along the course of the masseter.

Intraoral assessment and treatment can be preceded by massaging and stroking the two temporalis muscles and masseters.

Perform intraoral assessment and treatment wearing a finger cot, provided that the child permits it and does not signal any resistance:

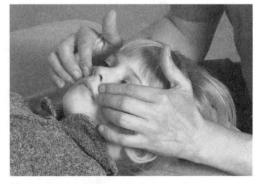

Figure 28.12. Palpating the maxilla and supporting it in harmony with the craniosacral rhythm.

- Test the sucking reflex and its strength.
- How free is the viscerocranium, in particular the maxilla, vomer, and palatine bones? (For a specific description, see the following section, 28.9.)
- To assess the viscerocranium and the cranial base together, how do the maxilla and palatine bones move in relation to the sphenoid and the SBS?
- Examine the facial bones for intraosseous compression.
- Using broad contact of the terminal phalanx of your index finger or little finger on the maxilla, offer light decompression anteriorly, up toward the ceiling if the child is supine.
- With one finger, make contact with the transverse palatine suture while your other hand touches the frontal bone. Listen to the interplay or the craniosacral rhythm of the vertical axis of the maxilla, palatine bones, vomer, ethmoid, and frontal bone, and support it.
- Palpate the flexion and extension of the facial bones as a whole, including the frontal bone; for example, position your index fingers on the maxilla, your middle fingers on the zygomatic bones, your third fingers on the zygomatic arches, and your thumbs on the frontal bone. Listen to the craniosacral rhythm and intentionally synchronize all the facial bones, inviting space, widening, and balance.
- What are the qualities of the craniosacral rhythm? How synchronous is it now in the region of the facial bones as a whole?

Integration of treatment in the head region:

- Use the cranial vault hold, or make contact with one hand at the occipital

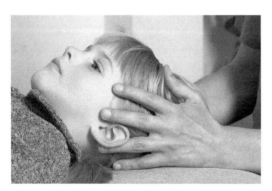

Figure 28.13. Cranial vault hold: evaluating and balancing the craniosacral rhythm.

bone and one hand at the frontal bone: gently "mold" the head in harmony with the motion of the craniosacral rhythm.

- How are the temporal bones moving in harmony with the craniosacral rhythm after assessment and release in the cranial sphere?
- Cranial vault hold: assess, integrate, and perform a before-and-after comparison.
- What is your impression of the condylar parts of the occipital bone, or of the posterior cranial base, following release of the neurocranium and viscerocranium?

Supporting head-torso integration:

- Place one hand transversely under the occipital bone, with two or three fingers of your other hand under the cervical region. Listen supportively.
- How free is the dural tube from the occipital bone as far as the sacrum following treatment of the neurocranium and viscerocranium?
- Perform integration using at least one position on the torso: for example, the diaphragm and solar plexus, cervical region and arm

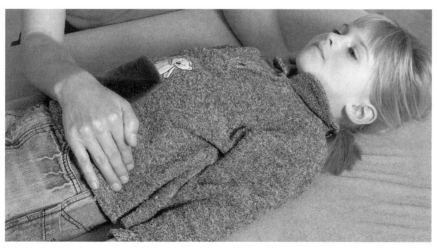

Figure 28.14. Hand contact in the cervical region and using an arm bridge spanning the pelvis to release the sacroiliac joints.

bridge spanning the pelvis, or sacrum and pelvic region. Your intention is balance and harmonization. Establish contact with a connective tissue area of your choice on the child's torso, and support the inherent motion of the tissue, listen with each hand to the structure as well as function and motion, and then listen between your hands: are there any micromovements? How do you perceive the fluids?

With the child lying on its back, front, or side, place one hand at the occipital bone and the other hand at the sacrum:

- Listen to establish whether side-bending or torsion is present at the occipital bone; listen to the motion patterns at the sacrum, and balance them.
- What are the qualities of the motion of the craniosacral rhythm?
- Test the mobility of the spinal column or dural tube; widen the occipital bone cranially and the sacrum caudally in harmony with the craniosacral rhythm.
- Is a stillpoint developing? If so, is it CV4 or EV4?
- Afterward, listen to the craniosacral rhythm or the mid-tide at the legs, knees, or feet, and perform a before-and-after comparison.

Overall comparison: What are the differences between the start of the session and now? In which structures or in which region has there been the greatest release or easing of tension? To what extent is the craniosacral rhythm more harmonious? Has there been or are there any spontaneous stillpoints, or has there been a change to the mid-tide, the fluid body?

Once the treatment session has ended, return the baby to its mother's arms.

After you have gained an overall impression of structure and function and of the self-regulatory capacity of the organism, using elements of the foregoing assessment and treatment options, start each subsequent session by gauging how much has changed since the last craniosacral session with the child. Afterward you can again draw on the wide range of options outlined above.

28.9. Specific Assessment and Treatment of the Viscerocranium

During the baby's journey through the birth canal, compression of varying intensity and duration is exerted in different ways on the baby's cranium and torso. Because of this, specific assessment and treatment of the entire neurocranium and viscerocranium is almost always indicated. Increasing experience will bring a greater sense of safety and trust and will shorten the treatment.

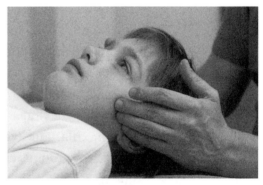

In dysfunctions of the SBS and the cranial base, the cervical and thoracic region and the hyoid bone should ideally be treated first. The masseters and temporal bones should also be included here; in preparation the masseters can be massaged or stroked along their course toward the mandible. Release the tension in the mandible and evaluate and balance the two temporal bones.

Figure 28.15. Massaging or stroking along the course of the masseters.

If possible, during the following assessment and treatment:

- Listen to the craniosacral rhythm or the mid-tide.
- Invite space, widening, and balance.
- Slowly widen your perceptual field from a local focus to adjacent areas, then to the entire head; the head including the cervical region; the head, cervical region, and torso; the whole body globally; and the body together with its biosphere.

- Allow the motion and the fluids, the "inner physician," to do the work.

A specific local assessment and treatment should take account of the following structures of the viscerocranium:

- The facial bones as a whole: palpate flexion and extension, including the frontal bone.
- Zygomatic bones: assess overall mobility and restriction. Are the zygomatic bones floating, or is one or both rigid? Perform release from the outside and from inside the mouth. Following blows to the zygomatic bone, this structure should be assessed and tensions released in order to prevent dysfunctions in the region of the temporal bones, sphenoid, and orbits.
- Nasal bones: assess overall mobility and restriction, listen to the physiological motion in external and internal rotation, and invite decompression.
- Ethmoid: palpate overall mobility and restriction and physiological motion in flexion and extension. Release tensions in the frontal bone, maxilla, and frontonasal suture. Then support and synchronize the craniosacral rhythm at the maxilla and frontal bone simultaneously.
- Lacrimal bones: assess overall mobility and restriction, listen to the physiological motion in external and internal rotation, and invite decompression.
- Orbits: assess overall mobility and restriction as well as physiological motion. Is there any reduction or increase in the size of either orbit in terms of length, breadth, or diagonal dimensions? Invite widening, for example diagonally at the frontal bone and zygomatic bone simultaneously.

Intraorally:

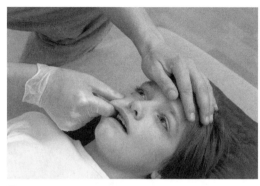

Figure 28.16. Intraoral release of the zygomatic bone.

- Use your index finger or little finger to release tension in the masseter and medial and lateral pterygoid muscles on both sides.
- Gently decompress both zygomatic bones one by one (see fig. 28.16).
- Gently decompress the maxilla, possibly at a forty-five-degree angle, so that the vertical and horizontal sutures gain more space to an equal extent.
- With one index finger or little finger, make contact with the transverse palatine suture while placing your other hand on the child's frontal bone. Next, encourage the interplay by listening to and going with the craniosacral rhythm of the vertical axis, which comprises the maxilla, palatine bones, vomer, ethmoid, and frontal bone, and synchronize and support the motion.
- At the maxilla, listen to and balance flexion and extension as well as external rotation and internal rotation.
- Perform decompression and release of the maxilla and vomer while simultaneously using one hand to stabilize the sphenoid at the greater sphenoid wings or at the frontal bone. Depending on the child's age, use the index finger or the little finger of your other hand to establish contact with the midline of the hard palate, and position the thumb of that hand outside the mouth immediately under the child's nose. Use gentle decompression and invite release.
- Using your index finger or little finger, establish contact with the hard palate at the midline of the maxilla or median palatine suture, and attune yourself to the motion of the vomer. With your other hand, span the child's frontal bone, for example, or contact the sphenoid wings with two fingers. Via the vomer, make contact, vertically upward or superiorly, with the rostrum of the sphenoid,

the body of the sphenoid, the pituitary in the sella turcica, and then via the pituitary stalk with the hypothalamus. Invite space and widening. The craniosacral rhythm supports this process in flexion/external rotation, the mid-tide in the inhalation phase.

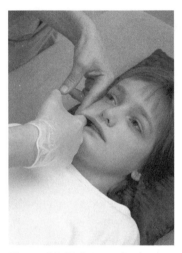

Figure 28.17. Intraoral release of the masseter.

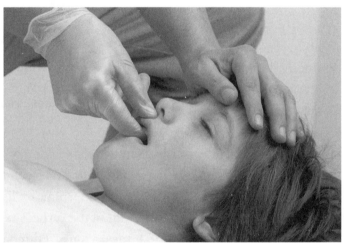

Figure 28.18. Intraoral release of the maxilla and vomer while stabilizing the frontal bone.

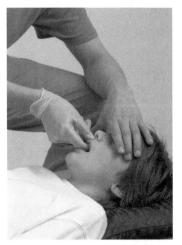

Figure 28.19. Intraoral release of the maxilla and vomer while stabilizing the sphenoid.

- Treat the left and right palatine bones individually. Make contact with the bone level of the palatine bone but do not under any circumstances apply compression toward the orbit. Using your index finger or little finger, begin by testing and improving lateral mobility; afterward, deliver subtle decompression in the direction of the maxilla or mouth. This creates more space between the palatine bones and the pterygoid processes, which also eases the tension on the pterygopalatine ganglion, among other things. Afterward, decompress the maxilla once again, as described above, or, if it is already released, balance it at once.

- Mandible: do not apply touch to the TMJs because they will be released together with the mandible. Start by listening to the spontaneous release of the mandible. If it is highly restricted, you can begin by releasing it using gentle decompression directed toward the point of the child's chin. As the restriction starts to be released, listen to the inherent motion of the mandible and go with it in an attentive and spacious way.

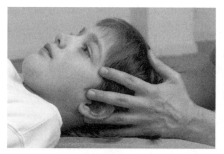

Figure 28.20. Cranial vault hold: integrating the neurocranium.

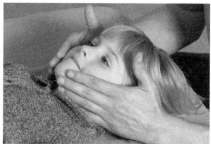

Figure 28.21. Releasing the mandible, suprahyoid muscles, and TMJs.

After specific treatment in the facial region, assess its effects on the neurocranium:

- Assess any symmetries or asymmetries of bones. Is there a balance of tension in the membranes? How do you sense the fluctuations of all bodily fluids together with the CSF?
- Integration: using the cranial vault hold, assess the head as a whole, perhaps molding and harmonizing with the motion of the craniosacral rhythm.
- Is a spontaneous stillpoint becoming established? If so, is it a CV4 or an EV4?
- Integrate the treatment at the torso, pelvis, and sacrum or at the feet. If a spontaneous stillpoint has not developed during the final quarter of the session, listen to the craniosacral rhythm or the mid-tide in the pelvic region or at the feet and invite a stillpoint.

28.10. Jugular Foramen and Occipitomastoid Suture Release

Releasing the temporal bones and the occipital bone from adhesions and compressions creates more space for the occipitomastoid sutures and the jugular foramina. About eighty-five percent of venous blood flows via the paired jugular foramina from the interior of the cranium to the sigmoid sinus, and then via the internal jugular veins toward the heart. Each jugular foramen also affords passage for cranial nerves IX, X, and XI as well as for blood vessels. Their function can be supported, among other things, using the gentle ear pull technique and subsequent specific jugular foramen release. These techniques are valuable in infants with sucking and swallowing disorders to support cardiac and pulmonary function and all autonomic processes, especially digestion. They can also be used where there are difficulties in the cervical or shoulder region and with head rotation.

28.10.1. Method

To release the two jugular foramina, position yourself at the child's head. In order to be able to perform the release technique with adequate subtlety, sit high up and sufficiently close to the end of the table. The child should be lying not too far down on the treatment table.

Place one hand transversely beneath the occipital bone and stabilize it without compressing any suture in the process. Place your other hand loosely on the table on the other side of the head, close to the child's ear.

Next release the jugular foramen using your hand beneath the occipital bone to slowly deliver subtle but clear lateral traction, while your other hand simultaneously performs a gentle ear pull, for example slightly posterolaterally. In this way greater space and widening is offered at the horizontal or transverse level on both sides. In the process the simultaneous traction that draws the occipital bone and ear apart should be even and steady; you may need to ask the child if it feels pleasant. During this release technique, again listen to the inherent motion of the structures. If the structure on one side or the other stops during widening, maintain steady traction: do not reduce or increase the lateral traction. Slowly disengage the bilateral sideways traction after about twenty to sixty seconds. Then perform release on the other side using the same technique.

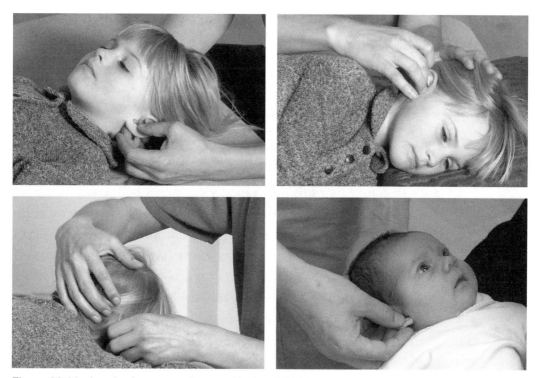

Figure 28.22. Jugular foramen release with the child lying on its back, front, or side, or in its mother's arms.

The gentle ear pull along with jugular foramen and occipitomastoid suture release on both left and right sides can also be performed with the child seated or lying in its mother's arms or in her lap. In that scenario, adjust your stance and hand position accordingly to meet the demands of the situation. Here too you should be attentive, flexible, and go with the possible head movements of the child.

In my practice, when using these two techniques, I also accept the possibility that the child might not like them or that they might be applied for only five to ten seconds instead of thirty seconds because the child is moving around too much. However, initial release can also be achieved after only a relatively short time. And it may be that further opportunities to release these structures will present themselves during the current or subsequent session. Under no circumstances should release techniques be performed for too long—especially if the structures are already free—because overstimulation must be avoided.

28.11. Releasing the Intracranial Membranes

Releasing the parietal bones, temporal bones, frontal bone, and occipital bone also eases the tension on the dura mater, the membranous structure that fills the cranial vault like a balloon. The intracranial membranes—the falx cerebri, falx cerebelli, and tentorium cerebelli—can be released even more specifically. The tentorium cerebelli will already have been released, for example, as you performed the gentle ear pull, released the two jugular foramina, and balanced the craniosacral rhythm at the temporal bones. The tension in the falx cerebri will already have been reduced by the frontal lift and parietal lift as well as release of the frontonasal suture; and tension in the falx cerebelli will have been eased by treating the occipital bone, for example by atlanto-occipital release and by spreading the occipital condyles.

The following techniques for releasing the intracranial membranes in children effects as a venous-sinus drainage, so that the used blood can better drain. This also increases the exchange of liquor. It can be applied to reduce, for example, headache, growth and developmental disorders, torticollis, scoliosis, and back problems. The balance of forces acting on the dural tube is also dependent on the balance of forces acting on the intracranial membranes, and vice versa. As envelopes protecting the CNS, the meninges also react to stress. For this reason, the specific release of membrane tension can also act to reduce cerebral and autonomic disorders. If the child finds treatment of the bony cranium unpleasant, the bone level may be touched only lightly, and intention can be directed toward release at the membrane level.

In infants the motility and mobility of the intracranial membranes helps to resolve cranial compression that may have arisen during the birth process. The bones are relatively soft, the fontanels are still open, and the sutures are starting to become increasingly developed. For this reason I do not use the following technique to treat the intracranial membranes in children who are less than one year old. In children less than one year old I assess and treat the cranium and membranes as a whole, possibly combined with jugular foramen release or other specific techniques, all of which are performed so gently that they constitute little more than a suggestion. Along with the other intracranial membranes, the tentorium cerebelli is also released, which consequently also eases the tension on the jugular foramen.

When you are treating infants and children, adapt your finger position to the size of the child's head. Of greater importance than pinpoint accurate positioning, however, are the prerequisites that the practitioner does not exert any pressure whatsoever, is personally relaxed, and has a very supple touch. You will treat predominantly using intention and perception.

For the following membrane release techniques, the child may be on its back, front, or side; infants may be held in their mother's arms or over her shoulder.

Preparation: if possible, assess and treat the sacrum, dural tube, diaphragm and solar plexus, superior thoracic aperture, and atlantooccipital joint. Various cranial release positions can also be used in preparation. Sacrum and cradle holds may also suffice as a simple preparatory step.

Practitioner's position: at the child's head, usually seated, or, exceptionally, standing to treat the most posterior part of the falx cerebri. Before taking up each finger position or contact, always check your optimal sitting position and height and your distance from the table.

Child's position: lying on its back, although lying on its front may be an alternative.

28.11.1. Releasing the Falx Cerebelli

Approaching from each side, insert your hands underneath the child's occipital bone. Lightly place the terminal phalanges of your fingers in broad contact on the external occipital crest, with the tips of your fingers touching. Start by positioning the terminal phalanges of your index fingers broadly on the occipital ridge. Then position the terminal phalanges of your other fingers so as to follow the anatomical structure of the occipital bone vertically along the course of the falx cerebelli. Your thumbs play no part and exert no pressure at all on the cranial base or cervical region. Using the broad placement of your supple phalanges, make a suggestion of contact via the scalp and bone with the structure of the falx cerebelli. Listen to the motion of the CSF and membranes, and invite release.

28.11.2. Releasing the Tentorium Cerebelli

From the head end of the table, insert your hands underneath the child's occipital bone in such a way that your terminal phalanges are positioned at the level of the external occipital protuberance laterally to the right and left. In this broad contact position, the terminal phalanges of your two little fingers touch each other on the external occipital protuberance, and your third and middle fingers are placed laterally along the attachment of the tentorium cerebelli to the occipital bone and the petrous part of the temporal bone. The soft tips of the terminal phalanges of your index fingers are the most laterally placed contact points. Once again make a suggestion of contact and invite release. Depending on the size of the child's head, treatment is usually given in two stages, working outward from the middle.

28.11.3. Releasing the Falx Cerebri

Before each new finger position, check your sitting position and height and your distance from the table. Treat the entire attachment surface of the falx cerebri from back to front as far as the crista galli. Take your hand position using an approach from the sides. Position the touching soft tips of your terminal phalanges broadly along the line of the falx cerebri. You can reach the posterior part, as close as possible to the external occipital protuberance, using the soft tips of the terminal phalanges of your index fingers, and possibly your middle fingers. In the first position, the child's head is lying on the treatment table and on your relaxed terminal phalanges in their broad placement. Following the curvature of the child's head, your other fingers are located correspondingly higher along the line of the sagittal suture. In the vicinity of the bregma point and frontal bone, support your elbows on the table at each side before you position the soft tips of your terminal phalanges along the line of the frontal or metopic suture.

This release of the intracranial membranes may be combined with release of the frontomaxillary or nasal suture, the gentle ear pull, and jugular foramen release. It may also be integrated, for example, with the cradle hold, release of the dural tube and sacrum, and stillpoint invitation or induction.

If you do not yet have any practical experience as a craniosacral practitioner in this area with adults, you are advised to attend an appropriate course, and it is not recommended that you apply these techniques in children. Other technical variations for release of the intracranial membranes can also be found in the textbooks by Torsten Liem.[2]

28.12. Tour of the Ventricles

The tour of the ventricles often improves the strength or force of the CSF, the fluid drive of the craniosacral system. It is used, for example, if the craniosacral rhythm or the mid-tide is relatively weak despite craniosacral system release—a phenomenon that may be encountered after pharmacological therapy, illness, inflammation, immunization, or surgical procedures. Among other things, the tour of the ventricles helps to remove waste materials from the brain. It can be employed in situations where CV4 as a fluctuation technique is contraindicated or is unpleasant for the child. Children with delayed development or with learning difficulties have also responded positively to the tour of the ventricles.

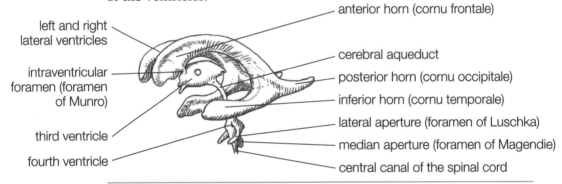

left and right lateral ventricles

intraventricular foramen (foramen of Munro)

third ventricle

fourth ventricle

anterior horn (cornu frontale)

cerebral aqueduct

posterior horn (cornu occipitale)

inferior horn (cornu temporale)

lateral aperture (foramen of Luschka)

median aperture (foramen of Magendie)

central canal of the spinal cord

Figure 28.23. Lateral view of the cerebral ventricles.

The more often you have used the tour of the ventricles yourself, the more readily you can undertake the tour in the child. It is helpful to possess detailed anatomical knowledge of the cerebral ventricles. The tour of the ventricles can begin at the fourth ventricle, the transitional point from the external to the internal CSF spaces, and then proceed up the cerebral aqueduct to the third ventricle, and then to the lateral ventricles in turn. Equally, the tour of the ventricles can be undertaken in the opposite direction: begin in the cerebrum by picturing one lateral ventricle with its central part, anterior horn, posterior horn, and inferior horn, then after retracing your steps via the interventricular foramen and the anterior superior roof of the third ventricle, proceed to the other lateral ventricle. The narrow but tall third ventricle in the diencephalon—with the terminal lamina, the anterior floor of the hypothalamus with contact to the optic chiasm and the pituitary stalk, and the interior walls of the two thalamic regions—has contact in its posterior part with the pineal gland; after this, semi-obliquely downward, comes the cerebral aqueduct, which leads to the fourth ventricle. This is situated between the pons, cerebellum, and medulla oblongata. It has various apertures: laterally are the two foramina of Luschka, and somewhat deeper is the median aperture, also called the foramen of Magendie. These three apertures form the connections between the internal and external CSF spaces.

In the tour of the ventricles, instead of specifically sensing or visualizing regions from the fourth ventricle upward or regions from the lateral ventricles to the third ventricle, you may also be surprised where your attention draws you once you start to sense or visualize your ventricular system. In his time, Sutherland was already instructing his students to imagine themselves as a minnow making its way through this system filled with fresh CSF. You might therefore also imagine a minnow that swallows old brain cells or nibbles away at the ventricle walls to remove deposits from previous inflammations as well as toxins, narcotics, and chemical medications. In this way you are able to clean up the walls of the ventricles. In addition, the liver and kidneys can be supported.

28.13. Contacting the Amygdalae

As a further variation, you might contact the corpus amygdaloideum, the amygdala: the inferior horn of the lateral ventricle, also called the cornu temporale, is located in the region of the temporal lobe. An extension of the most anterior part of the inferior horn, the amygdala forms the inferior arcuate terminal part of the hippocampal formation. From the anterior part of the inferior horn, you can attune to the amygdala. Once you have this in your consciousness, invite space and widening. You are ready to receive and waiting relaxed in the neutral. Attune yourself to the craniosacral rhythm or the mid-tide and Long Tide while you watch to see whether there are any changes in the child. Perhaps it is breathing in and out more deeply, or the atmosphere in the room becomes more peaceful. There may be a spontaneous discharge in the form of a twitch and then deeper relaxation; a stillpoint is established, or the fluid drive of the craniosacral rhythm or the mid-tide becomes more clearly perceptible. Here it is important for you as practitioner to regulate your distance appropriately: under no circumstances should you be positioned too closely or intentionally induce impulses in the amygdala from outside.

28.14. Evaluating Stress in Infants

Mother and child build up a symbiotic relationship during pregnancy that persists for some time after childbirth due to the total dependence of the baby on the mother. This relationship changes gradually as the child develops. Because of this shared intimate period and the child's dependent status, many children react verbally and nonverbally during the initial interview when the mother is asked whether anything of note occurred during the period covering conception, pregnancy, the birth itself, and the immediate postnatal phase. During the general assessment of the overall situation or the craniosacral-specific assessment of the child, if the mother is recounting a very uncomfortable topic, the emotional burden and stress factors in the child may be revealed in the following ways:

- Breathing may become more superficial or more rapid, falter, stop, or suddenly change in some other way.
- There may be a very rapid change in gaze and body tonus.
- The craniosacral rhythm may stop—due to stress, rather than due to a stillpoint resulting from reorganization.

These are indications that the child is physically or psychologically stressed by the topic being addressed and is showing a strong physical reaction.

28.15. The Child's Capacity for Self-Attachment

Provided that self-attachment has not been disturbed immediately after birth, this resource will support the child on a somatic, psychological, and neurophysiological level. In concrete terms this expresses itself in the baby in intact sleeping and sucking patterns, optimal digestive function, coordinated movements, and a greater facility and effectiveness in learning from new experiences.

The cause of stress for the baby may lie in the interruption of self-attachment, which is the ability to sense "inwardly" and thus to remain connected, or in poor bonding with its immediate caregivers. Disturbance of self-attachment produces confusion or shock in the baby and consequently leads to symptoms that may admittedly be superficially treated by pharmacological means but whose root cause may often remain hidden.

For example, if you notice that the child's crawling movements lack coordination and that afterward it loses all contact and starts to scream, this may point to problems in self-attachment. It is quite possible, for example, that because she was given analgesics or an anesthetic, the mother may no longer recall the first hour after delivery and is therefore unable to provide any information. However, the child's body, as well as its subconscious, does not forget what has interrupted the instinctive drive to round off an essential need.

In your treatment, as you consider the immediate needs of the child and hold the topic of self-attachment after birth in your perceptual field, you can offer the child opportunities to explore that will encourage both its self-attachment as well as its contact with the mother.

At that time the baby may initially want to express its disquiet by screaming; afterward, as dictated by its need, it may want to sense belly-to-belly skin contact with the mother and later to be breast-fed for a sufficiently long period. The practitioner supports the baby's efforts and also communicates with the mother in the process. With the support of the practitioner and the mother, over the course of one or more sessions, the child can resume and harmoniously round off, complete, and deepen the previously interrupted process of self-attachment. Anyone who has not already witnessed this on several occasions may perhaps find it hard to believe that as a result, many of the child's symptoms can be alleviated or resolved within a few hours or days. In particular, Raymond F. Castellino and William Emerson have made valuable contributions in this area in terms of our under-standing of these primary dynamics and their repercussions.[3]

28.16. Rounding Off the Birth Process Properly

The particular therapeutic processes that unfold during a series of craniosacral treatment sessions and the intensity with which this may happen depend on a variety of factors: the momentary state of the child, for example drowsy or upset; its temperament; and its trust in the surroundings and in the practitioner—but also on how greatly the child has been affected by the birth process as a whole, from the first contractions through to the bonding phase after delivery. With-out prompting, many babies very quickly seek to repeat unwinding movements similar to those undertaken during the birth process. I have also witnessed this phenomenon in infants and school-age chil-dren, and even in adults, if they relax and let go or evidently come into contact with the cause of their primary pain. Everyday situations that have a similar dynamic to the birth process, such as excessive pressure or pushing, a sense of constriction, no longer being able to make headway, can—albeit subconsciously—remind babies and sensitive children or adults of the threshold experience of birth and activate its content or intensity.

With resource-oriented support, this rounding off does not retraumatize but can act in a liberating way. There is the opportunity both for the child and the adult to experience anew the birth-related issues of the past, but this time in a safe therapeutic setting. In this process, with a gesture or with unwinding that emanates from within, they can experience their own birth in a new and more rounded way (see figs. 28.24 and 28.26).

Incessantly crying babies in particular frequently become calm if, in conjunction with cranial release, the dural tube is allowed to unwind, bringing a reduction in the intensity of traumatic activation during the birth process.

As a practitioner you should watch to see whether there are any micromovements, resulting from impulses of the cell memory, that develop into movement patterns that are consistent with unwinding.

If the child enters a birth process during the craniosacral session, support this in a resource-oriented way, for example by helping to determine the correct tempo with brief pauses, or sometimes verbally supporting the child and thus guiding it through its therapeutic process. As stated earlier, the journey from the treatment table to the floor mattress during a session can symbolize the passage through the birth canal; for example, it activates the balance function and cranial nerve VIII, which is responsible for hearing and balance. If the mother's self-attachment is sufficiently strong, if she is sufficiently connected with her own resources and not overwhelmed by the situation, the practitioner can involve her in the therapeutic process for a time.

If a baby cries protractedly during the session and there is no change, do not allow the baby to go on crying for too long; instead, help it in its orientation by speaking to it, seeking eye contact, offering it a finger, and adjusting the quality of your touch. If the situation continues unchanged and the baby cries or screams incessantly, take deliberate action to modify the situation. For example, assist the child

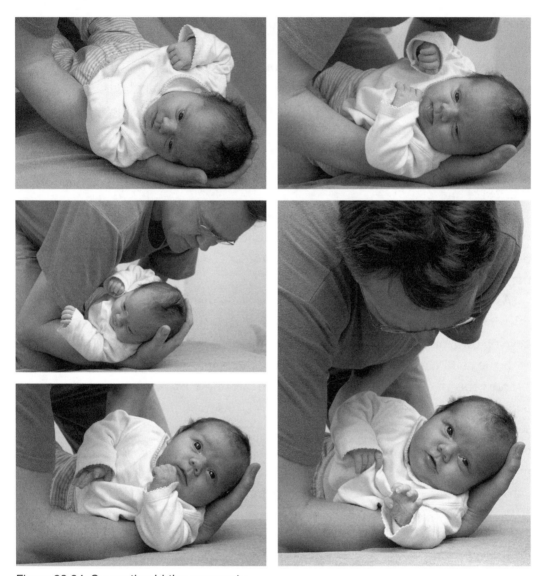

Figure 28.24. Supporting birth movements.

into a more agreeable body position, or give the child to the mother to cradle in her arms and speak to or to soothe by rocking in its carriage. Take care not to expose the child to too many new stimuli by implementing too many changes.

As the craniosacral practitioner, you do not always have to be in hands-on contact with the child; however, you must remain in emotional and energetic contact with the child and the mother. At the same time, continuously regulate your distance to make sure it is correct. The child must be able to sense the neutral presence and benevolent support of the practitioner so that:

- It can shed tears over its difficult delivery.
- Cell memories can resolve spontaneously with spiraling unwinding movements.
- Inertial fulcrums and dysfunctions can resolve during a stillpoint or in the stillness.
- Homeostasis is strengthened, and the craniosacral rhythm and midtide become more balanced.

Would the child like to slide down from the treatment table onto the floor? In this playful sliding down from the table onto a mattress on the floor, aside from the play element, the child also has the opportunity to engage with a certain amount of excitement. In this game the child can explore its agility and sense of balance and face the novelty of a challenge that might perhaps also entail just a hint of fear. I support the child like a plane touching down, as it lands safely on the mattress "runway" and, having landed, experiences release and relaxation. The sliding down from the table game also simulates the birth process, in which the head is directed downward and balance and gravity play a role. It often happens that children want to repeat the experience several times. I then invite the child to try out a number of variations and to consciously experience the different phases with me. At the start of this exercise, I demonstrate it as I would do it, and then leave it up to the child whether to imitate me or to do it in its own way.

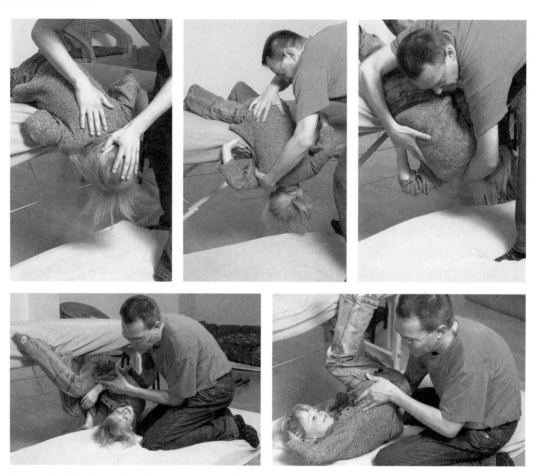

Figure 28.25. Playfully sliding down from the treatment table.

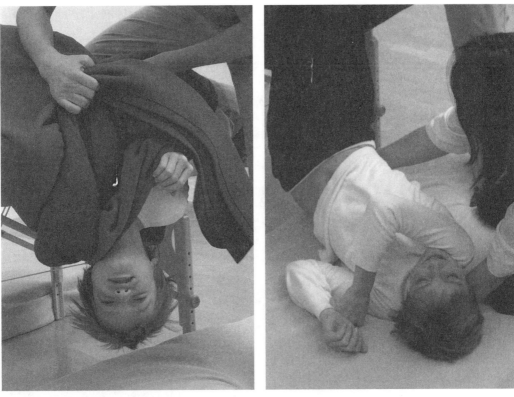

Figure 28.26. Playfully sliding down from the treatment table: rounding off the birth process properly.

28.17. Offering Rebonding

In the right circumstances the craniosacral practitioner can set the scene again for various forms of bonding. For example, the mother-child encounter involving slow, undisturbed skin-to-skin contact can be reenacted and can make an essential contribution to healing for both parties. The child lies with its belly exposed on the naked belly of the mother, who caresses it lovingly. Touching, skin-to-skin contact, and the pressure and warmth on the bellies of the mother and the child cause oxytocin levels in the brains of both to rise. This "love hormone" stimulates in the baby a readiness to explore and search for its mother's breast, while the mother's blood pressure falls and she becomes calmer as she devotes herself intensively to her child. This enables intimate mother-child contact to take place or to become even more profound.

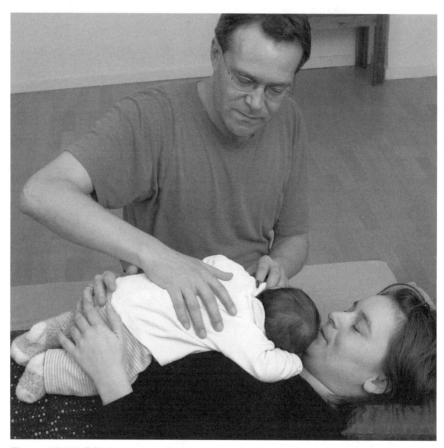

Figure 28.27. Offering rebonding.

HEALING TOUCH FOR CHILDREN WITH PHYSICAL OR MENTAL DISABILITIES

29

A physical or mental disability that is present from birth onward is almost always of genetic origin or attributable to problems that arose during pregnancy or the birth process. It may also be the result of an accident or illness. Disabilities may have detrimental effects on the craniosacral system. Conversely, a poorly functioning craniosacral system may also be counted among the causes of disability. When stress develops later, the nervous system reacts increasingly with impairment or malfunction.

In terms of the diagnosis of conditions that become apparent only later in life, we are faced with the question of when an individual can be deemed "ill." Such an assessment may well be important for pathogenesis, medical diagnosis, and disability insurance. For me, as a craniosacral practitioner, people with what might be termed a disability are simply different. They enable healthy adults to face up to differentness and to gauge how tolerant and compassionate we truly are in our behavior toward these different people. In this process, "normal" adults are challenged both in terms of their patience and the authenticity of their compassion. "Disabled" people rarely bear a grudge and very often display a refreshing spontaneity and a quite considerable capacity for love that can be immensely attractive.

Disabled children should be supported at the earliest possible stage with Craniosacral Therapy provided by a fully qualified practitioner, and where feasible, this should be done during the initial months of life. However, this is no substitute for conventional allopathic medical treatment and will not cure Down syndrome or other serious forms of disability. However, long-term Craniosacral Therapy during the first four years of life provides enormous support for the child's overall development and helps it to build up and establish adequate resources at an early stage. Even after age four, eight, or twelve, children with a disability can be helped in terms of their essential condition and development. Treatment given at a later age serves primarily to support autonomic processes, reflected in the child's well-being, calmness, and joy. All this strengthens the child's immune system so that any infections developed are less frequent and of shorter duration.

Children with congenital or acquired disability often have functional impairments with regard to breathing, sucking, chewing, and swallowing (see sections 19.3 and 20.5 for more on the subject of sucking and swallowing disorders). Depending on the type of disability, these children may have a tendency to kyphosis, an abnormal rounded curvature of the spine, or scoliosis, which is lateral curvature of the spine. For example, the thoracic spine may show an excessive and permanent forward curvature. Certain conditions such as cerebral palsy, poliomyelitis, and rickets tend to lead to weak or unilaterally developed musculature and to postural anomalies, and hence to changes in individual vertebral bones, resulting in scoliosis. Dysfunctions involving the sphenoid, occipital bone, and sacrum also have repercussions on the dural tube and may give rise to postural problems. The craniosacral practitioner needs to assess and treat the regions in question. In cases where there is a tendency to childhood autism, it is necessary in particular to include the entire cranial base together with both temporal bones. During and after the session, a freer craniosacral rhythm and a more harmonious fluid body will assist the bodily structures to start to achieve greater balance from the inside out.

Young children with Down syndrome, also called trisomy 21, often have generally poor and floppy muscle tonus that is frequently reflected in sucking problems. Interdisciplinary collaboration with a physiotherapist, occupational therapist, or speech therapist is helpful in this context. Children with Down syndrome present with a broad spectrum of disability. The degree of disability cannot be predicted at birth. Sometimes the tongue protrudes from the mouth, perhaps indicating a cranial problem, such as deformity of the occipital bone and its condyles. Regular craniosacral sessions will increase the child's oxygen supply, making mouth-breathing less necessary.

Children with Down syndrome and other disabilities often also have a narrowing of the facial and nasal region and small nostrils. Nasal breathing therefore needs to be encouraged. Comprehensive treatment of the viscerocranium will include the maxilla, palatine bones, vomer, frontonasal suture, zygomatic bones, and the orbits. In addition, the entire respiratory supply system should be supported by releasing access to the pharynx, the cervical region, and the shoulder-neck region, and by providing visceral treatment for the lungs. The mandible, floor of the mouth, and hyoid bone should also be released in craniosacral sessions. When treating the front of the body, you should also release the neck region—and once you have treated the top, you should also include the bottom. In this way you will integrate the changes simultaneously. See section 21.3 for information about the social nervous system and section 30.26 on Sinusitis.

The earlier and the more regularly a child with a disability receives Craniosacral Therapy, the more advantageous this will be for the development of the structures mentioned. This has a huge effect on the child's health because the easier it is to deliver a proper air supply, the less danger there will be of oxygen deficiency—during sleep, for example—which might lead to further brain damage.

The needs of the child must be respected. It is often the case that a disabled child is not able communicate clearly in words. You must therefore pay attention to body language and to the autonomic responses to treatment. The body tells you how the child is doing, for example, by changes in breathing, muscle tonus, or temperature. If you are present with all your senses open, you can perceive the overall state and mood of the child and are able to gauge from the autonomic responses whether your touch is still desirable.

KEY POINT

In principle, in cases of disability, the point of Craniosacral Therapy is to alleviate the accompanying symptoms. As a result the child's potential is more likely to be set free, and its physical, mental, and spiritual development will be promoted. The child is then supported in learning to cope better with functions that may be absent or disturbed.

In cases of severe disability or distress, Craniosacral Therapy can be used in an attempt to improve quality of life so that the child can become more contented and increasingly able to make contact with its surroundings.

29.1. Healing Touch at One Single Body Site

Children with physical or mental disability sometimes cannot cope with treatment that lasts for longer than fifteen minutes, and they often find it disagreeable to be touched at multiple body sites. They react to this with restlessness, by adopting a defensive posture, or with an altered (slowed or accelerated) breathing pattern.

The voluntary participation of the child and the calm attitude of the practitioner are crucially important. Have faith in the capacity for self-regulation instead of trying to force something specific. This will also enable your touch to be perceived by the disabled child as pleasant and as bringing healing. When choosing the body site to be touched first, remember that locations that are most affected by the disability are less suitable. However, you might begin by slowly and gently touching a knee, a hand, a place on the back, a shoulder, or the shoulder-neck region. Ask the child for permission to touch this site or give notice of your intention to touch. The contact of your hand should be clear as well as stabilizing and spacious. As you apply your touch, pay attention to the reaction of the child and of the body site you are touching. Often the child will sense your touch for a few moments and will assess instinctively whether this might be agreeable or disagreeable. The breathing pattern and autonomic reactions will indicate how the child is feeling. If there is no clear sign that your touch is being rejected, continue with it.

Allow yourself and the child sufficient space and time. For the next three to ten minutes while you are applying touch, it may be that nothing obvious is happening or changing, or that the child reacts with its individual therapeutic process of activation-buildup and deactivation-release. It may be that the site you are touching becomes harder initially before softening later, or it may grow very warm or begin to pound—a sign indicative of a therapeutic pulse. The child may reveal its feelings or its difficult situation more clearly; it may tremble briefly or communicate through spontaneous sounds. Go with the child as it oscillates naturally back and forth between buildup and discharge, tension and release. Afterward, something will have changed both at the physical level and at the mental-spiritual level.

In order to anchor this new state, continue with your touch contact for a few moments longer. You will then probably give the child some advance notice before slowly disengaging your touch. After the initial back-and-forth and balancing, this process of self-regulation may reveal itself a second time. Go with it again until it is rounded off and established. However, it is imperative to watch for a suitable moment to disengage your touch contact at the right time: under no circumstances should you induce too much. You should facilitate maximal self-regulation using minimal stimulation and support instead of taking the child into deeper processes that might overwhelm or frighten it.

Even after you have ended your touch contact and have physically introduced some distance, remain with your heart and your perception for a few more moments with the child. What is your self-perception like now? How is the child? How is its body posture and mood now? Your subsequent verbal contact and your invitation to the child to take notice of its surroundings or to drink something will help the child to orient itself well in the outside world.

This short treatment can be very relaxing and releasing for the child. For the craniosacral practitioner it can serve as a gateway to treating the disabled child.

SELECTED INDICATIONS, WITH POINTERS FOR CRANIOSACRAL THERAPY

30

I have often asked myself whether short illustrative examples of indications commonly encountered in pediatric Craniosacral Therapy are helpful or whether they perhaps cause practitioners to focus too much on specific scenarios. There is no universally standardized treatment schedule for individual complaints. Fundamentally, treatment in Craniosacral Therapy addresses the whole person and not merely the symptom and the disease. In Craniosacral Therapy we therefore operate primarily in a systems-related manner rather than with a symptom-oriented approach. At the same time we are in direct contact with the child as a whole, and there are various approaches to release that we can use. This also includes stimulating the power of imagination and self-awareness, for example, using dialogue or imaginary journeys during the session.

In no way am I suggesting that pediatric Craniosacral Therapy always helps in all these indications. Nevertheless, I want to include some brief notes on structural associations. The following short sections will broaden your understanding of how craniosacral practitioners can assess and treat structure and function as connected elements. Craniosacral Therapy is both an intuitive and a scientific or empirical method. The greater your understanding and experience of the interrelated nature of the craniosacral system, anatomy, and neuroanatomy, the less you will need a rigid schedule.

At the Sphinx Craniosacral Institute, practitioners are taught not to treat a dysfunction in isolation. After tuning in globally, the common practice is to perform local treatment on the individual regions involved prior to rounding off the treatment again globally. This approach makes it more difficult for the novice, but after years of practice and experience, it becomes all the more worthwhile.

For example, anxiety-related disorders, which affect some ten percent of children in Switzerland, are very often the cause of physical symptoms such as bed-wetting and enuresis, stomachache, and loss of appetite. These complaints may be triggered by unresolved issues with siblings; by problems with school subjects, teachers, and fellow students; or by situations that are perceived to be threatening.

It is important to note that even though a number of selected indications will be addressed specifically in the following pages, the whole body should be assessed, because it is a functional unity. Uneven tensions in the body and in the cranial sphere in particular, due to the birth process, for example, commonly also cause the cerebral vessels to be displaced, twisted, or squashed and compressed. Pressure and traction in the region of the cranial base causes cranial nerve irritation, often adversely affecting cranial nerve function. This can lead to digestive problems with flatulence, vomiting, torticollis and plagiocephaly, or squint. Babies who scream and regurgitate a lot, for example, are often found to have irritation of cranial nerves IX, X, and XI.

What is the position and motion of the sphenoid like? Does the SBS show a particular motion pattern? How free is the cranial base as a whole? It is important that dysfunctions in the body as a whole and in the craniosacral system are released. If incipient functional disturbances do not become too anchored in the child's osseous structures, dental malocclusion, scoliosis, or other dysfunctions are less likely to develop later.

The petrous part of the temporal bone can be regarded as a demarcation line for the mapping and distribution of the cranial nerves. Cranial nerves I to VI are principally affected by functional disorders arising in the anterior half of the cranial base. Disorders involving cranial nerves I to VI frequently occur in conjunction with functional disturbances in the region of the viscerocranium, frontal bone, and sphenoid. Some sections of cranial nerves VII and VIII travel through the petrous part of the temporal bone and can be detrimentally affected by functional disturbances in the various parts of the temporal bone. Cranial nerves IX to XII are commonly affected in functional disturbances of the posterior cranial base.

How free is the motion of the sphenoid, the most central of the cranial bones? Is its motion robust and firm, or is it lightly levitating instead? If it is robust, the bone level is seeking to be preferentially addressed, and if it is levitating, the flexibility and mobility of the membrane level seem primarily to be revealed. How free are the various constituent parts of the cranial base, specifically the SBS, which is a main fulcrum in the craniosacral system?

For ease of reference, the following indications are arranged in alphabetical order.

30.1. ADHD and Difficulties with Concentration and Learning

Blood flow in the frontal part of the brain is often believed to be compromised in ADHD. In any Craniosacral Therapy you should therefore pay particular attention to the position and craniosacral rhythm of the frontal bone and its adjacent structures, including the falx cerebri. In accordance with the holistic nature of treatment, do not focus solely on individual structures but evaluate how the entire craniosacral system and its rhythm is becoming more balanced, and to what extent the child is also prepared to permit treatment using the biodynamic approach.

The dopaminergic system in chaos: from the mesencephalon, important dopaminergic systems ascend to the diencephalon. The mesencephalic zone can be stimulated indirectly using the CV4 technique. Dopamine from neurons in the territory of the third ventricle influences the pituitary. This territory can be supported via the more balanced craniosacral rhythm around the sphenoid and by undertaking a tour of the ventricles. Because dopamine is also involved in the perfusion of the abdominal organs and especially in renal function, these areas can be supported with visceral treatment in an attempt to balance the dopamine system indirectly. By treating the "second brain," especially the gut, as well as the liver and spleen, you will be encouraging areas that are involved in serotonin production, and this can have a mood-elevating effect. For this reason it is valuable always to include the abdominal region in any craniosacral session. Serotonin production also occurs in the hypothalamus, which lies close to the third ventricle and is also stimulated when the craniosacral motion of the sphenoid becomes more balanced.

The intracranial tension membranes are often problematic zones. Moreover, dysfunctions such as torsion are encountered in the region of the occipital bone, the SBS is usually compressed, the temporal bone trapped in internal rotation, and the frontal bone inertial or restricted—overall, patterns such as these are mostly to be treated in the cranial sphere. These patterns often lead to a fascial imbalance in the thoracic region and to dysfunctions involving the sacrum and sacroiliac joints.

From the foregoing remarks, the following possible short treatment sequence emerges: sacrum including arm bridge for the sacroiliac joints, abdominal organs, cervical spine (C1, C2, C3), occipital bone including condyles and atlanto-occipital release, SBS, cranium overall including frontal bone, viscerocranium, followed by rounding off and integration at the head, torso, sacrum, and feet.

Bite abnormalities, via compression, may lead to temporal bone dysfunctions, with potential repercussions on the cortical regions located there.

A range of foodstuffs, especially candy and sweetened beverages, may give rise to metabolic disorders that have implications for the internal organs and to diminished cerebral metabolism in the regions of the cortex and subcortex. To minimize reactions to food additives, the function of the liver and pancreas, kidneys and bladder, lungs, and heart can be stimulated using visceral treatment that serves to promote the mobility and motility of these organs. For a theoretical discussion of this topic, see section 20.9.

30.2. Allergies, Skin Rash, Hay Fever

Once a conventional allopathic medical diagnosis has been made and appropriate allergy tests have been conducted, craniosacral practitioners can support the relevant symptom areas. In addition, it is recommended that the lymphatic system, pulmonary respiration, the function of the large and small intestine, and specifically all dietary processing systems (ingestion, identification, digestion, and excretion of food) and the entire detoxification system be strengthened. Support the immune system by strengthening the release of the parasympathetic nervous system, liver, and spleen. The effect of possible environmental toxins should also be elucidated in the causation of allergies.

Pay particular attention to the free function of the sphenoid, SBS, cranial vault, and facial bones, and perform release on the intracranial membranes as well as on the cervical and upper thoracic vertebrae.

30.3. Asthma

Asthma is a common chronic disease of childhood. The condition is episodic in nature and is initially characterized by cough and rapid breathing, and later even by respiratory distress, and there is a typical wheeze on exhalation. Embryologically, the bronchial and intestinal mucosa both derive from the endoderm. Intestinal dysfunctions may affect the lungs via the diaphragm. If the child does not want to lie on its back, treatment is also possible with the child lying on its front or side. Rather than applying your touch to the child's front right away, you might want to begin by touching the sides of the thorax. If the supine position is possible, slip both hands underneath the child's shoulder blades. Assess the thoracic region, including the lungs, diaphragm, ribs, and vertebrae, as well as the intestinal region for possible functional disorders, and treat accordingly. Also pay attention to the region of T3–T5 and C3–C4.

Because the lungs and heart share the thoracic cavity, visceral treatment can be given.

30.4. Atopic Dermatitis

This is the most common dermatological condition of childhood. Craniosacral Therapy can be used to support lymphatic flow and drainage and to promote function of the liver, stomach, spleen, small intestine, large intestine, and kidneys. In addition, assess and treat the anatomical course of the vagus nerve, which is cranial nerve X, from the jugular foramen via the shoulder region to below the diaphragm.

30.5. Bladder and Sphincter Problems, Bed-Wetting, Enuresis

In cases of incontinence, assess and treat the joints of the locomotor apparatus, especially those of the feet, knees, and hips, which are often found to be restricted. Then, before attempting in the pelvic region to balance the position and craniosacral rhythm of the sacrum and the sides of the pelvis, apply just a suggestion of slow stretch on both thighs in an anterocaudal direction to perform preparatory release of the entire pelvic and abdominal segment and of the iliopsoas muscles that lead up to the lumbar vertebral region and the diaphragm. Due to the release of connective tissue, and especially with visceral treatment of the liver, kidneys, gallbladder, spleen, ureters, and bladder, the forces acting on these organs as well as on the entire pelvic and abdominal segment become more balanced. Tensions or postural anomalies can be treated additionally using deep-acting structural techniques, for example Myofascial Release.

Eutony exercises or contracting and relaxing the pelvic muscles can give the child a greater sense of security or a feeling of improved control. Because the body functions as a unity, you should, of course, also treat and release the shoulder-neck region, the cervical spine, and the atlanto-occipital region and harmonize the craniosacral rhythm in the neurocranium and viscerocranium. Holding tight and letting go also have a great deal to do with the masticatory muscles. Consequently, the masticatory muscles as a whole and the mandible, although they are remote from the problem zone, sometimes turn out to be indirect starting points for a far-reaching chain of release that has a pleasant streaming and flowing effect extending via the pelvis and legs down to the feet.

30.6. Cardiac Arrhythmias

In cardiac arrhythmias, the heartbeat may be introduced by a premature contraction, or else the heart rate may be abnormally increased overall. This possibly points to the existence of heart defects, heart disease, or inflammation of the myocardium, or it may occur after a surgical procedure. The precise cause often cannot be identified.

There are many options open to the craniosacral practitioner for assessment and treatment; for example visceral treatment of the suspensory systems of the heart; treatment for the diaphragm (is there upward-directed tension, or is there too little tension? If so, why?), the occipital bone, and, as the center for cardiac activity, the brain region around the fourth ventricle, as well as the ANS, which also regulates the involuntary heartbeat. In addition, also give consideration to the superior thoracic aperture; the suboccipital region, as the function of the phrenic nerve that controls the diaphragm may be disturbed in the area of the cervical spine; the cranial base; and at the cranial base, especially the lateral components of the occipital bone and the jugular foramen—cranial nerve X, also called the vagus nerve. The heart and lungs share the thoracic cavity, and therefore visceral treatment can be given to the lungs and pericardium. The remarks provided in section 30.3, above, may also be helpful.

30.7. Chronic Bronchitis

Recurrent, usually bacterial infections of the respiratory tract are often the cause of true chronic bronchitis. The craniosacral practitioner may well have recourse to fluctuation techniques such as CV4. Beyond that, you can strengthen the immune system: lymphatic pump via the feet and legs; or lymph drainage, especially in the cervical region. Then release the tissue directly above the clavicles, and perhaps gently support the mobility of the clavicles and sternum. The mobility and motility of the lungs and thorax should be supported overall.

30.8. Concentration or Learning Difficulties

See section 20.8 as well as section 30.1, above.

30.9. Constantly Crying Babies

For constantly crying babies, the underlying cause is often both in the compression of bodily structures as well as in a prenatal and perinatal state of shock or inadequate bonding after birth. The craniosacral practitioner can assess the situation on multiple levels and accompany the process by offering balancing corrections. Treatment is largely the same as in section 30.20, below. For theoretical remarks on this topic, see section 19.4.

30.10. C-section

For theoretical remarks on this topic, see section 15.2.3. The pressure caused by contractions in the birth canal and subsequent release constitute stimulation for the connective tissue that delivers important growth impulses. In a C-section, this stimulation is reduced or almost totally absent. Likewise, the stress hormones secreted in response to a natural birth that dilate the bronchi, for example, or elevate blood pressure are absent in cases of primary C-section. The expression of the amniotic fluid from the lungs by the contractions is also absent or occurs only to an inadequate extent. Consequently, babies delivered by C-section are almost always found to have "wet lungs," meaning too much amniotic fluid in their lungs, and this sometimes has to be removed by aspiration. Respiratory distress disorders or pneumothorax are frequently encountered after delivery by C-section.

If a secondary C-section becomes necessary, as in cases when labor is arrested for a prolonged period or the birth process become life-endangering, the baby's head has usually advanced as far as the pelvis, where contractions subject it to marked compression, especially on the birth lie side, without bringing any forward progress. This leads to the development of typical cranial shapes and fixed head tilt, torticollis, or plagiocephaly, and it reduces the newborn's vitality. By the time the C-section is performed, the baby's cervical spine may well have been exposed to pronounced tensile and torsional forces.

As the craniosacral practitioner, you should perform a comprehensive assessment of compression as it affects the cranium, cervical region, and torso before delivering treatment. You will also frequently palpate and then balance tensions, traction, and torsion in the meninges covering the brain and spinal cord. Support the baby's pulmonary function. The natural biological birth process can be relived and rounded off appropriately. You will be able to reduce or release the intensity of the shock state experienced in the course of a C-section.

30.11. Dental Occlusion Anomaly

A dental occlusion anomaly has an adverse effect not only on chewing but also on swallowing and speech. Craniosacral Therapy should be started as early as possible and continue on a regular basis during and after growth spurts. No later than age seven and before age ten, treatments are important because that is the period when the upper and lower jaws start to develop more fully. Thoroughly assess and support the mobility of the structures around the cranial sutures, zygomatic bones, maxilla and mandible, hyoid bone and cervical region, temporal bones, occipital bone, and shoulder girdle. See also section 30.30, below, and the theoretical remarks in section 20.7.

30.12. Digestive Problems (Diarrhea, Vomiting, Constipation)

When acute inflammation is suspected or when inflammation has been diagnosed, the regions listed below should not be treated. In cases where digestive problems have subsided or are chronic, perform assessment and offer visceral treatment on the esophagus, stomach, duodenum, and small and large intestines. You should also assess the hormone-regulating organs: the liver, gallbladder, pancreas, and kidneys. It may be that the vagus nerve, which is cranial nerve X and which supplies the viscera, has experienced some irritation in the cranium or cervical spine region, or perhaps there has been some umbilical trauma during the birth process. You can release the diaphragm and the shoulder-neck region, widen the occipital condyles, use atlanto-occipital release, and ease jugular foramen tensions. The hormone-producing parts of the digestive apparatus, and hence those parts that are responsible for regulating the gastric juices, as well as the regions around the pituitary and hypothalamus should be supported specifically in their function. See also section 30.20, below.

30.13. Disorders of Speech and Tongue Function

See section 20.5.

30.14. Eye Inflammation (Sticky Eye)

This condition may be caused by a difficult birth during which individual bones of the cranium or face have been compressed or displaced. Support the mobility of the surrounding cranial bones and membranes so that the tear-duct mucosa is better stimulated in harmony with the craniosacral rhythm and becomes better perfused. Harmonize the craniosacral rhythm of the viscerocranium, neurocranium, and sacrum, and possibly release the intracranial membranes. However, there may also be a compensatory cause, for example transmission of unilateral tensile forces or compression from the torso and cervical region via the muscles and ligaments to the cranium.

30.15. Forceps Delivery

This topic is discussed in section 15.1.

30.16. Growth Disturbances

You should assess and treat the structures that are involved in the regulation of growth. The best results are achieved if you support all three levels of the craniosacral system: bone, dural membranes, and CSF. In the cranial sphere, pay particular attention to the position and free functioning of the sphenoid so as to harmonize the activity of the pituitary. If the motion of the sphenoid is freer and more balanced, this will stimulate the third ventricle and hence also the hypothalamus and the pineal gland. Since the sphenoid should not be dealt with in isolation, also treat the SBS, the entire cranial base including the jugular foramina, the cranial vault, and the viscerocranium.

Frequently you will detect too much tension in the meninges and around the foramen magnum, and this adversely affects the brain, especially the brain stem, and hence growth. Consequently, treat the region of the foramen magnum, including the atlanto-occipital and cervical spine regions, and then accompany the meninges, including the intracranial membranes, into a more balanced state.

Use visual and palpatory findings also to assess and treat restrictions in the areas around the shoulder-neck, spinal column, clavicles, sternum, thorax including the diaphragm, pelvis, and sacrum. Combination with visceral treatment of the liver, kidneys and adrenal glands, gastrointestinal tract, and solar plexus will support the areas and functions that regulate growth.

30.17. Headache, Migraine

As in adults, headache in children may be linked to a variety of causes. You should assess and treat the entire craniosacral system, especially the pelvis, diaphragm, shoulder-neck region, cervical and thoracic spine, and muscles of the cranial base including atlanto-occipital release, the bone and membrane level, and the frontal bone with the attachment of the falx cerebri. You should possibly also treat the intracranial membranes, as well as the ethmoid via the frontonasal suture; and decompress the maxilla and palatine bones in order to release the pterygopalatine ganglion. Fluid intake (is the child drinking enough through the course of the day?) and diet, exercise, and psychosomatic stress factors should also be taken into account.

30.18. Hip Dysplasia, Hip Joint Dislocation

The development of the hips can be determined to a major extent by whether the child lies unfavorably in the womb. Hip problems occur more commonly with breech deliveries because the differing position of the hips probably has an adverse effect on the development of the hip joint structures after birth. In particular, the craniosacral practitioner can help to promote the better development of the hips by balancing the hips and pelvis, including the sacrum and lumbar-torso region, as well as the occipital bone.

30.19. Hydrocephalus

The cause of hydrocephalus is a disparity between CSF-producing elements, such as the blood supply, venous plexuses, or the ependymal layer, and elements that absorb CSF, such as the arachnoid villi or venous sinuses; this disparity causes intracranial hypertension. An example is when one lateral ventricle is blocked and becomes enlarged while the free side does not.

In the condition known as communicating hydrocephalus, CSF absorption is diminished due to an issue such as meningitis, and the CSF reaches the lumbar part of the spinal canal; the pressure is equally high in the internal and external CSF space. Obstructive hydrocephalus often happens because of a tight or interrupted cerebral aqueduct due to an issue such as compression, herniation, or a tumor. The CSF is unable to reach the external subarachnoid space, and the brain is pressed against the neurocranium.

The CSF outflow system may be impaired in several areas. If there is narrowing of the interventricular foramen, also called the foramen of Monro, CSF buildup occurs in the associated lateral ventricle. If the third ventricle is narrowed, buildup occurs in both lateral ventricles. If the cerebral aqueduct is narrowed or interrupted, CSF buildup occurs in the third ventricle and the lateral ventricles. If the foramen of Luschka and the foramen Magendie in the region of the fourth ventricle are obstructed, then all four ventricles become enlarged. The pressure-associated symptoms may lead to vomiting, poor feeding, or seizures. The condition is diagnosed by computed tomography or ultrasound. If hydrocephalus fails to improve, surgery is performed to drain the CSF via a shunt.

The conventional allopathic medical diagnosis is important for the craniosacral practitioner: if hydrocephalus is caused by acute meningitis, treatment of the head region is contraindicated. In general, where intracerebral pressure is high, do not use the CV4 or other structural techniques. Treatment in hydrocephalus demands a high level of experience so that the symptoms and the underlying cause do not deteriorate to become life-threatening.

Once conventional allopathic medical experts have confirmed that hydrocephalus is minor or manageable, or following removal of a shunt, the craniosacral practitioner may support the child in its self-regulation without using invasive techniques. If the lateral ventricles are affected, you will frequently encounter side-bending or torsion of the sphenoid, which is causing constriction of an interventricular foramen and thus disturbing CSF outflow from the associated lateral ventricle. If the third or fourth ventricles are involved, an EV4 performed without pressure can encourage drainage into the external CSF space.

We can listen and give space for jugular foramen (see section 27.6) and support the venous-sinus drainage with functional release of the intracranial membranes (see section 28.11).

30.20. Infantile Colic

For theoretical remarks on this topic, see section 19.4. The condition may be caused by a prenatal disorder, for example the psychological state of the mother, who may have secreted increased levels of stress hormones that were absorbed via the hormonal link with her unborn child during pregnancy. Umbilical trauma, caused by cutting the umbilical cord too early, and the associated shock reaction may be a further cause of infantile colic. Umbilical trauma often gives rise to existential anxiety that can take root as a reflex phenomenon in the abdominal region. Commonly the cause is to be found in compression or displacement phenomena in the cervical and thoracic spine or cranial base, adversely affecting the function of the cranial nerves. See also section 30.12, above.

Assess and treat the cranium for bone displacement. Assess the position of the four constituent parts of the occipital bone and spread the lateral components, thus also creating more space for the foramen magnum. Support the parts of the temporal bones adjacent to the occipital bone by supporting the craniosacral rhythm at the temporal bones and performing the gentle ear pull and jugular foramen release. You can also perform release on the suboccipital region and the shoulder-neck region. Also assess and treat the balance of tension in the dural tube, cerebral meninges, and especially in the intracranial membranes.

30.21. Internal Rotation of the Legs

If left untreated, this condition can lead to joint damage and postural harm. Here you proceed in a similar manner as for hip problems, but specifically you assess and balance the tension state in the lower abdominal region. This may have caused the legs to rotate inward via the action of the associated muscles, fasciae, and fascial chains. For example, the condition may be due to hypertonus of the iliopsoas muscle, the upper components of which extend to the spinal column below the diaphragm. You should therefore perform a full assessment and treatment of the body as a whole. It may be that the internal rotation of the legs is a psychosomatic pointer to a felt need for protection, or shame, or profound unease.

30.22. Otitis Media

Assess and treat the temporal bones. Encourage their motility and mobility by balancing the craniosacral rhythm, and in particular treat the sutures, tentorium cerebelli, jugular foramina, cervical spine including the fascia, thoracic spine, and thorax including the diaphragm. Your assessment and treatment should also take account of the TMJs and the muscles and ligaments that have attachment to the temporal bones, especially the sternocleidomastoid, splenius capitis, and digastric muscles. A high palate, possibly encouraged by thumb-sucking, as well as a predominant or chronic practice of mouth-breathing may also have repercussions on the eustachian tube. The

vomerovaginal canal affords passage to a branch of the sphenopala-
tine artery, the nerve fibers of which travel from the pterygopalatine
ganglion to the eustachian tube. Narrowing of this canal may also be
a contributory cause of otitis media. Harmonization of the viscerocranium, including release of the palatine bones from the maxilla and the
pterygoid processes of the sphenoid, is therefore advisable. The ear,
nose, and throat region as a whole should be assessed and balanced.
The immune system may be strengthened via the liver and spleen. As
supplementary measures, for example, use the recoil technique in the
thoracic region and the lymphatic pump via the legs.

30.23. Plagiocephaly, Torticollis, KISS Syndrome

Plagiocephaly and torticollis are deformities of the newborn caused
by an incorrect or restrictive intrauterine environment, such as deep
pelvic lie during pregnancy or a taut maternal psoas muscle; by a
complicated birth or external application of force during the birth
process; by C-section; or by the use of forceps or a ventouse (see
section 15.1). Plagiocephaly may also be caused by floppy head syndrome, the baby's one-sided sleeping position, or scoliosis. In such
circumstances the child can often only be breast-fed successfully on
one side. A suboccipital restriction is often encountered in the vicinity
of C2–C3. However, the cause may also be in tension or a lesion at
the cranial vault, at the cranial base, or in the viscerocranium. This
not only causes plagiocephaly but also affects the cranial base and the
balance of forces acting on the meninges covering the brain and spinal
cord. Both anatomically and neurophysiologically, the occipital bone
and the suboccipital region are closely associated with autonomic
regulatory centers in the medulla oblongata.

The receptivity of this region to sensory input and stimulation
has a major influence on the development of the postural and supportive motor systems. The short neck muscles are twice as densely

populated with receptors as the muscles of the hands. Moreover, a dysfunction in this area leads to reduced information and energy flow between the body and the brain. Pressure on the child's head during the birth process also commonly leads to a cervical spine syndrome. The majority of these children feel unwell, and they communicate this by excessive crying. On the other hand, some reduce their contact with their surroundings, become increasingly withdrawn, and resign themselves to their pain.

Plagiocephaly and torticollis should be confirmed by conventional allopathic medical diagnosis and only then treated using Craniosacral Therapy. In torticollis the allopathic physician may be able to provide a more precise diagnosis after an X-ray. In patients with plagiocephaly or torticollis, and in the kinetic imbalance due to suboccipital strain (KISS) syndrome, treatment should be given as early as possible—ideally before or during the next growth spurt. From the mechanical-structural standpoint, treatment should address the cervical spine, particularly the territory of C1, C2, and C3, among other aspects. It is also important always to include the condylar parts and the basilar part of the occipital bone in your assessment and treatment. The structures in close proximity, such as the hyoid bone, the entire shoulder-neck region, and the superior thoracic aperture, including the clavicles and sternum, should be assessed and balanced.

During assessment and during and after treatment, monitor or gently test the motion restriction of the head: what degrees of rotation to left and right are possible before, during, and after treatment? Check the head rotator muscles on both sides, and assess the position of the two mastoid processes and the symmetry of the ears. If the temporal bone is tilted or compressed, this may result in positional anomalies of the TMJs. During your assessment, seek out and treat the cause of the imbalance, such as an irritated cranial nerve due to jugular foramen narrowing. Also assess and treat the other cranial nerves and the atlanto-occipital junction.

My personal experience in treating children with plagiocephaly and torticollis shows that the sessions are even more effective if balancing is performed not only on the areas mentioned, but if you also identify those body sites or zones where the shock, stress, pain, or fear—for example, of further compression—have been stored. This is frequently the case in the region of the neck, the diaphragm, and the solar plexus. You can also identify in which body segments emotions have been trapped, or which segments are hypertonic or hypotonic. When the restricted structures are released, the child may experience feelings of helplessness, being overwhelmed, or other emotions from the past that had been stored in the treated segments; you should then accompany the child through the process of release. If you are able to discover where the body and the craniosacral system reflect the physical trauma, where too much or too little buildup is present, and how much emotional support the child needs, the healing process will be encouraged comprehensively and relatively quickly. On the other hand, if release involves only the structural level and you neglect the emotional-energetic level, it is more likely that an unprocessed residual memory or psychosomatic block will remain stored in the body.

The practitioner and parents can support the corrective process by encouraging the child to use its neck muscles more often and in a more balanced way. The child should be placed on its belly more often, should not just sleep on its back, and should be breast-fed and addressed from both sides so as not to further reinforce the one-sided pattern.

30.24. Preterm Birth

A preterm birth is one that occurs between week twenty-four and week thirty-seven of gestation. Among other things, the tauter uterine cervix may produce lesions in the region of the baby's occipital bone because this area is not as resistant to pressure and is therefore still highly vulnerable. Often artificial ventilation is necessary, and this may cause injury in the region of the pulmonary bifurcation. Your role as craniosacral practitioner is to release any compression and to support pulmonary function. It is important to stimulate the child's development as a whole and to create as much space for the organism as possible so that the newborn can develop optimally on all levels. For further details, see section 15.2.5 for theoretical aspects and section 27.1 for practical aspects of supporting pulmonary function.

30.25. Scoliosis

As long as scoliosis is still a postural anomaly, the craniosacral practitioner can be very effective in preventing a structural deformity. Later, your efforts will be directed at ensuring the spinal column remains mobile so that the scoliotic curve causes no pain or as little pain as possible. Perform regular release of the dural tube via the sacrum and occipital bone, and support unwinding.

30.26. Sinusitis

Infants in particular are relatively susceptible to inflammation of the ethmoid air cells, a condition known as ethmoidal sinusitis. This may lead to raised intraocular pressure; headaches, especially between the eyes; facial pain; and tiredness or exhaustion. Sinusitis may affect a number of different paranasal sinuses. The mucosa becomes swollen. It almost always leads to a pronounced irritative cough, and possibly to a yellowish-green discharge from the nose.

As the craniosacral practitioner, assess and improve the mobility of the facial bones and of the cranial base as a whole, in particular the sphenoid and temporal bones. The temporal and zygomatic bones may hold the maxilla tight, massively restricting its motion as well as that of the frontal bone and ethmoid. The ethmoid is a central point for the attachment of the facial bones. The two adjacent nasal conchae transport the inspired air into the olfactory region and into the respiratory tract and are therefore also important for pulmonary respiration. If the ethmoid is tilted and its craniosacral rhythm is restricted, the cause may also lie in torsion or side-bending of the SBS. In this case the entire cranial base should be comprehensively treated and its mobility synchronized. The ethmoidal spine of the sphenoid is particularly important for transferring the motion of the sphenoid to the ethmoid. Releasing the frontonasal suture is always helpful in sinusitis. The craniosacral rhythm that has become more balanced as a result of treatment is consequently better able to drain the frontal and paranasal sinuses. Additionally, the circulation of the blood and lymph is improved, and this alleviates congestion, edema, and inflammation.

30.27. Squint

In this condition it can be helpful to release tensions in individual cranial bones that may possibly be irritating cranial nerves. In the process you may treat the SBS, sphenoid, and orbital bones, including the maxilla. Intracranial membrane release (see section 28.11) may also bring therapeutic success in children with squint.

30.28. Sucking Problems, Nipple Confusion

For a theoretical discussion of this topic, see section 19.3.

30.29. Surgical Procedures (Before and After)

Before and after surgery, for example for cleft palate or synostosis, Craniosacral Therapy is appropriate to support the general health of the child and therefore its immune system. Support the craniosacral system and lymph flow, release the occipital bone with its four component parts and the jugular foramina, provide visceral support for liver and spleen function, and possibly invite the mid-tide and the fluid body to undergo a holistic shift. It is frequently better not to treat the site directly but to facilitate greater motility and mobility in its immediate proximity. This may reduce the traumatic effect of surgery and encourage wound healing afterward. In the case of serious conditions such as cerebral hemorrhage, do not treat the affected head region; instead support the child peripherally, for example via the feet, using the functional or biodynamic treatment approach.

30.30. Tooth and Jaw Problems

For theoretical remarks on this topic, see section 20.7. In all circumstances relating to the maxilla or mandible, dental occlusion anomalies, and TMJ problems, you should at the very least treat the structures from the thorax and vertebra T5 up as far as the cranial base because the cervical and jaw muscles travel upward from there. Prior to that, you should have assessed and treated the hips, sacroiliac joints, and sacrum: postural problems, in particular skeletal factors and the compensatory configurations they evoke, have a relatively pronounced effect on growth patterns in the jaw region. Past injuries in the shoulder-neck region, caused by overzealous pulling on the arm or fracture of the clavicle during the birth process, may often be forgotten but may exert a compensatory effect on the hyoid bone, TMJ, and the cranial base as a whole. The two temporal bones should move evenly in external and internal rotation. If this is not the case, the angle of inclination of one or both temporal bones might contribute to TMJ problems or to malocclusion. In addition, some brief yet clear intraoral work should be performed on all the accessible facial bones to achieve release.

Everything that has already been said relating to the specific assessment and treatment of the viscerocranium (see section 28.9) may be helpful. For example, check how freely mobile the two halves of the maxilla are. Specifically, where the upper and lower jaws are narrow, encourage their intraosseous mobility. Also palpate and treat all the muscles and ligaments in the vicinity of the floor of the mouth, mandible, suprahyoid and infrahyoid muscles, cervical and pharyngeal region, and shoulder-neck region, including the clavicles and sternum. Often the goal is creating space, and to this end we can deliver impulses to the structure with our treatment.

Crooked dental alignment can be reduced by improving the mobility of the teeth: you can make contact with individual teeth and support them in their relative mobility, which may result in spontaneous unwinding movements of individual teeth. In addition, check and balance the tension of the masticatory muscles as a whole. Any imbalance of the masticatory muscles or in the anterior facial region in turn provokes compensatory configurations around the mastoid process and in the suboccipital region, commonly around the occipital ridge, atlas, cervical spine, and below. For this reason treatment is not limited to the directly affected structures but also includes functionally and anatomically associated regions.

I have achieved particularly good success when I have specifically used gentle structural techniques in the neurocranium and viscerocranium, including intraoral Craniosacral Therapy, in conjunction with visceral and myofascial treatment:

- Before tooth and jaw corrections, I release these structures so that they are as free as possible and have to undergo less compensation during the corrective process.
- During corrections, I treat the surrounding territory.
- Afterward, I again treat all structures with the objective that the corrected regions again move increasingly in harmony with the craniosacral rhythm and that overall mobility is supported.

Once the child is more relaxed and ready, I more frequently use the functional or biodynamic treatment approach. I tend to start out by working with the structural approach because physical restrictions, such as areas of substantial compression, can often be released relatively simply on the structural level in a few sessions. If the craniosacral system and the body are free from the thoracic segment upward, functional Craniosacral Therapy can be used to balance the membrane tension, and afterward the fluid body and potency can be supported in the biodynamic field.

Depending on the child's constitution, sessions may last thirty to forty-five minutes each. At the end of this time it is not unusual for the child to prefer to play again or to engage in some different activity. However, if a child is deeply relaxed (sometimes the mother may also easily drop off to sleep), if a more prolonged stillpoint has become established, or if spontaneous self-corrections are taking place due to the mid-tide or Long Tide, then rather than disturbing this process, I extend the session by ten to twenty minutes. The next session may then last for only thirty minutes.

30.31. Upper or Lower Brachial Plexus Paralysis

From its origins in the cervical region, the brachial nerve plexus travels beneath the clavicle toward the arm. Strong traction or twisting actions on the head or strain placed on the nerve plexus due to shoulder dystocia may cause paralysis of the arm or hand. In upper brachial plexus paralysis, motor and sensory fibers from C5 and C6 are affected: the arm dangles flaccidly, but the fingers can still be moved. In lower brachial plexus paralysis, the fibers from C8 and C9 are involved: the shoulder can be moved, the forearm dangles down, and the hand and fingers cannot be moved—the grip reflex is absent or there is a claw-hand deformity. As the craniosacral practitioner, you may assess and release the fascia around the clavicle, cervical spine, thorax, and arms because these structures, like the plexus itself, may have been strained and the nerve supply may no longer be optimal.

Assess the organism as a whole, release any disorders present, and thus stimulate the self-healing forces.

30.32. Ventouse Delivery

Ventouse (vacuum device) delivery entails stress for the still soft cranial bones and the membrane system beneath them. This stress is then stored by the tissues, often resulting in intraosseous dysfunctions. For theoretical remarks on this topic, see section 15.1.

PART FOUR

Treatment Examples

The following treatment examples have been drawn from my routine work in Craniosacral Therapy practice over the past decade. They are subjective accounts and have deliberately not been written using a standard template or format. These examples are intended first to form a practical bridge to the theoretical sections of this book, and second to illustrate the various procedures, release approaches, and treatment options available in pediatric Craniosacral Therapy. My intention is in no way to set out a standardized treatment protocol—such a thing is nonexistent in holistic therapies. My assessments of the overall situation of parents and children are never set in stone, nor do they constitute a diagnosis or a prognosis; instead they provide a snapshot in time. I always factor in an element of the unknown, an indefinable something that I or my client may perceive only imperfectly, if at all, and that perhaps wants to remain hidden. I know that I am unable to simultaneously recognize all the parallel emerging therapeutic processes on the physical, emotional, energetic, and mental-spiritual level—and indeed, I do not have to, because I have absolute faith in the primordial principle of self-regulation, which unfolds continuously as a natural law.

In my assessments as they are presented in these illustrative treatment examples, I have neither judged the children and parents nor given them a pathological label. However, the impression gained by the practitioner is important when making an initial evaluation in order to gauge any changes that occur during the individual sessions and over the course of treatment as a whole. All names in these illustrative examples have been changed to protect the identities of the individuals concerned.

A Mother in Month Eight of Pregnancy

During the first trimester of her pregnancy, Michelle had received two craniosacral treatment sessions from a friend, and she had found the experience to be pleasantly relaxing. Six weeks before her due date she developed major bleeding that entailed a risk of infection for both mother and baby. A visit to a gynecologist revealed that the opening of the cervix was still closed and the mucus plug had not yet been discharged. I decided to attend to the client at home, and took my portable massage table and an ample supply of soft positioning aids such as floor cushions and blankets. Her two other children—ages two and a half and four years—were playing in their room and occasionally checked that all was well by looking into the living room where I was treating their mother. As she had mentioned over the phone, she briefly confirmed again in our initial dialogue what she was hoping for from the treatment: greater relaxation, reduced stress levels following her previous scare, and that the unborn child would remain in the womb and thus be carried to term for a further six weeks.

After taking a brief history and asking the client to let me know how she was feeling during the session, I positioned Michelle comfortably on her back. Before applying touch I took a few moments to sense my own body and emotions, and then the entire room, and the situation at that moment. I was again aware that my treatment of the mother would also indirectly affect her unborn child, and so I again allowed myself a few moments to attune my emotional, mental, and energetic distance from both individuals, and to listen to the beauty of the stillness. I then performed a brief assessment of various bodily structures in the mother, and in the process I also differentiated the qualities of the craniosacral rhythm. The entire right-hand side of her body was clearly more permeable and freer, while the left side of the pelvis and the left shoulder appeared to be restricted and firm; the client confirmed this. Next we took sufficient time to find the optimal side-lying position for her. Two firm cushions placed in front of her thorax eased the tension on the client's upper body and shoulder-neck region in such a way that her arm was able to rest relaxed on the two cushions. With my left hand I touched her neck region so that my soft, warm touch would support and ease the tension in this zone, which is so vulnerable to stress. Very soon she was breathing in and out more deeply. The tissues seemed to slowly blend with my hand and became warmer. She also told me that she was feeling noticeably more relaxed, but then she again became aware of a familiar occasional stabbing pain in the region of her right costal arch.

I then placed my other hand, initially with the fingers slightly spread, in broad contact over her lower lumbar region so that I was touching her sacrum and sacroiliac joints. Here I also listened and supported the total structure in its fine self-corrective processes. After just a short time, she slipped into deeper relaxation. Suddenly a spontaneous stillpoint established itself. Deep in-breaths and out-breaths and clearly audible gastrointestinal sounds signaled to me the change in the ANS. After the stillpoint, the craniosacral rhythm could be sensed more strongly, but its balance was not yet improved. With one hand I palpated the neck region and with the other the region of the L5-sacrum-sacroiliac joints, and I attuned myself to the torso region in between: I was attentive to the respiratory movements; the permeability of the pelvic, abdominal, and thoracic segment; and the mobility of the dural tube, and I remained open to whatever wanted to enter my perceptual field. I sensed ever more clearly the link from the left-side neck region to the left shoulder and from there to the right costal arch, which in turn was clearly connected with the sacroiliac joint on the left side. I suspected a compensatory restrictive link, and for the moment did not apply any structural technique. I continued listening to establish whether and how this inertial line started to change with regard to the respiratory rhythm and the craniosacral rhythm.

At that moment Michelle informed me that the mild stabbing in the region of her right costal arch was growing stronger. In my right hand, placed at the sacrum, I sensed a strong pounding, a therapeutic pulse. Intuitively I slowly intensified the contact of this hand with the tissue slightly so that contact was not lost, thus signaling to the tissue that it was still being supported in the local release process that was emerging. Again I had the impression that the client's left shoulder and her left sacroiliac joint were extremely restricted. Now, however, the connecting region in between started to become increasingly balanced. At the precise moment when I wanted to ask Michelle how the stabbing sensation now felt, whether she would like me to apply touch to her costal arch or whether I should continue my contact at the neck and pelvic region, she spontaneously breathed deeply in and out twice. A powerful jerk in her left sacroiliac joint followed, from which something resembling a hot piercing arrow was discharged outward through my hand. The astonished client's reaction was, "Oh, an old forgotten weak spot from a riding accident when I was young has just surfaced again. It feels exactly like it did when the accident happened."

After this release in the left sacroiliac joint region, the sacrum and occipital bone clearly started to move increasingly in harmony with the craniosacral rhythm, and further self-corrections of the bodily structures ensued. During the first ten minutes my left hand in the neck region was an important anchor, a point that communicated a pleasant sense of being held, while very pronounced processes were at work in the region of the pelvis and right costal arch. I therefore continued to apply my touch in the neck region while my right hand gently touched the inferior thoracic aperture. As Michelle's thoracic space started to clearly and continuously widen, I placed my right hand higher at the superior thoracic aperture, where I further supported the release of the thoracic segment. By the time this had become established for a sufficiently long period of time, not quite twenty minutes had elapsed and the client wanted to change her position.

When she was lying comfortably on her back, I sensed the craniosacral rhythm at various cranial bones. The temporal bone, sphenoid, and occipital bone showed evidence of definite motion restriction on the left side, especially in terms of amplitude and spectrum. With her head in the cradle hold I then spent about two minutes performing release in the region of the atlanto-occipital joint. Gateways to release appeared to open up here as well, as if they had simply been waiting for this moment: the pronounced hypertonus on the left side abated within a short time and it was soon possible for me to gently insert my supple finger pads at the occipital ridge. Once again, the mood in the room became calmer and more peaceful. Although the client was already relaxing deeply in herself, her entire upper cervical region together with all the structures of the head again began to be released at a deeper level—as if everything were becoming wider, lighter, and heavier all at once. After a spontaneous deep breath, Michelle said, "It's like a light has been switched on in my head. My whole body is completely relaxed, and I feel as if I'm at a health spa."

Again I refrained from inducing a stillpoint, and I knew that it was time now to round off the short treatment sequence with the client supine. I allowed some time for this relaxed state to become more deeply anchored with Michelle now in the side-lying position. I listened to the craniosacral rhythm at the occipital bone and sacrum and was surprised how exquisitely balanced it had now become. Just before I intended to disengage my hands, a stillpoint lasting for about three minutes established itself spontaneously. During the stillpoint I had the impression that I was sensing in the mother a different, slightly faster craniosacral rhythm than before, and I assumed that this was the craniosacral rhythm of her unborn child.

After the stillpoint, the craniosacral rhythm also became more balanced throughout the left side of the client's body. She had forgotten about the mild stabbing pain in the region of her right costal arch. I allowed her sufficient time to sit up and reorient herself in the room. She felt very refreshed and seemed surprised about recalling the riding accident. She was even more impressed that she could sense how very tense she had been in the shoulder-neck region and that this tension and tautness had been transformed in such a short time into all-embracing light—even though, as she admitted, she had no interest whatsoever in esoteric things. Michelle was looking forward to a further treatment session in the coming week with her friend, who had attended courses at our Sphinx Craniosacral Institute. I subsequently learned from the friend that the client had had no further worrying bleeds and that her third child was also born healthy.

A Baby with Plagiocephaly

At the end of a training course day, a couple came to us with their six-week-old baby, who had plagiocephaly following a difficult birth. Various investigations had been performed in the pediatric clinic. As well as plagiocephaly the baby was able to move its head only to the left and with a very small radius of movement of just an inch or so. Because its head was always in the same position when it was lying down, the baby had already developed a flattened and tilted occipital bone. I welcomed the baby, which was placed on the massage table by its mother. I then began gently to support it by positioning one hand on its sacrum-pelvis region and the other holding its occipital-neck region, using my touch to offer safety, stability, and space for spontaneous inherent motion. The baby exhibited micromovements relatively quickly, both where my hands were giving support and in the territory of the spinal column and dural tube between my hands where I went with the spontaneous inherent contraction and widening.

I encouraged the baby with my attentive touch, and occasionally also verbally, to continue with this impulse. Its legs and feet now started to thrash and kick. I touched its feet with my knee. The baby accepted this contact at once, as demonstrated by the fact that it became visibly and perceptibly calmer, made eye contact with me, and started to free itself from tensions in the pelvic region using clearly coordinated inherent unwinding movements. While this was going on I sensed that the pronounced restriction in the region of the cervical vertebrae slowly started to release itself. After about two minutes there was a marked reduction in the motion at the pelvis. Instead the baby started to scream and cry, and there were strong contractions around the diaphragm. I slowly disengaged my hand from beneath the sacrum, and I told the baby that I was able to sense its powerful emotions and that I would continue to accompany it through the process, and then placed my hand softly and clearly over the area of its diaphragm and solar plexus. Using my hand in the shoulder-neck region, I made even clearer contact with the upper dorsal region, in response to which arrhythmic unwinding movements became apparent along the entire spinal column.

The baby's diaphragm and solar plexus became extremely warm. I felt my way into the child's tensions and releases on the physical and emotional level and supported it clearly and spaciously at the same time. Using my hand in the diaphragm, abdomen, and solar plexus region, I went with these tension states. This was even more helpful for the cervical region as it underwent release because the baby was by now moving its head far more clearly than five minutes earlier. I suspected that the physical trauma in the cervical region and the emotional-energetic trauma in the diaphragm and solar plexus had been stored up and that both were starting to be released.

The baby now clearly cried less, but its screams had become more powerful, and it increasingly started to vary its supine and side-lying positions. With my support it then also moved on to its belly, started to make definite crawling-type movements, and attempted to propel itself forward. I again supported this impulse using my knee, which the baby successfully used to push off from. The baby paused briefly from time to time and ceased its movements. I asked the parents to position themselves to one side of the table on the floor mattress because the child was now making its way in that direction. I invited the baby verbally and by touch to take more time and to allow itself pauses so as not to overtax itself. But it would not be held back, and soon it reached as far as the edge of the table, where, crying and screaming, it stretched with its head toward the floor. I then gave the parents a brief word of explanation ("This will now probably be followed by a further phase symbolizing the birth process") and I accompanied the baby safely down from the table using spiraling movements. Mother and father were waiting down below. The baby was received by its mother and lovingly taken into her arms while the father embraced the mother from behind and also welcomed the child.

The students attending the course observed the session compassionately and silently. I also allowed myself to take a short break. After the rebonding phase between the parents and the baby on the floor mattress, all three reoriented themselves again increasingly in the room.

When the mother stood next to the table again, holding her baby, for the first time it started to make eye contact with some of the course delegates, looked around, and, lightly supported by its mother's hand in the neck and occipital region, slowly moved its head to the left, to the right, and back again. Everyone in the room saw that the baby could now move its head in both directions and that the radius of movement was relatively wide. I was surprised how much obvious improvement had been possible in this treatment session, which lasted about forty-five minutes. The parents too could hardly believe it and were visibly relieved. By the time they left the baby was already asleep against its mother's body—and no wonder, as this had been a powerful session, and sleep beside its mother was now the best medicine of all.

A Constantly Crying Baby with Infantile Colic and Disturbed Sleep

Peter was not quite three months old when his mother brought him to my practice. The reason she brought him to Craniosacral Therapy was that Peter cried a great deal, had difficulty calming down, slept very poorly, and sometimes woke up with a start. His mother described him as rather difficult to get through to and contact-averse.

In this first session I took sufficient time to record a careful initial history, during which I observed the mother and the child for most of the time and attuned myself to the overall situation. According to the pediatrician's report, Peter was suffering from infantile colic and episodes of atopic dermatitis. The birth had been extremely difficult. In the clinic there had been a total of five induction attempts over two and a half days. The amniotic fluid was in short supply, and the baby's heart sounds were so alarmingly reduced that an emergency C-section was required as a life-saving measure: the umbilical cord had been wrapped several times around Peter's neck. I gained the impression that his mother was perceptibly affected during her description of the birth and was neither suppressing nor exaggerating anything. She had already faced up to and adequately dealt with her own situation. Her descriptions all sounded congruent and reflected the ability to emotionally sense and hold on to both joy and sorrow.

Session 1: on the treatment table Peter responded immediately with eye contact, and there was an intensive mutual exchange. Peter was alert, and his grip and sucking reflexes were very good. When the child turned its head, an action that I supported with my touch in the head and neck region, I saw and sensed that Peter's cervical spine showed no major restrictions, even though head rotation to the left stopped sooner than to the right. His motor skills overall were fine, and the slower and more rapid movements of his extremities were smooth and rounded. All these observations indicated to me that the eleven-week-old Peter was doing relatively well after his difficult birth because infantile colic and atopic dermatitis are also encountered in children after more straightforward deliveries. In the first ten minutes, during which I supported Peter in his movement impulses, especially the spinal column, dural tube, and the costal arch, and was briefly able to assess the head and pelvis, he repeatedly looked at me while smiling and babbling away—he was in an extraordinarily calm yet attentively alert phase at the same time.

But that suddenly came to an end. Peter started to whine and to thrash wildly with his legs. Very soon he arched his torso, which was accompanied by increasingly violent screams. His mother confirmed to me that his screaming episodes always started this way and that he was almost impossible to calm down. I addressed Peter and told him that I sensed his discomfort and suffering and that my hands, in his diaphragm region, would also accompany him through this unpleasant experience. A brief increase in his body-arching and screaming signaled the climax of this intense agitation; Peter calmed down extremely quickly, which was the usual pattern, according to his mother, and then soon fell into a relaxed sleep. I then treated his mother, who had requested some release of tension in her shoulder region while Peter slept on her belly.

After about ten minutes, he woke up. He seemed to be out of sorts, no longer wanted to lie on his mother's belly, and did not respond to her negotiated contact. He began to turn away from her, and I accompanied him gently through a second phase of body-arching and screaming. From moment to moment my two hands adapted to Peter's tonus and movement impulses. In the process I occasionally encouraged him verbally in his expression of discomfort and pain. Beneath my hands I was aware of gastrointestinal rumblings that conjured up a picture of an impending thunder-and-lightning storm. Because the experience of the physiological birth process is absent in cases of C-section but can be rounded off later as a relived experience, I gave advance warning of what I was about to do and then started to take on Peter's intense movement impulse. Slowly and safely I accompanied him in his spiraling movements from the treatment table down to the blanket on the floor. This experience seemed to please him, and the maximum buildup of agitation gradually started to subside. While he sucked his fingers, the sound of his mother's and my voice seemed to have a calming effect on Peter. His body-arching and his screaming and crying quickly and clearly diminished.

Session 2: Peter's mother reported that since the first craniosacral session Peter had screamed far less often and for shorter periods. He was able to fall asleep more easily in the evenings, even though he woke up during the nights. I told her that I was happy for both of them. Peter looked at me, took hold of my fingers, squeezed them, and started to move around, appearing to want to play with me. I supported this by placing one hand on his belly and costal arch, while with my other hand I complied with his desire for contact with his hands and feet and simultaneously tested whether he was seeking out resistance. In the process we engaged in affectionate eye contact. Peter smiled at me, and I asked his mother, "How was your contact with Peter immediately after he was born?" At the time she had been utterly exhausted and at the end of her tether—which I could fully understand.

This was followed by a series of movements down from the table intended to round off the incomplete birth dynamics. Peter very much enjoyed playfully giving himself over to his spontaneous releasing movements and being safely supported in it by me. I paid very close attention to his timing and to his rhythm of active forward propulsion and passive resting in himself to enjoy the ongoing effects. After the five induction attempts and his feeling of being trapped by the umbilical cord, I could imagine only too well that it was now liberating and essential for Peter that he experience himself freely in response to his own impulses and in harmony with his own rhythm so that he might move forward in life. When Peter—accompanied by me in his birth movements down from the table—arrived on the floor with the soft blanket with a nursing pillow, he was welcomed and affectionately touched by his mother and me.

Mother and child engaged in prolonged intimate eye contact as if they were looking at each other for the very first time and wanted to size each other up. The familiarization and bonding processes that had not been possible immediately after birth, and had in fact been absent up until that day, could now be made good without any problem whatsoever. I stayed with the mother and child and was simply present, perhaps representing the father in this position, and as the practitioner I ensured a safe space so that this time around Peter was able to reexperience a straightforward birth process, and the bonding with his mother could now begin in a completely new way.

We were happy that Peter was so alert and present. Since another critical factor for Peter during the birth had been the very short supply of amniotic fluid, I spontaneously suggested to his mother that when they got home she might bathe together with Peter in warm water and let him feel skin-to-skin contact with her, allowing him time and responding to his impulses.

For the moment, however, after this birth reenactment and bonding phase in the second session, mother and child seemed to want to rest. Both were lying comfortably on the treatment table. After they had relaxed together for a short while, a new cycle of activation-buildup and deactivation-release started: Peter started to whine, resisted contact, and began to scream and cry exactly as at the start of the first session, and unmistakably and energetically pushed himself away from his mother. Was this perhaps symbolic of the situation of separation during the emergency C-section?

Since Peter was thrashing wildly and uncontrollably for a few seconds, repeatedly trying to push himself away, and evidently distraught and screaming, I held him in a clear way that he could sense, offered him my finger, and encouraged him verbally to sense his own strength and my support. Once again Peter emitted a loud primal scream, and this was followed by marked somatoemotional relaxation with brief trembling; then the agitation curve seemed to ebb gradually. Now was the right time to offer mother and child contact again. Slowly I placed Peter—who was still holding tightly to my finger and was being securely held by me—in his mother's lap without disengaging my contact with him. Both mother and child reacted with release and sighing in response to this body contact. Soon Peter began to scramble upward toward his mother's breast. I did not force anything, I simply gave Peter a little nudge on his way at his legs and pelvis from time to time so that he did not become too frustrated and expend too much strength. I suggested to his mother that she sense her heart and her child, and that she could now sense all the feelings that she had not experienced after the birth, and in so doing, allow her child to sense her heart connection and her respiratory movements. When I saw how tenderly both of them were able to do this, I knew that my job was done and that bonding was now underway, as should have happened after the birth.

Meanwhile—mostly using his own strength—Peter had arrived at his mother's breasts, and the mood in the room was characterized by contentment, clarity, and love. I suggested that she allow plenty of time now to breast-feed Peter properly and to enjoy the intimate togetherness. I told her that I would leave the treatment room now and would look in again later. After fifteen minutes I knocked on the door, and on entering the room found the blissfully smiling Peter fast asleep, and a visibly and profoundly impressed mother. "In the twelve weeks since he was born, Peter has never been able to lie quietly on top of me. Now I've been privileged to experience this for such a long time and so intimately." The follow-up dialogue was relatively brief because the session spoke for itself and I did not want to diminish the intimate mood by switching to the level of the intellect. To enable her to process the birth herself, she was thinking about having a few further sessions with a craniosacral practitioner known to both of us.

Session 3: His mother told me that Peter was again doing better. His digestion was improved, and he was settling down at night more quickly than he had previously. He would wake up briefly in the night crying but was quickly comforted and fell asleep again. The idea of bathing together had been a great success. Peter had been very happy about this and gave lots of squeals of delight. In the past two days his two older step-brothers had visited and there had been a great deal going on in the home—almost too much for Peter, who was now in very high spirits. In this third session Peter would often lie on his mother's belly—something that he had not previously enjoyed at all. My application of touch was not met with restricted tonus or stressed breathing. Consequently I was able to treat Peter on a structural level in the region of his neck, back, spinal column, and sacrum, and especially the dural tube.

The region around T12–L1 was abnormally restricted. When I offered empathic contact and hence more support and space there with my hand, various release phenomena and autonomic reactions occurred: Peter's breathing changed relatively quickly, there was twitching and release, a softening of internal organs, and increased peristaltic activity throughout the abdominal and pelvic region. In and around

Peter's head I gently widened the region of the occipital condyles, then listened in a cranial vault hold to the craniosacral rhythm, and molded the cranial base and cranial vault in harmony with the rhythm. I also treated the tentorium cerebelli using the gentle ear pull technique and jugular foramen release left and right. The tentorium cerebelli repositioned itself over a two-minute period and afterward moved in a more balanced way in harmony with the craniosacral rhythm, the falx cerebri, and the dural tube. While Peter enjoyed the ongoing effects, I used the intervening time to treat his mother. During the last fifteen minutes of the session I listened to the craniosacral rhythm and a spontaneous stillpoint in mother and child. The mid-tide could be sensed in both of them, and the inherent treatment plan was at work.

After this session a detailed follow-up dialogue would also have been somewhat disruptive, because mother and child were very relaxed and connected. She was so pleased that she and her husband had decided to spend the coming vacation not in the mountains but at home.

Seven weeks later I received a thank-you card from Peter's mother. Peter had become increasingly released from his inconsolable "curled-up hedgehog" state and had since become very much more calm and contented. The episodes of screaming had virtually ceased, and he settled down at night on his own. The colic had disappeared, and the atopic dermatitis now occurred only rarely and in mild form.

Digestive and Sleep Disorders, Constant Screaming

Session 1: Kate, a mother of three, had been given my address by her physiotherapist. At short notice we arranged an initial appointment for Laura, who was not quite nine months old. As had been the case with Kate's first two children, Laura had major digestive problems. Regardless of whether it was water, milk, or different kinds of baby cereal, everything caused regurgitation, vomiting, or diarrhea. Her two siblings had also already received Craniosacral Therapy while they were still living in Canada. Kate had had difficult births with two of her children. The pregnancy with Laura went beyond the due date, and labor had been pharmacologically induced in the hospital. However, when only three contractions occurred in four hours, the decision was made to use epidural anesthesia, and then the birth proceeded rapidly.

She seemed to be visibly fully extended in looking after her three children and running the home. On top of that, she and Laura had hardly slept the previous night because Laura had been screaming a great deal and was almost inconsolable. Exhaustive investigations into Laura's digestive and sleep problems had yielded no evidence to indicate any abnormalities, and in terms of conventional allopathic medicine, everything had been checked and was fine. Laura seemed to be strong, with good motor skills and good balance. I addressed her and was able to make a start with supporting her on the treatment table in her movements. And she enjoyed it.

With both hands I went with her spontaneous movements in her entire torso region, especially at the midline in the region of the cervical and thoracic spine. In this process I noted extreme diaphragmatic tension that began to diminish steadily after a few minutes as a result of my clear and yet spacious contact. After the first part of the session, during which Laura, sitting and lying down, seemed to unwind out of her discomfort, there followed a treatment sequence with Laura lying down during which I was able to treat her entire thoracic and cervical region up as far as the cranial base. After eight months it could still be seen and sensed clearly that Laura's left clavicle had been broken at birth and that understandably, she had not yet come to terms with this. Afterward I listened to the craniosacral rhythm at several cranial bones, then gently released two mild compressions, and attuned myself increasingly to the tension states in the cerebral and spinal meninges, including the intracranial membranes, which were nevertheless able to show a minor improvement in balance. During the final third of the session, Laura fell asleep and, after a spontaneous stillpoint, the process of self-regulation continued at the level of the mid-tide.

Session 2: Kate related that there had been no improvement after the first Craniosacral Therapy session, but a week's vacation in the snow had done the whole family good. Laura smiled at me at the start of the session and then, to her mother's amazement, fell asleep. After briefly assessing and releasing the dural tube, I used both hands to ease the tension in the diaphragm, solar plexus, and kidneys, and then again in the entire thoracic region to reduce the effects on Laura of the broken clavicle and to make this zone increasingly accessible again to the body as a whole. Laura sighed and breathed very irregularly a few times in her sleep. Her self-regulation was already strengthened after just five minutes, as signaled by subtle release processes both around the midline and in the extremities. I treated the suboccipital region and then comprehensively addressed the area around the atlanto-occipital joint, the entire cranial base, and also briefly the cranial vault. In this way all the groundwork was prepared then to specifically release the left and right jugular foramina.

While this was happening, gastrointestinal sounds began to give a concert of very special quality: the various regions of Laura's "second brain" started to emit a range of sounds that became increasingly rich in variation and volume. To conclude I used the cranial vault hold to harmonize the craniosacral rhythm at the head and attuned myself to the membrane and fluid level. After a spontaneous stillpoint the qualities of the craniosacral rhythm were definitely more balanced than before, except that the left side still seemed to be a little more inertial compared with the right side. However, I knew that there had already been sufficient release in the cervical and head region, and I did not want to overtax the system in any way. Instead of becoming bogged down on the left side, I was convinced that both the already released and newly integrated structure as well as the various slow rhythms would help the now clearly reduced restrictions on the left side to undergo further release. I therefore integrated the session in the abdominal and pelvic region and then remained seated for the last ten minutes at the side of the treatment table, where I placed one hand broadly in the area of the navel, and the other in the area around the shoulder and neck along with the occipital bone. I observed the holistic shift, and then in parallel with the stillness I sensed how the inherent treatment plan took further steps toward greater balance, while the fluid drive became clearly more pronounced.

Session 3: after the second session, Laura began to regurgitate less often, and her digestion improved—above all, however, she was awake for less time at night and she fell asleep more easily. Kate seemed to show less emotional and nervous agitation. During this third session I listened and treated Laura briefly in the same regions as in the second session, including the atlanto-occipital region, the occipital condyles, both jugular foramina, the left shoulder region, and the left clavicle. Laura seemed to greatly enjoy my applied touch. Her mother, with whom I occasionally had a quiet word during the sessions, also confirmed that Laura was extraordinarily quiet and was not showing any refusal to comply, in contrast to her usual behavior.

Then a more active phase of the session got under way so as to address issues related to the birth process. Laura alternately cried and screamed. I supported her little crawling movements as far as the end of the table and then the spiraling unwinding movements from the table down to the floor. In this process I attuned myself especially to Laura's emotional and energetic state and made certain that while she felt my company in the process sufficiently clearly, I did not proceed too intensively. Here I supported Laura in her individual timing—both in her phases of forward movement and in her rest phases—using my comprehensive touch, my heart, and my sympathetic approach as well as addressing her verbally. Laura cried and screamed, sometimes falteringly, sometimes forcefully. Throughout the entire symbolic birth process I took care to ensure that her left shoulder, the clavicle that had been fractured at birth, was not compressed. This first journey from the table down to the floor was relatively brief. Once Laura had arrived on the floor mattress, her mother welcomed her and took her lovingly and intimately into her embrace.

After this first birth process it was still not possible for Laura to sense her mother calmly; Laura's agitation was intense, and she expressed it with considerable volume. Afterward my clearly perceptible hand over the diaphragm and solar plexus region had a calming effect on Laura, with the result that eye contact with her mother was possible. After this brief rebonding phase Laura began to cry again and twisted her entire torso as if she were trying to escape from something uncomfortable. It appeared that in reliving her birth process the intensity of the difficult birth experience had started to be released, but that Laura was still tormented by discomfort and painful memories. Her mother placed the child on the treatment table again, and I supported Laura again in her movements. In response she cried less and instead visibly gained strength. I found this very demanding: on one hand I was exclusively supporting Laura's inner movement impulses, and on the other she occasionally needed clear but not excessive resistance to be able to use her own strength to free herself from her previously restricted state.

The first journey from table to floor, symbolizing the birth process, had gone relatively quickly and Laura had given the impression of being helpless and disoriented. The second journey took longer and was characterized by much more strength, contact, orientation, and more harmonious timing, with active phases combined with plentiful quieter phases in which Laura enjoyed the ongoing effects and gathered her strength. When Laura landed on the mattress, mother and child greeted each other immediately and then enjoyed an intensive rebonding phase. While I was in the process of considering the various options for integration and rounding off the session, with astonishing speed the peaceful togetherness between mother and child faded: Laura again began to intensively unwind her torso and to whine. Her regurgitation became more marked, and she thrashed with her legs and feet. When I offered her a finger to hold, she grasped it to herself and demonstrated in a dynamic way that she still possessed a great deal of strength and endurance.

Because Laura had clearly been able to build up resources during her first two attempts at this birth game, and her mother had accompanied both in a harmonious way, I supported Laura again a third time in her symbolic birth process. This time Laura's movements and the sounds she emitted were very different compared with the first two occasions. Laura sometimes made little burps and farts, and more dramatically her movements showed vibrancy and strength, and she was extremely present, attentive, and alert. Instead of crying, this time she gave voice to powerful shouts and seemed to find this liberating. The subsequent rebonding of mother and child this time also included a bottle-feed. I suggested to her mother that she position Laura in such a way that they could look into each other's eyes during feeding. I also encouraged her now to grant herself permission in the following moments to be there entirely for herself and Laura and to maintain the heart connection and eye contact with her daughter, including vocal expression. Her mother asked me to apply my touch to her own shoulder-neck region, and she perceptibly and visibly relaxed in response. At a slight distance from the body I then briefly sensed along Laura's back and touched her in those places where my hand felt drawn.

When her mother wanted to move from her position on the floor, I suggested that she make herself comfortable with Laura on the soft treatment table and simply enjoy the experience. Her mother was deeply touched that Laura—for the first time since she had been born—was now willing to rest contentedly on her belly and doze off. Inwardly I was deeply connected with my heart and with the dynamic stillness. I was able to clearly sense the inhalation and exhalation phase of the mid-tide, and I widened my perceptual field beyond the room (Zone C) as far as the horizon (Zone D). Time seemed to stand still because when I glanced again at the clock in the treatment room, exactly fifty-five minutes in total had elapsed. I sensed that it was imperative to leave the mother and child on their own for a few more moments to enjoy the ongoing effects. After this session I was certain that it had helped not just Laura but also her mother to discard the unwanted ballast of worries, to strengthen mutual contact, and to find life in general a little easier to handle.

Session 4: Laura smiled at me, and her mother told me with visible amazement that her daughter had slept through four whole nights for the first time since her birth nine months earlier. Her digestion had also improved again, and her mother could put up with the more frequent farting because it bore no comparison with Laura's torment before she started the sessions. The intense regurgitation of fluids and baby food now occurred only rarely, especially perhaps when there was generally too much activity in the home. Her mother also appeared to be visibly more relaxed than even a week earlier. Understandably she was overjoyed at no longer having to be stressed out for hours each night listening to her daughter screaming, but instead to be able to get more rest.

During the first third of this fourth session I again assessed and treated Laura's thoracic region, clavicles and superior thoracic aperture, cervical region, atlanto-occipital joint, SBS, cranial base, and right and left jugular foramina. Afterward Laura alternated between active expressive phases and passive phases in which she was very much connecting and sensing inwardly. There was no longer any impulse for the birth game, as in the two previous sessions. Instead Laura slipped into a very contented and relaxed state, with the result that during the first half of the session I was able to harmonize the craniosacral rhythm while the process at the level of the fluid body and mid-tide continued and deepened. Following the automatic shift, the inherent treatment plan went into operation in a way that defies description. Laura's mother had fallen asleep in the interim. After the session we left it that this would be the last one for the time being and that her mother could contact me again at any time as necessary. The fourth session had presumably stabilized Laura's improved state of health, and the biodynamic treatment level had additionally deepened all impulses toward healing.

Infant Following Ventouse Delivery

This example describes the case of eighteen-month-old Tobias, who had had an extremely difficult birth and was now being treated in the setting of a pediatric Craniosacral Therapy training course. His mother had already received several craniosacral sessions, and Tobias had received two. She was now forty years old and in her sixth month of pregnancy. This session therefore concerned the health and well-being of three people, with the particular treatment objective of supporting Tobias in his development. A full conventional allopathic medical diagnosis was available. While taking a brief case history I simultaneously established resonance with the mood of the mother and the child. Her pregnancy with Tobias had been planned, and there had been no problems. Because she was relaxed, I asked her at this point what then had been the most beautiful phases of her pregnancy so that these could be made accessible to her as a resource. She then related to me that at the time of the birth she had been admitted to the hospital as an emergency case. She and her baby had been taken to the limits of their endurance because labor had lasted for thirty hours. In the end Tobias could be delivered only with the aid of a ventouse (vacuum device).

His health afterward gave cause for concern: Tobias suffered a stroke and had a pneumothorax, for which he underwent percutaneous aspiration. He then received potent analgesics and was artificially ventilated and tube-fed for a week. I knew that for both mother and child this would be a highly charged traumatic experience, and I mentioned with great appreciation the enormity of the achievement of both of them in completing this birth process. While she was able to accept this, she then showed consternation and anger at the diagnoses and prognoses offered over the past eighteen months by some conventional allopathic physicians who had given her son only a minimal chance of survival—and even then, only with major disabilities. I was able to empathize with the various emotions of his mother and confirmed for her that thankfully these prognoses had failed to materialize because, despite his difficult start in life, Tobias was doing relatively well.

I now turned to Tobias, greeted him, told him my name, and said that I and the group of students in the room had a benevolent attitude toward him and his mother, and that I would support him in whatever way might be helpful. Even before this Tobias had been looking around the room with interest, seeking eye contact with individuals, and showed himself to be extremely present and balanced throughout the entire session whenever contact was offered. He found his bearings, looked at the play corner, went to get his favorite book that he had brought along, and accompanied his mother into the play corner. I praised Tobias: "You're already tall and very independent for your age." His mother told me that her current pregnancy was more stressful than the first, that she had digestive problems and rapidly felt exhausted. In the meantime Tobias scrambled up his mother's front and then wanted to slide head-first down her back. I made sure that there was a sufficiently soft mat and blanket on the floor to provide a comfortable enough landing for Tobias's experiment, and quick as a flash, Tobias was already sliding down his mother's back toward the floor. He laughed, looked at his mother, looked at me, and then repeated the exercise. This time he even rolled away on the mat. Then he took a time-out.

While he was doing this I was able to place my hands at his neck and cervical region and sacrum; I listened and then moved my hand at the sacrum to Tobias's dorsal region, where I palpated both pulmonary lobes and the diaphragm. I shared my impressions with everyone present: "Tobias's breathing is free and can be easily sensed." I intuitively placed my upper hand slightly higher on his occipital bone. "Tobias is pushing himself subtly yet clearly toward my hands, probably indicating where there is tension and where he needs support," I announced to his mother and the group. His mother was astonished at how Tobias allowed himself to be touched and lay there calmly, because this was unusual for him with people he did not know.

While I was applying my touch to Tobias, he was able to move freely at any time, and I went with any small and large movements that he spontaneously made. The right side of his body was extremely present and powerful; sometimes his left side did not seem to be as important to him, and here there was a degree of potential for encouragement and development. I offered Tobias a finger, which he took hold of, and he gave me an insistent look. With one hand I established broad contact on Tobias's back over his thoracic spine while placing my other hand on his front over his abdomen and solar plexus; listening continuously I adapted myself to the structures and their inherent motion. Tobias next touched my hand as if he was trying to tell me, "Yes, that's good. Stay there; I like that, and hold me tightly to you." Perhaps it was also simply just a sign of contact, affection, and trust. After he gave a very deep out-breath I gained the impression that Tobias's thorax became laterally wider, fuller, and broader for about thirty seconds. His breathing was now more rounded and even.

Next it was time for a short break, a pause. I announced that I was about to disengage my hand contact. Tobias stayed quietly on his left side, alert and relaxed, and made eye contact with his mother. I asked her later whether she would also like treatment; to her great delight a craniosacral practitioner in the course started to treat the region of her sacrum and the junction of the thoracic and lumbar spine. While this was happening Tobias lay beside her on the mat, close enough to watch his mother.

Although a ventouse had been used toward the end of the delivery process, the shape of Tobias's head eighteen months later was no longer abnormal. In the cranial vault position I listened at several cranial bones simultaneously. The right sphenoid wing felt like it was emitting sparks. I then treated the right-side torsion and the side-bending with right-side convexity by molding the cranial bones several times very gently in harmony with the craniosacral rhythm, and then made a before-and-after comparison of the craniosacral rhythm. I then placed one hand below Tobias's cervical region while inserting my other hand from a cranial direction so far beneath his head that my soft fingertips were palpating the occipital ridge and establishing touch contact there for a prolonged time—without pressure and with my fingers adapting to the structure and not vice versa. Tobias gave the impression of being strongly contented and looked at me with big eyes. I reminded him: "Simply enjoy it. Your mother, everyone else here, and I are relaxed and enjoying this. You can also change your position at any time or ask for something different."

In the cervical region I sensed various releases, discharges, and micromovements. The cervical region and occipital bone let go for several minutes into my supple hands. With my fingers at the occipital ridge I sensed a permanent softening of the tissue, with the result that I was able to make clearer contact with the two condylar parts of the occipital bone and sense their position. The result was consistent with my assessment of the SBS and the occipital squama, and with my overall impression of the cervical spine.

I was able to detect various compressions and then gently began to slightly spread the occipital ridge as my supple terminal phalanges became wider, fuller, and broader. I invited the atlanto-occipital joint, including the fine ligaments, to become freer and wider from the inside out. Afterward Tobias's cervical region and occipital bone had a floating and relaxed feel. The motion of the occipital squama in harmony with the craniosacral rhythm was now more clearly perceptible, and I had the impression that the region as a whole was starting to become more balanced. The tissue was now working increasingly from the inside and revealed the release pathway, which I went with as I gave my support. I moved the hand that had been over the cervical region and now placed it over Tobias's upper abdomen so that I could sense or address the inferior thoracic aperture, the diaphragm, the thorax as a whole, the stomach, the transverse colon, and the solar plexus as desired.

Later I integrated the session by also including the torso and pelvis. Tobias, meanwhile, had fallen asleep on the mat in the play corner. His mother announced that her unborn child was now moving and active. The other practitioner treated her in the region of the sacrum and hip and released a compression in the lumbosacral joint. Tobias gave two deep sighs. The inner physician was simply at work in him, at various body locations simultaneously: sometimes a foot would twitch, followed by the left side of his body. Tobias carried on sleeping for a while. His body showed small, fine micromovements. I quietly announced to Tobias that I was about to disengage my hand contact. When he woke up, his mother entered into warm, intimate contact with him, showed him how pleased she was, and took him into her arms. After this rebonding phase Tobias and his mother left.

Tobias is now three years old. He has developed splendidly, and I am happy to report that none of the horrendous prognoses offered after he was born have come to pass.

Problems with Social Contact and Behavioral Discipline

Session 1: Three-year-old Selina was extremely aggressive toward her mother and would not accept any behavioral discipline whatsoever. This prompted her mother to visit my practice at the Sphinx Craniosacral Institute with her daughter on four occasions. Her mother told me how Selina had "got stuck for a very long time" during labor, and apparently no one had noticed how far advanced the birth process already was. Selina was very restless, especially at night, was always tearing her blanket off, and frequently developed colds. She liked the large seminar room, which she explored closely. Behind the curtain she discovered the knee roll pillows, the colors of which she could name, and she placed them on the massage table. Afterward she decorated the floor mattress with a large number of floor cushions and said, "There—that's done." Later she practiced the "sliding down from the table" game several times with great delight.

I treated the mother's kidney region and the area of her abdomen and solar plexus. As she relaxed more deeply, Selina climbed up onto the massage table and held my fingers. After I had eased the tension in her mother's lumbar region, I continued with her shoulder-neck area. While I was doing this, Selina often climbed up onto the table, sat down, and lay on top of her mother before climbing down again after a while. Suddenly, however, Selina lay lower down over her mother's pelvis and thighs and demanded that her mother make more space for her. When her mother gave her more space, this was followed by absolute silence. I was astounded that this position was so similar to the situation of giving birth. After three minutes Selina slid down from the table again and contentedly looked at her picture book while I rounded off her mother's treatment.

Session 2: Her mother reported that communication with Selina had improved considerably after the first craniosacral session. She was proud of her daughter. In addition, on the day after the session, her mother had had a swollen abdomen, and her body felt as it had at the time when she was recovering from pregnancy. At the start of the second session Selina sat on her mother's lap and rested for about ten minutes while I treated her mother. Later, Selina crept up higher against her mother and rested with her face against her mother's breast, which reminded me of the bonding process after birth.

Session 3: Once again Selina explored the room while I treated her mother. After a while she again scrambled up onto the massage table, sat with her mother, and then laid her head against her mother's breast. Selina became quiet and very peaceful. After I had released the tense back of the supine mother, I spotted Selina's bottle on the window sill and asked them if they would like it. Mother and child both said "yes," and while Selina drank from the bottle, her mother exposed her breast as when breast-feeding so that Selina could feel the skin-to-skin contact. I held back and was amazed how Selina, without any active help from me, had aptly rounded off her own birth process in three sessions.

The craniosacral sessions brought an enormous improvement in the mother-child relationship. They helped the mother to relax more and to be proud of her daughter. Compared with beforehand, Selina hardly ever removed the blanket at night and only rarely suffered with colds. She also only rarely failed to follow her mother's instructions relating to behavioral discipline.

Developmental Delay

The parents of five-year-old Lara told me that her hearing was poor and that she spoke little. Conventional allopathic medical examination revealed, however, that her hearing was averagely developed. Lara seemed to me to live in an almost inaccessible world that was cut off from her surroundings. At birth there had been a knot in her umbilical cord. While I began by treating the father during Session 1, Lara removed her shoes and so signaled her willingness to be treated. Her legs and pelvis were visibly rotated to the right, and her shoulder and head to the left. Her whole body seemed to be a little rigid. Lara often had the fingers of her left hand in her mouth.

In Session 2 it struck me again that Lara showed prominent abdominal breathing but hardly any thoracic breathing, and it was often faltering. While the release of her parietal bones was pleasant for her, Lara found the application of touch to her frontal bone to be disagreeable. At that point the parents remembered that their daughter, at the age of eighteen months, had fallen onto her forehead and required stitches. Since that time her developmental disorders had become clear. I released the structures around the frontal bone, and at the end of the second session I had the impression that the membrane level was also more balanced, which would have further repercussions on the frontal bone.

During Session 3 I again released the dural tube, the atlanto-occipital joint, the condylar parts of the occipital bone, and the SBS by decompressing the sphenoid. On this occasion Lara also permitted touch contact at the frontal bone.

During Session 4 Lara wanted to lie with her mother on the massage table. I was able to treat the child's dorsal area and supported the subtle unwinding movements in the torso and sacral region. While this was going on Lara frequently jabbed at her mother's zygomatic bones. Was this pure coincidence, or was Lara trying to signal something? I was subsequently able to treat her head region and both zygomatic bones. Afterward her head and mandible no longer jutted so far to the left as in the previous sessions. Lara slept during the final quarter of this session. Her left shoulder, arm, and hand twitched repeatedly, as if a great deal of retained tension was being discharged in these areas.

At the start of Session 5, Lara appeared to me to be definitely more open, more sociable, and more coordinated in her movements. Her mother reported that her daughter had made clear progress on all fronts, was more open, and was much more amenable to being taught how to do things by her parents. I treated Lara's torso and head again, especially her frontal bone, zygomatic bones, temporal bones, and other parts of the cranial base. According to information received from her mother, Lara again showed very positive changes after her next growth spurt.

Mild Developmental Delay and Hyperactive Tendency, Social Contact Problems in Kindergarten

I visited and treated five-year-old Julian on five occasions in his home. His parents were concerned because he was allegedly lagging a little behind in his development, he showed hyperactive traits, and he was about to undergo assessment before starting school. His mother was present during Session 1, which was conducted on the massage table in Julian's room. At the end she said she had the feeling from having watched that she would also like to be treated herself. I suggested that she should also receive treatment during my next visit to the house. She worked part-time as a physiotherapist, and during this craniosacral session, as well as experiencing the release of tension she also briefly relived an abrupt landing that she had sustained in the past while paragliding. Julian also enjoyed Session 2.

Before Session 3 the father told me that Julian had expressed fears that he might fall out of bed. I noticed that Julian's bed was less than eighteen inches off the ground, and I suspected an experience that was related to a loss of balance or was linked to his birth experience. I took this as a cue to invite him at the start of the session to slide down from the table to the floor. I showed him how to do it and then allowed him plenty of time to make various attempts. During the session that followed Julian calmed down again from the agitation that he had experienced previously.

At the start of Session 4, Julian presented me with a drawing. It showed a house in a brightly colored garden. Visible on the roof were six enormous chimneys from which belched large quantities of smoke. I let him know that I was pleased and thought to myself that during and after the three Craniosacral Therapy sessions he had probably been able to let off a great deal of steam. His parents told me that Julian was no longer afraid at night and was now also happier about going to kindergarten and visiting friends.

At the end of Session 5 Julian seemed to me to be better connected to himself and much more confident in his movements.

Developmental Delays, Learning Difficulties

Ten-year-old Bruno was attending additional language development classes because he suffered from dyslexia. He did not enjoy reading and writing, but made up for this by excelling in geometry and math. He did not start talking until he was three years old. Labor had been very prolonged: in the hospital his mother had been given medication to help her sleep, and she had been left on her own all night. In the morning the baby had to be delivered by ventouse. Bruno's head had an extremely elongated shape. During Session 1 he enjoyed all applications of touch to the head, except at the parietal bones, where the ventouse suction device had been attached. At the start of each of the following sessions Bruno was always highly attentive and he would comment on any change in the room: for example, an orange candle had been burning last time, and this time the candle was white, or the soft positioning aids were arranged differently from last time.

At the beginning of Session 2, Bruno's pelvis and torso tended slightly to the left, and his upper body and head tended markedly to the right. For his pollen allergy I treated his thorax with broad percussion, gave visceral treatment to his liver and spleen, and also treated his frontal bone and nasal bone and released the frontonasal suture. At first Bruno declined my suggestion that he slide down from the treatment table to the floor. Later, however, he felt he wanted to try it: coming out of a gentle unwinding, he moved slowly toward the table edge. He stretched his head down over the edge but then went no further. Suddenly he let both arms and legs drop and stopped moving—as if he was playing possum. Was this a sign that he was reliving his birth situation, the epidural anesthesia phase, or the shortage of oxygen supply? I asked him how he was feeling. "It's fine," he whispered. After a little time had elapsed Bruno had an impulse to move forward slowly. I helped him in this by supporting him with my hands as he slid head-first down from the table.

In Session 3 I treated the thorax again, performed jugular foramen release, and was able to balance somewhat the torsion to the left with side-bending. His head had a very solid, compact feel. Bruno liked the application of firm touch to his head. I therefore released his parietal and temporal bones while decompressing with clear traction, which he enjoyed. Bruno's maxilla was very narrow, and his teeth were very crowded. Using slight lateral mobilization I released the fixed zygomatic bones. In this my aim was also to achieve greater mobility for the maxilla and, via the zygomatic bones, also for the cranial base and the greater wings of the sphenoid. Afterward, Bruno embarked on an imaginary journey in which he found himself in a violent tempest on the high seas, and then he was back on dry land again. Before the end of the session he wanted to slide down from the table to the floor mattress on his own, after which he was visibly satisfied and proud.

At the beginning of Session 4, his mother reported that during the past three months and now after three Craniosacral Therapy sessions, Bruno had made huge strides forward in his development. For the moment he needed no further language development classes, was more open, and was better able to stand up for himself. Bruno had again been greatly looking forward to today's session. In this final session before the summer vacation, I also treated Bruno in the side-lying position, both at the sacrum and occipital bone, as well as along his spine and especially in the region around T7, T8, and T9. To free the cranial base from compression even more, I also performed cranial base and jugular foramen release, and again treated the SBS torsion. By the end the dural tube also felt clearly more flexible and wider.

Two more sessions followed during the autumn. With my support, Bruno greatly enjoyed making spontaneous rotatory movements on the table and also away from the table. The balance and reaction exercises on the tuning board and another balancing disk were a big challenge for him, but they gave him pleasure. The motion patterns in the cranial region were clearly reduced compared with the findings in the spring and summer. In both autumn sessions it was principally a question of releasing tensions and compressions in the torso and pelvis and in the dural tube. Afterward these areas became significantly softer and more balanced. Bruno had emerged from his defensive attitude and gave greater expression to his feelings. This also included better anger management and the ability to see things through to completion.

At the end of the final session, as a special gift, Bruno performed for me on his recorder.

Dental Braces, Occasional Headaches

At her own request, eleven-year-old Samantha occasionally received craniosacral treatments from her mother, a physiotherapist and craniosacral practitioner. She had heard from her mother about the Sphinx Craniosacral Institute and now wanted to receive treatment from me. An open-minded girl, Samantha had been wearing dental braces for about a year and had since experienced occasional headaches that had been kept to a minimum with the help of Craniosacral Therapy. I assessed and treated Samantha's feet, knees, hip joints, sacrum and dural tube, diaphragm, and thoracic segments, and in the cervical region her hyoid bone and the atlanto-occipital joint. Via her arms I also performed release for her shoulders and the cervical region as far as the occipital ridge. I then treated her neurocranium and viscerocranium. The SBS accepted my invitation into decompression, and in response to subtle lifting of the frontal bone, the orbital sutures and the coronal suture were released.

Samantha asked for the intraoral session to be kept brief. I therefore decided to take just one single contact position inside her mouth, at the midline of the hard palate. There, via the maxilla and vomer, I performed minimal decompression on the vertical connection up as far as the rostrum, crest, and ethmoidal spine of the sphenoid, while using two fingers of my other hand to stabilize the two greater wings of the sphenoid. In this process I also gave consideration to the space between the palatine bones and the pterygoid processes so that the pterygopalatine ganglion would also be decompressed. I applied this subtle release technique for about one minute. It was very effective because afterward the motion of the sphenoid was clearly stronger and more balanced. Then, working from the outside, I performed a lateral spread of the two halves of the maxilla and the zygomatic bones. For a short time I also listened at the mandible and went with its widening motion. To conclude, at the head I supported both temporal bones into external rotation, listened in the cranial vault hold, and integrated the session in the pelvic region.

Three weeks after the session, Samantha's mother reported back to me that her daughter had not experienced any more headaches. It had been important for her that I had kept my promise and not given extensive intraoral treatment; otherwise this would have reminded her of past visits to the dentist, where, on each occasion, she had had to endure more prolonged intraoral treatment than had been stated beforehand.

Note: The treatment examples above illustrate that minor and major miracles are possible with just one session, or a few follow-up sessions, of pediatric Craniosacral Therapy. However, their inclusion here is not intended to set the bar of parental and practitioner expectation so high that this generates stress during the session. There are many children who require several sessions before the first changes become evident, and it may even take eight to twelve more sessions to achieve the effect described in these treatment examples.

APPENDIX: CRANIAL NERVES

Cranial Nerve I: Olfactory Nerve

FUNCTION
- sense of smell

INNERVATION
- nasal mucosae

PATHOLOGY
- complete loss of sense of smell
- disturbed sense of smell

CRANIOSACRAL-SPECIFIC STRUCTURES
- sphenoid
- ethmoid
- Cranial nerve I traverses the cribriform plate of the ethmoid.

Cranial Nerve II: Optic Nerve

FUNCTION
- vision

INNERVATION
- retina

PATHOLOGY
- visual field defects
- diplopia (double vision)

CRANIOSACRAL-SPECIFIC STRUCTURES
- body of sphenoid
- lesser wing of sphenoid
- tentorium cerebelli
- Cranial nerve II traverses the optic canal.

Cranial Nerve III: Oculomotor Nerve

FUNCTION
- raising and lowering eyes
- medial movement of eyes, constriction of pupils
- muscles of accommodation
- raising the upper eyelid

INNERVATION
- all ocular muscles except lateral rectus and superior oblique

PATHOLOGY
- divergent strabismus
- ptosis (drooping eyelid)
- mydriasis (dilatation of pupil)
- diplopia (double vision)

CRANIOSACRAL-SPECIFIC STRUCTURES
- lesser and greater wing of sphenoid
- tentorium cerebelli
- Cranial nerve III traverses the superior orbital fissure.

Cranial Nerve IV: Trochlear Nerve

FUNCTION
- lowering of gaze, abduction, intorsion

INNERVATION
- superior oblique muscle

PATHOLOGY
- diplopia (double vision)
- divergent strabismus
- limitation of eye movement downward and outward

CRANIOSACRAL-SPECIFIC STRUCTURES
- temporal bone
- spinal dura mater
- C1, C2
- Cranial nerve IV traverses the superior orbital fissure.

Cranial Nerve V: Trigeminal Nerve

FUNCTION
- mouth sensation
- facial sensation
- masticatory muscles

INNERVATION
- general sensory supply of face, paranasal sinuses, teeth
- motor supply of masticatory muscles

PATHOLOGY
- defect of trigeminal ganglion and of the three subdivisions:
  - cranial nerve V1 (ophthalmic nerve)
  - cranial nerve V2 (maxillary nerve)
  - cranial nerve V3 (mandibular nerve)
- masticatory muscle paralysis
- neuralgia

CRANIOSACRAL-SPECIFIC STRUCTURES
- temporal bone
- spinal dura mater
- C1, C2
- Cranial nerve V traverses:
  - superior orbital fissure (V1)
  - foramen rotundum (V2)
  - foramen ovale (V3)

Cranial Nerve VI: Abducens Nerve

FUNCTION
- lateral movement of eyeball

INNERVATION
- motor supply of lateral rectus muscle

PATHOLOGY
- convergent strabismus
- diplopia (double vision)

CRANIOSACRAL-SPECIFIC STRUCTURES
- sphenoid
- temporal bone
- Cranial nerve VI traverses the superior orbital fissure.

Cranial Nerve VII: Facial Nerve

FUNCTION
- facial expression
- glandular secretion
- sensation of anterior two-thirds of the tongue

INNERVATION
- special sensory:
  - anterior two-thirds of the tongue
  - soft palate
- motor:
  - facial muscles
- secretory:
  - sublingual glands
  - submandibular glands
  - lacrimal glands

PATHOLOGY
- facial nerve palsy: disturbance of muscles of facial expression
- undifferentiated hearing, hypersensitivity to sound

CRANIOSACRAL-SPECIFIC STRUCTURES
- geniculate ganglion
- TMJ
- Cranial nerve VII traverses:
  - internal acoustic meatus
  - stylomastoid foramen

Cranial Nerve VIII: Vestibulocochlear Nerve

FUNCTION
- balance
- hearing

INNERVATION
- special sensory:
  - vestibular part
  - cochlear part

PATHOLOGY
- vestibular dizziness due to ear disease
- deafness
- nystagmus

CRANIOSACRAL-SPECIFIC STRUCTURES
- TMJ
- temporal bone
- Cranial nerve VIII traverses the internal acoustic meatus.

Cranial Nerve IX: Glossopharyngeal Nerve

FUNCTION
- taste
- salivary gland secretion
- swallowing

INNERVATION
- special sensory:
  - posterior one-third of the tongue
  - tonsils
  - middle ear
- motor:
  - stylopharyngeus muscle
  - pharyngeal constrictor muscles

PATHOLOGY
- disturbances of swallowing
- disturbances of taste
- dry mouth

CRANIOSACRAL-SPECIFIC STRUCTURES
- occipital bone
- temporal bone
- Cranial nerve IX traverses the jugular foramen.

Cranial Nerve X: Vagus Nerve

FUNCTION
- lowers heart rate
- increases intestinal peristalsis

INNERVATION
- special sensory:
  - heart
  - lungs
  - bronchi
  - trachea
  - larynx
  - pharynx
  - gastrointestinal tract
  - external ear
- motor:
  - pharynx, heart
  - lungs, bronchi
  - gastrointestinal tract
- secretory:
  - glands
  - gastrointestinal tract, respiratory tract

PATHOLOGY
- ipsilateral paralysis of the soft palate
- disturbances of swallowing
- speech disturbances

CRANIOSACRAL-SPECIFIC STRUCTURES
- occipital bone
- temporal bone
- Cranial nerve X traverses the jugular foramen.

Cranial Nerve XI: Accessory Nerve

FUNCTION
- head rotation
- shoulder lifting

INNERVATION
- motor:
  - sternocleidomastoid muscle
  - trapezius muscle

PATHOLOGY
- torticollis

CRANIOSACRAL-SPECIFIC STRUCTURES
- temporal bone
- occipital bone
- Cranial nerve XI traverses the jugular foramen and foramen magnum.

Cranial Nerve XII: Hypoglossal Nerve

FUNCTION
- tongue movement

INNERVATION
- motor:
  - muscles of the tongue
  - infrahyoid muscles

PATHOLOGY
- tongue deviation to the affected side
- atrophy or wasting of the tongue

CRANIOSACRAL-SPECIFIC STRUCTURES
- occipital bone
- SBS
- Cranial nerve XII traverses the hypoglossal canal.

GLOSSARY

ADHD: Attention deficit/hyperactivity disorder

afferent: Conveying from the periphery toward the center, for example from a sensory organ to the CNS

amygdala: The corpus amygdaloideum, an almond-shaped structure within the tip of the temporal lobe of the brain; part of the limbic system

ANS: Autonomic nervous system, the totality of nerve and ganglion cells not subject to the control of the will and the conscious mind

anteflexion: Forward curvature

anterior: Toward the ventral surface of the body, from the middle

anteversion: Forward tipping or tilting

A-O release: Releasing tensions in the atlanto-occipital joint

atlanto-occipital joint: The articulation between the atlas and the occipital bone

birth lie side: In the womb, the side of the baby that is conjunct with the mother's spine

bonding: The formation of close emotional ties between people, especially between mother and child

brachial plexus: A network of nerves that conducts signals from the spinal cord to the shoulder, arm, and hand

brachial plexus paralysis: Paralysis of the shoulder, arm, or hand due to injury to the brachial nerve plexus

branchiogenic organs: Glands with internal secretion, for example the thymus, thyroid, and epithelial buds

Breath of Life: The symbol and expression of the invisible, timeless, and unidirectional element that releases creative existential forces

cell memory: The capacity of the body's cells to store the memory of past events

cephalhematoma: A collection of blood under the scalp of a newborn, caused by pressure during birth

cerebral aneurysm: Widening of a cerebral artery or vein due to a change in the vessel wall

cerebral aqueduct: A narrow channel carrying CSF from the third to the fourth cerebral ventricle; also known as the mesencephalic duct

choroid plexus: Infoldings of blood vessels of the pia mater, which produce CSF

cingulate gyrus: Arch-shaped convolution closely related to the surface of the corpus callosum; part of the limbic system

CNS: Central nervous system, that portion of the nervous system consisting of the brain and spinal cord

compensation: Restoring balance following organic dysfunction or its sequelae

contraindication: Any circumstance that makes undesirable the use of a particular medicine or diagnostic or therapeutic procedure

cortisol: A stress hormone synthesized in the adrenal cortex

cranial: Upward, toward the top of the head

craniosacral rhythm: An expression of the Breath of Life, with a slow rhythmic motion of six to twelve cycles per minute; abbreviated as CSR

craniosacral system: A system comprising the cranial bones, spinal column and sacrum, the meninges covering the brain and spinal cord, and the CSF

C-section: Cesarean section, incision through the abdominal and uterine walls for delivery of a fetus

CSF: Cerebrospinal fluid, the fluid contained within the four ventricles of the brain, the subarachnoid space, and the central canal of the spinal cord

CV4: Literally, "compression of the fourth cerebral ventricle," a still-point in extension, internal rotation, or exhalation

cyst: A fluid-filled cavity or sac; a cyst may contain one small space or multiple small spaces and may be walled off

cytoplasm: All the contents outside the cell nucleus and enclosed within the cell membrane

decompression: Relief of pressure, for example by direct release in the opposite direction to compression

dissociation: A state of detachment, being out of touch with the here and now

dopamine: A hormonal biochemical precursor of norepinephrine and epinephrine

dorsal: Toward the back, posterior

dura mater cranialis: The toughest of the three membranes covering the brain

dura mater spinalis: Toughest of the three membranes covering the spinal cord

dynamic stillness: A symbol of universal, all-embracing presence beyond the horizon; the eternal source or foundation of all life force; an external fulcrum that is the source of greatest healing potential

dysfunction: A disturbance, impairment, or abnormality of function

ectoderm: Outermost of the three primary germ layers of the embryo

endoderm: Innermost of the three primary germ layers of the embryo

endorphin: A morphine-like endogenous hormone

ependymal layer: Fine lining membrane of the brain and central canal of the spinal cord

epidural anesthesia: The administration of an anesthetic into the space between the dura mater and the internal surfaces of the vertebral arches, usually performed in the lumbar region

ER: External rotation

ethmoid bone: A light, sponge-like bone located between the orbits in the anterior part of the cranial floor

EV4: Literally, "expansion of the fourth cerebral ventricle," a still-point in flexion/external rotation or inhalation

extension: Stretching; drawing apart

falx cerebelli: The small fold of dura mater in the midline of the posterior cranial fossa

falx cerebri: The sickle-shaped fold of dura mater extending downward in the longitudinal cerebral fissure

fascia: Sheets or bands of connective tissue that cover and support all the structures in the body, providing stability and flexibility

fetus: The unborn child from the beginning of month three of gestation until birth

flexion: Bending

foramen, interventricular: Channel carrying CSF from the paired lateral ventricles to the third cerebral ventricle

foramen, jugular: Paired opening on the cranial base between the occipital bone and mastoid process on each side

foramen magnum: The large opening in the anterior and inferior part of the occipital bone

foramen of Luschka: Paired lateral aperture of the fourth cerebral ventricle

foramen of Magendie: Median aperture of the fourth cerebral ventricle

frontal bone: Cranial bone forming the forehead, the roofs of the orbits, and most of the anterior part of the cranial floor

fulcrum: A point around which motion takes place

holistic matrix: Whole-body matrix of connective tissues and the fluids contained in them

homeostasis: Dynamic state of balance between an organism and its surroundings

hydrocephalus: Dilatation of the cerebral ventricles with accumulation of CSF within the skull

hyoid bone: A bone located in the neck and suspended from the styloid processes of the temporal bones by ligaments and muscles for example

hypothalamus: The ventral part of the diencephalon, the center controlling and integrating the ANS; regulates all internal and external stimuli as well as body temperature, hunger, and hormones such as oxytocin

iliopsoas muscle: A blending of two muscles, the psoas major and the iliacus, as they travel toward their common insertion site above the inguinal ligament

indication: A sign or circumstance suggesting a remedial course of action, a reason for using a particular diagnostic or therapeutic procedure

inferior vena cava syndrome: Supine hypotensive syndrome

infrahyoid: Below the hyoid bone

instroke: The inwardly directed movement of biological energies from the periphery to the core

intention: The intense and concentrated focusing of the intellect and emotions toward a particular healing-related objective

interaction: The quality, state, or process of two or more things acting on each other

intracranial membranes: In particular, the vertical and horizontal membranes or meninges that envelope the brain

intraoral: Inside the mouth

IR: Internal rotation

lateral: To the side, away from the midline of a structure

lesion: Any pathological or traumatic disturbance or loss of function

ligament: A band of fibrous tissues that connects bones or cartilages

limbic system: The "emotional brain," part of the brain that is involved in the regulation of behavior and emotions

living matrix: See *holistic matrix*

locus coeruleus: A region of the brain stem that regulates alertness and relaxation, a bluish-gray eminence at the anterior lateral edge of the rhomboid fossa

Long Tide: An expression of the Breath of Life, with a rhythmic motion of about one cycle per one hundred seconds

lordosis: The anterior concavity in the curvature of the lumbar and cervical spine, as viewed from the side; abnormally exaggerated lordosis = hollow back

mandible: Lower jaw

masseter: Muscle that raises the mandible and closes the jaws

mastoid process: A conical process projecting forward and downward from the external surface of the petrous part of the temporal bone, just behind the external acoustic meatus

maxilla: One of the paired bones that form the upper jaw, part of the face, and the lower part of the orbits

medial: Toward the midline of a body or structure

mesoderm: The middle layer of the three primary germ layers of the embryo

micromovement: Inherent movements on the smallest level, for example from a tissue or joint, sometimes as a sign that a release has happened in the body

mid-tide: An expression of the Breath of Life, with a rhythmic motion of two to three cycles per minute

mobility: Movement of one structure in relation to another

morphology: The science of the form and structure of organisms

motility: Inherent motion

motor: Producing or subserving motion

neurocranium: The part of the cranium that encloses the brain

neuroendocrine: Pertaining to the secretion of neurohormones

neurotransmitter: Any of a group of chemical substances that forward messages at the synapses in the CNS and in peripheral nerves

nociception: The perception of pain

nociceptor: A sensory receptor for pain, such as free nerve endings and polymodal fibers

norepinephrine: A stress hormone formed in the adrenal medulla and throughout the sympathetic nervous system

occipital bone: Bone forming the posterior part of the base of the cranium

occipital condyle: One of two oval processes on the lateral portions of the occipital bone, on either side of the foramen magnum, for articulation with the atlas

occlusion: Degree of closure achieved by the contact surfaces of the teeth in the upper and lower jaws

olfactory bulb: The bulb-like expansion of the olfactory tract on the undersurface of the frontal lobe of each cerebral hemisphere

opioids: A group of endogenous substances with morphine-like activity

ossification: The formation of bone

osteoblastic: Bone-forming

outstroke: The outwardly directed movement of biological energies from the core to the periphery

oxytocin: A peptide formed in the hypothalamus; stimulates contractions in labor, milk ejection, and bonding, hence the popular designation "love hormone"

palpate: To examine by touch, or sensing by touch

palpation: The act of sensing and assessing through the hands and fingers

parietal bone: One of the paired bones forming the greater portion of the sides and roof of the cranial cavity

pathological: Indicative of or caused by disease or illness

peptide: Chemical compound consisting of amino acids linked by peptide bonds

peripheral nervous system: The link between the CNS and the organs, meaning the nerves and ganglia outside the brain and spinal cord

peristalsis: The wave of contraction passing along the alimentary canal, and the sounds associated with it

perpendicular plate of ethmoid bone: A thin bony plate that descends from the inferior surface of the cribriform plate of the ethmoid bone and participates in forming the nasal septum

phenomenology: The analysis of subjective processes and events; the science of phenomena, also called existential philosophy and metaphysics

phrenic nerve: Long nerve that travels from the cervical region to the thoracic cavity as far as the diaphragm

phylogenetic: Pertaining to the developmental history of a type or group of living creatures

placenta: A fetomaternal organ responsible for metabolism and hormone production; in embryological terms, part of the unborn child

placental insufficiency: Inability of the placenta to perform its metabolic function

posterior: Toward the dorsal surface of the body, from the middle backward

potency: Strength, force, or power; also the potency in the fluid body, acting like charged biophotons or prana

primary respiration: Expression of the Breath of Life, a universal force that generates slow rhythms; also associated by many authorities with the Long Tide and mid-tide

prolactin: A hormone that stimulates and sustains lactation after birth

prostaglandins: A collective term for a group of hormonelike substances

protoplasm: The entire substance of living human, animal, or plant cells that is surrounded by the cell membrane

protuberance, external occipital: The most prominent point on the outer surface of the squama of the occipital bone

psoas major muscle: Greater psoas muscle that flexes the thigh or torso

pubic symphysis: A fibrocartilage joint formed by the union of the bodies of the pubic bones in the median plane

pulmonary surfactant: Surface phospholipid that aids the development of pulmonary alveoli in the newborn. Part of the protective and self-regulatory system of the bronchi; its absence leads to shock lung and pulmonary edema.

reflex: An involuntary, stereotypical response of the nervous system to sensory input

resource: A source of positive strength or help that supports health and balance

reticular system: The ascending reticular activating system, located in the reticular formation of the brain stem

round ligament pain: Pain in the round ligament of the uterus, experienced in the pelvic and lumbar region

sacroiliac joint: The joint between the sacrum and the iliac bone of the pelvis on both sides

sacrum: A wedge-shaped bone formed usually by five fused vertebrae lodged dorsally between the two hip bones

SBS: Sphenobasilar synchondrosis or sphenobasilar joint; an important articulation between the sphenoid and the basilar part of the occipital bone; the main fulcrum on the cranial base

self-attachment: The ability to sense inwardly and to remain connected with oneself

sensory: Involving or referring to the senses

serotonin: A hormonelike substance produced in the hypothalamus and gut that regulates various organ functions

SomatoEmotional Release®: Release of emotion that has been retained, suppressed, and isolated within the body; developed by John Upledger as an ability to explore emotions in using dialogue.

sphenobasilar synchondrosis or sphenobasilar joint: See *SBS*

sphenoid: A single wedge-shaped bone lying at the middle part of the cranial base and articulating with most of the other cranial bones

spinal anesthesia: Anesthesia delivered close to the spinal cord; regional anesthesia

stacking: A special treatment technique in which the restricted patterns and free movements are stacked, and tissue tension is reduced or released as a result

stillpoint: A temporary pause in the craniosacral rhythm and in the mid-tide

suprahyoid: Above the hyoid bone

suture: A specialized joint of the bones of the cranium

suture, flat: A type of cranial suture with simple apposition of the contiguous surfaces, without interlocking of the borders of the participating bones

suture, serrated: A type of cranial suture in which the participating bones are united by interlocking processes resembling the teeth of a saw

suture, squamous: A type of cranial suture formed by overlapping of the broad beveled edges of the participating bones

symptom: Evidence of illness, a pathological change that is characteristic of a particular disease or belongs to a particular condition

temporal bone: One of the paired bones forming the inferior lateral aspects of the cranium and part of the cranial floor

tentorium cerebelli: The process of dura mater that supports the occipital lobes of the brain and covers the cerebellum

thalamus: A large ovoid mass in the posterior part of the diencephalon forming most of each lateral wall of the third ventricle; the "gateway to consciousness"

transverse: Horizontal or side-to-side

trauma: An event or series of events caused by danger or injury: violation of borders, physical or psychological

trochanter, greater: A broad flat process at the upper end of the lateral surface of the femur

unwinding: Involuntary movements of the tissue to release tensions and entanglements

ventral: From the midline toward the front of the body

ventricular system, cerebral: The four cerebral ventricles and the cerebral aqueduct, containing the CSF

vertical strain: the sphenoid displaced upward (superiorly) or downward (inferiorly) in relation to the occipital bone at the SBS

visceral: Pertaining to the internal organs or viscera

viscerocranium: The facial bones of the skull

visualize: To picture something in the mind's eye

vomer: The unpaired flat bone that forms the inferior and posterior part of the nasal septum

zygomatic arch: Arch formed by the articulation of the zygomatic (cheek) bone with the temporal bone

zygomatic bone: Quadrangular cheek bone

ONLINE RESOURCES

Jaap van der Wal's phenomenological embryology: www.embryo.nl

Stephen W. Porges's polyvagal theory: www.stephenporges.com

Marshall Rosenberg's Nonviolent Communication: www.cnvc.org

Dr. Robert Schleip, who provides a wealth of interesting topics and links: www.somatics.de

Dr. Peter A. Levine's Somatic Experiencing® trauma healing: www.traumahealing.com

Karlton Terry: www.karltonterry.com

Raymond F. Castellino: www.raycastellino.com

William Emerson: www.emersonbirthrx.com

Daniel Agustoni: www.craniosacral.ch

NOTES

Chapter 3: Craniosacral Therapy

1. Daniel Agustoni, *Craniosacral Rhythm: A Practical Guide to a Gentle Form of Bodywork Therapy* (Edinburgh: Churchill Livingstone, 2008).

2. William Garner Sutherland, *Teachings in the Science of Osteopathy* (Fort Worth, TX: Sutherland Teaching Foundation, 1991).

3. Andrew Taylor Still, *The Philosophy and Mechanical Principles of Osteopathy* (Kansas City, MO: Hudson-Kimberly, 1902), 39; William Garner Sutherland, *Teachings in the Science of Osteopathy* (Fort Worth, TX: Sutherland Teaching Foundation, 1991).

4. Daniel Agustoni, *Harmonizing Your Craniosacral System: Self-Treatments for Improving Your Health* (Forres, UK: Findhorn Press, 2008). *Harmonizing Your Craniosacral System: 17 Exercises for Relaxation and Self-Treatment,* compact disc (Forres, UK: Findhorn Press, 2008).

Chapter 4: The History of Craniosacral Treatment for Children

1. Andrew Taylor Still, *Autobiography of Andrew T. Still, with a History of the Discovery and Development of the Science of Osteopathy* (1897; repr. New York: Arno Press, 1972), 182.

2. Andrew Taylor Still, *The Philosophy and Mechanical Principles of Osteopathy* (Kansas City, MO: Hudson-Kimberly, 1902), 39.

3. William Garner Sutherland, *Contributions of Thought: The Collected Writings of W.G. Sutherland* (Portland, OR: Rudra Press, 1998); Sutherland, *Teachings in the Science of Osteopathy.*

4. Sutherland, "Bent Twigs," in *Contributions of Thought.*

5. Sutherland, *Contributions of Thought,* 216.

6. Rollin E. Becker, *Life in Motion: The Osteopathic Vision of Rollin E. Becker, DO* (Portland, OR: Rudra Press, 1997); Rollin E. Becker, *The Stillness of Life: The Osteopathic Philosophy of Rollin E. Becker, DO* (Portland, OR: Stillness Press, 2000).

7. Beryl E. Arbuckle, *The Selected Writings of Beryl E. Arbuckle* (Camp Hill, PA: National Osteopathic Institute and Cerebral Palsy Foundation, 1977).

8. Rebecca Conrow Lippincott, *A Manual of Cranial Technique* (Ann Arbor, MI: Edwards, 1948).

9. Hollis H. King, ed., *The Collected Papers of Viola M. Frymann, DO: Legacy of Osteopathy to Children* (Indianapolis: American Academy of Osteopathy, 1998).

10. Ibid.

11. Wilhelm Reich, *Character Analysis,* 3rd ed. (New York: Farrar, Straus & Giroux, 1980); Wilhelm Reich, *Children of the Future: On the Prevention of Sexual Pathology* (New York: Farrar, Straus and Giroux, 1983).

12. Otto Rank, *The Trauma of Birth* (Eastford, CT: Martino Fine Books, 2010).

13. Ronald D. Laing, *The Divided Self: A Study of Sanity and Madness* (London: Tavistock, 1960); Frank Lake, *Mutual Caring: A Manual of Depth Pastoral Care* (Lexington, KY: Emeth Press, 2009); Geoffrey Victor Whitfield, *The Prenatal Psychology of Frank Lake and the Origins of Sin and Human Dysfunction* (Lexington, KY: Emeth Press, 2007).

14. David Chamberlain, *Babies Remember Birth: And Other Extraordinary Scientific Discoveries about the Mind and the Personality of Your Newborn* (New York: Ballantine, 1989).

15. Thomas Verny, *The Secret Life of the Unborn Child: How You Can Prepare Your Unborn Baby for a Happy, Healthy Life* (New York: Dell, 1982).

16. Frédérick Leboyer, *Birth without Violence,* rev. ed. (Rochester, VT: Healing Arts Press, 2002).

17. Peter A. Levine, *In an Unspoken Voice: How the Body Releases Trauma and Restores Goodness* (Berkeley, CA: North Atlantic Books, 2010).

Chapter 6: What Is the Purpose of Craniosacral Treatment for Children?

1. Sutherland, *Teachings in the Science of Osteopathy,* 111; Sutherland, *Contributions of Thought,* 327–33.

Chapter 9: The Unfulfilled Desire to Have Children

1. Michel Odent, *The Scientification of Love,* rev. ed. (London: Free Association Books, 1999).

Chapter 10: The Pregnancy

1. Agustoni, *Craniosacral Rhythm.*

Chapter 11: The Prenatal Period: From Conception to Mature Fetus

1. Jaap van der Wal, *The Embryo in Us: A Phenomenological Search for Soul and Consciousness in the Prenatal Body,* 2012, www.portlandbranch.org/march-2012-newsletter; Julien Offray de La Mettrie, *Machine Man and*

Other Writings, ed. Anne Thomson (New York: Cambridge University Press, 1996); Julien Offray de La Mettrie, *Man a Machine; and Man a Plant,* trans. Richard A. Watson and Maya Rybalka (Indianapolis: Hackett, 1994).

2. Rupert Sheldrake, *A New Science of Life: The Hypothesis of Formative Causation* (Los Angeles: Jeffrey P. Tarcher, 1981).

Chapter 12: Bonding during Pregnancy

1. Athanassios Kafkalides *The Knowledge of the Womb: Autopsychognosia with Psychedelic Drugs* (Bloomington, IN: AuthorHouse, 2005).

2. Stanislav Grof, *Beyond the Brain: Birth, Death and Transcendence in Psychotherapy* (Albany, NY: State University of New York Press, 1985); Stanislav Grof, *The Cosmic Game: Explorations of the Frontiers of Human Consciousness* (Albany, NY: State University of New York Press, 1998).

3. Alessandra Pointelli, *Twins: From Fetus to Child* (London and New York: Routledge, 2002).

Chapter 14: How the Child Experiences Birth

1. Grof, *Beyond the Brain;* Grof, *The Cosmic Game.*

Chapter 15: Difficult Births

1. Bradycardia was once considered to indicate fetal distress, but the situation is now understood to be more complex; it can be a protective shock reaction. No hasty decision is made to perform a C-section if the fetus subsequently recovers and heart sounds continue to be normal.

2. William Emerson, "Birth and Life: The Hazy Mirrors," *European Journal of Humanistic Psychology* 6 (1978): 17–23; William Emerson, *Infant and Child Birth Refacilitation* (Guildford, UK: University of Surrey Press, 1984).

Chapter 17: Bonding after Birth and during Child Development

1. Versions have been recorded by Van Morrison, Richie Havens, The Young Gods, Eric Burdon, Tom Jones, and others.

Chapter 18: Anatomy, Neuroanatomy, and Neurophysiology for Craniosacral Work

1. King, *Collected Papers of Viola M. Frymann.*

2. Sutherland, *Teachings in the Science of Osteopathy;* Sutherland, *Contributions of Thought.*

3. Agustoni, *Craniosacral Rhythm.*

4. Torsten Liem, *Cranial Osteopathy: Principles and Practice* (Edinburgh: Churchill Livingstone, 2004); Torsten Liem, *Cranial Osteopathy: A Practical Textbook* (Seattle: Eastland Press, 2009).

5. Candace Pert, *Molecules of Emotion: The Science behind Mind-Body Medicine* (New York: Simon & Schuster, 1999).

6. Kerstin Uvnäs Moberg, *The Oxytocin Factor: Tapping the Hormone of Calm, Love, and Healing* (Cambridge, MA: Da Capo Press, 2003).

7. Sue C. Carter, *The Integrative Neurobiology of Affiliation* (New York: New York Academy of Sciences, 1996).

8. Stephen W. Porges, *The Polyvagal Theory: Neurophysiological Foundations of Emotions, Attachment, Communication, and Self-Regulation* (New York: W. W. Norton, 2011).

Chapter 19: Treatment of Mother and Child after Birth

1. Murray Enkin, Marc J. N. C. Keirse, James Neilson, Caroline Crowther, Leila Duley, Ellen Hodnett, and Justus Hofmeyr, *A Guide to Effective Care in Pregnancy and Childbirth,* 3rd ed. (Oxford, UK: Oxford University Press, 2000).

Chapter 20: Further Considerations during the Child's Development

1. Gerald Hüther and Helmuth Bonney, *Neues vom Zappelphilipp: ADS verstehen, vorbeugen und behandeln* (Mannheim, Germany: Patmos, 2010).

2. Donna McCann, Angelina Barrett, Alison Cooper, Debbie Crumpler, Lindy Dalen, Kate Grimshaw, Elizabeth Kitchin, et al., "Food Additives and Hyperactive Behaviour in 3-year-old and 8/9-year-old Children in the Community: A Randomised, Double-Blinded, Placebo-Controlled Trial," *The Lancet* 370:9598 (November 2007), 1560–67. See also Marvin Boris and Francine S. Mandel, "Foods and Additives Are Common Causes of the Attention Deficit Hyperactive Disorder in Children," *Annals of Allergy* 73:5 (May 1994), 462–68.

3. Swiss Agency for Therapeutic Products (Swissmedic), personal communication with the author.

4. "Hyperaktive Kinder im Pillenrausch," *Der Spiegel,* May 25, 2007.

5. Lisa Nienhaus, "Ritalin Die Karriere einer Pille," *Frankfurter Allgemeine Zeitung* (Frankfurt), October 2, 2007.

6. Heiner Frei, Regula Everts, Klaus von Ammon, Franz Kaufmann, Daniel Walther, Shu-fang Hsu-Schmitz, Marco Collenberg, et al., "Homeopathic

Treatment of Children with Attention Deficit Hyperactivity Disorder: A Randomised, Double Blind, Placebo Controlled Crossover Trial," *European Journal of Pediatrics* 164:12 (December 2005), 758–67. See also Heiner Frei, Klaus von Ammon, and André Thurneysen, "Treatment of Hyperactive Children: Increased Efficiency Through Modifications of Homeopathic Diagnostic Procedure," *Homeopathy* 95:3 (2006), 163–70; Heiner Frei, Regula Everts, Klaus von Ammon, Franz Kaufmann, Daniel Walther, Shu-fang Hsu-Schmitz, Marco Collenberg, et al., "Randomised Controlled Trials of Homeopathy in Hyperactive Children: Treatment Procedure Leads to an Unconventional Study Design. Experience with Open-label Homeopathic Treatment Preceding the Swiss ADHD Placebo Controlled, Randomised, Double-Blind, Cross-Over Trial," *Homeopathy* 96:1 (2007), 35–41.

7. King, *Collected Papers of Viola M. Frymann.*

8. Joseph Egger, C. M. Carter, J. Wilson, M. W. Turner, and John F. Soothill, "Is Migraine Food Allergy? A Double-blind Controlled Trial of Oligoantigenic Diet Treatment," *The Lancet* 2:8355 (1983), 865–69; Joseph Egger, C. M. Carter, P. J. Graham, D. Gumley, and John F. Soothill, "A Controlled Trial Oligoantigenic Diet Treatment in the Hyperkinetic Syndrome," *The Lancet* 1:8428 (1985), 940–45; Joseph Egger, Adelheid Stolla, and Leonard M. McEwen, "Controlled Trial of Hyposensitisation in Children with Food-induced Hyperkinetic Syndrome," *The Lancet* 339:8802 (1992), 1150–53; Joseph Egger, "Möglichkeiten von Diätbehandlungen bei hyperkinetischen Störungen," in *Hyperkinetische Störungen bei Kindern, Jugendlichen und Erwachsenen,* 2nd ed., ed. Hans-Christoph Steinhausen (Stuttgart, Germany: W. Kohlhammer, 2000).

9. Emmy E. Werner and Ruth S. Smith, *Journeys from Childhood to Midlife: Risk, Resilience, and Recovery* (Ithaca, NY: Cornell University Press, 2001); Emmy E. Werner and Ruth S. Smith, *Overcoming the Odds: High Risk Children from Birth to Adulthood* (Ithaca, NY: Cornell University Press, 1992); Emmy E. Werner and Ruth S. Smith, *Kauai's Children Come of Age* (Honolulu: University of Hawaii Press, 1977).

Chapter 21: The Miracle of Self-Healing

1. Alfred Pischinger, *The Extracellular Matrix and Ground Regulation: Basis for a Holistic Biological Medicine* (Berkeley, CA: North Atlantic Books, 2007).

2. James L. Oschman, *Energy Medicine: The Scientific Basis* (Edinburgh: Churchill Livingstone, 2000); Kenneth J. Pienta and Donald S. Coffey, "Cellular Harmonic Information Transfer through a Tissue Tensegrity-Matrix System," *Medical Hypotheses* 34:1 (January 1991), 88–95.

3. Aaron Antonovsky, *Health, Stress and Coping* (San Francisco: Jossey-Bass, 1979).

4. Porges, *Polyvagal Theory.*

5. Michael D. Gershon, *The Second Brain: A Groundbreaking New Understanding of Nervous Disorders of the Stomach and Intestine* (New York: HarperCollins, 1998).

6. Giacomo Rizzolatti and Corrado Sinigaglia, *Mirrors in the Brain: How Our Minds Share Actions and Emotions* (Oxford, UK: Oxford University Press, 2008).

7. Antonio Damasio, *The Feeling of What Happens: Body and Emotion in the Making of Consciousness* (New York: Houghton Mifflin Harcourt, 1999).

8. Michael J. Meaney, "Nature, Nurture, and the Disunity of Knowledge," *Annals of the New York Academy of Sciences* 935 (May 2001): 50–61; Bruce H. Lipton, *The Biology of Belief: Unleashing the Power of Consciousness, Matter and Miracles* (Santa Rosa, CA: Mountain of Love, 2005); Bruce H. Lipton, *An Introduction to Spontaneous Evolution,* DVD (Carlsbad, CA: Hay House, 2012); Bruce H. Lipton and Steve Bhaerman, *Spontaneous Evolution: Our Positive Future (and a Way to Get There from Here)* (Carlsbad, CA: Hay House, 2009).

9. See also Sharon Begley, *Train Your Mind, Change Your Brain: How a New Science Reveals Our Extraordinary Potential to Transform Ourselves* (New York: Ballantine Books, 2007).

Chapter 22: Principles of Noninvasive Craniosacral Therapy for Children

1. Agustoni, *Craniosacral Rhythm.*

2. Will Davis, "An Introduction to the Instroke," in *The Radix Reader,* eds. Linda Glenn and Rudolf Müller-Schwefe (Albuquerque: Radix Institute, 1999).

3. Sutherland, *Teachings in the Science of Osteopathy,* 14.

4. See Levine, *In an Unspoken Voice;* and Peter A. Levine and Maggie Kline, *Trauma through a Child's Eyes: Awakening the Ordinary Miracle of Healing* (Berkeley, CA: North Atlantic Books, 2006).

5. See Richard Bandler and John Grinder, *Patterns of the Hypnotic Tech-

niques of Milton H. Erickson, MD, vol. 1 (Capitola, CA: Meta Publications, 1975); Richard Bandler and John Grinder, *The Structure of Magic, Vol. 1: A Book About Language and Therapy* (Palo Alto, CA: Science and Behavior Books, 1975).

6. See Hal Stone and Sidra Winkelman, *Embracing Our Selves: Voice Dialogue Manual* (Los Angeles: De Vorss, 1985).

7. Still, *Philosophy and Mechanical Principles of Osteopathy.*

Chapter 23: General and Craniosacral-Specific Assessment

1. Gerda Boyesen, "The Primary Personality," *Journal of Biodynamic Psychology* 3 (1982).

Chapter 24: Differing Treatment Approaches and Different Rhythms as Expression of the Breath of Life

1. Sutherland, *Teachings in the Science of Osteopathy.*

2. Charles Ridley, *Stillness: Biodynamic Cranial Practice and the Evolution of Consciousness* (Berkeley, CA: North Atlantic Books, 2006); Michael J. Shea, *Biodynamic Craniosacral Therapy,* vol. 1 (Berkeley, CA: North Atlantic Books, 2007); Michael J. Shea, *Biodynamic Craniosacral Therapy,* vol. 2 (Berkeley, CA: North Atlantic Books, 2008); James Jealous, *The Biodynamics of Osteopathy: An Introductory Overview,* compact disc (Apollo Beach, FL: Marnee Jealous Long, 2001).

Chapter 25: Approaches to Release Following Shock and Trauma

1. Reich, *Character Analysis.*

2. Gerda Boyesen, *Entre psyché et soma: introduction à la psychologie biodynamique* (Paris: Payot, 1985).

3. Levine, *In an Unspoken Voice.*

4. Levine and Kline, *Trauma through a Child's Eyes.*

5. Patch Adams, *Gesundheit!: Bringing Good Health to You, the Medical System, and Society through Physician Service, Complementary Therapies, Humor, and Joy* (Rochester, VT: Healing Arts Press, 1993).

6. Norman Cousins, *Anatomy of an Illness as Perceived by the Patient: Reflections on Healing and Regeneration* (New York: Norton, 1979).

Chapter 26: Basic Principles and Practice Tips

1. Agustoni, *Craniosacral Rhythm.*

Chapter 28: For Fully Qualified Craniosacral Practitioners

1. Becker, *Life in Motion*, 182–83.

2. Liem, *Cranial Osteopathy: Principles and Practice;* Liem, *Cranial Osteopathy: A Practical Textbook.*

3. Raymond F. Castellino, http://www.raycastellino.com;William Emerson, http://emersonbirthrx.com/.

BIBLIOGRAPHY

Adams, Patch. *Gesundheit!: Bringing Good Health to You, the Medical System, and Society through Physician Service, Complementary Therapies, Humor, and Joy.* Rochester, VT: Healing Arts Press, 1993.

Agustoni, Daniel. *Craniosacral Rhythm: A Practical Guide to a Gentle Form of Bodywork Therapy.* Edinburgh: Churchill Livingstone, 2008.

———. *Harmonizing Your Craniosacral System: Self-Treatments for Improving Your Health.* Berkeley, CA: North Atlantic Books, 2011.

———. *Harmonizing Your Craniosacral System: 17 Exercises for Relaxation and Self-Treatment.* Compact disc. Forres, UK: Findhorn Press, 2008.

Almaas, A. H. *The Inner Journey Home: Soul's Realization of the Unity of Reality.* Boston: Shambhala, 2004.

———. *The Unfolding Now: Realizing Your True Nature through the Practice of Presence.* Boston: Shambhala, 2008.

Antonovsky, Aaron. *Health, Stress and Coping.* San Francisco: Jossey-Bass, 1979.

Arbuckle, Beryl E. *The Selected Writings of Beryl E. Arbuckle.* Camp Hill, PA: National Osteopathic Institute and Cerebral Palsy Foundation, 1977.

Arnold, Anthony P. *Rhythm and Touch: The Fundamentals of Craniosacral Therapy.* Berkeley, CA: North Atlantic Books, 2009.

Bandler, Richard, and John Grinder. *Patterns of the Hypnotic Techniques of Milton H. Erickson, MD.* Vol. 1. Capitola, CA: Meta Publications, 1975.

———. *The Structure of Magic, Vol. 1: A Book About Language and Therapy.* Palo Alto, CA: Science and Behavior Books, 1975.

Barral, Jean-Pierre. *Manual Thermal Evaluation.* Seattle: Eastland Press, 2005.

Barral, Jean-Pierre, and Alain Croibier. *Manual Therapy for the Cranial Nerves.* Edinburgh: Churchill Livingstone, 2008.

Barral, Jean-Pierre, and Pierre Mercier. *Visceral Manipulation.* Seattle: Eastland Press, 1988.

Becker, Rollin E. *Life in Motion: The Osteopathic Vision of Rollin E. Becker, DO.* Portland, OR: Rudra Press, 1997.

———. *The Stillness of Life: The Osteopathic Philosophy of Rollin E. Becker, DO.* Portland, OR: Stillness Press, 2000.

Begley, Sharon. *Train Your Mind, Change Your Brain: How a New Science Reveals Our Extraordinary Potential to Transform Ourselves.* New York: Ballantine Books, 2007.

Blechschmidt, Erich. *The Ontogenetic Basis of Human Anatomy: A Biodynamic Approach to Development from Conception to Birth*. Berkeley, CA: North Atlantic Books, 2004.

Boris, Marvin, and Francine S. Mandel. "Foods and Additives Are Common Causes of the Attention Deficit Hyperactive Disorder in Children." *Annals of Allergy* 73:5 (May 1994), 462–68.

Boyesen, Gerda. *Entre psyché et soma: introduction à la psychologie biodynamique*. Paris: Payot, 1985.

———. "The Primary Personality." *Journal of Biodynamic Psychology* 3 (1982).

Calais-Germain, Blandine. *Anatomy of Movement*. Rev. ed. Seattle: Eastland Press, 2007.

Carlson, Richard, and Benjamin Shield, eds. *Handbook for the Heart: Original Writings on Love*. New York: Little, Brown, 1996.

———, eds. *Handbook for the Soul*. New York: Back Bay Books, 1995.

———, eds. *Healers on Healing*. New York: Jeremy P. Tarcher/Putnam, 1989.

Carreiro, Jane E. *An Osteopathic Approach to Children*. Edinburgh: Churchill Livingstone, 2003.

———. *Pediatric Manual Medicine: An Osteopathic Approach*. Edinburgh: Churchill Livingstone, 2009.

Carter, Sue C. *The Integrative Neurobiology of Affiliation*. New York: New York Academy of Sciences, 1996.

Chaitow, Leon. *Cranial Manipulation: Theory and Practice*. Edinburgh: Churchill Livingstone, 2005.

———. *Palpation and Assessment Skills: Assessment and Diagnosis through Touch*. Edinburgh: Churchill Livingstone, 2003.

Chamberlain, David. *Babies Remember Birth: And Other Extraordinary Scientific Discoveries about the Mind and the Personality of Your Newborn*. New York: Ballantine, 1989.

———. *The Mind of Your Newborn Baby*. Berkeley, CA: North Atlantic Books, 1998.

Cousins, Norman. *Anatomy of an Illness as Perceived by the Patient: Reflections on Healing and Regeneration*. New York: Norton, 1979.

Damasio, Antonio. *Descartes' Error: Emotion, Reason, and the Human Brain*. New York: G. P. Putnam, 1994.

———. *The Feeling of What Happens: Body and Emotion in the Making of Consciousness*. New York: Houghton Mifflin Harcourt, 1999.

Davis, Will. "An Introduction to the Instroke." In *The Radix Reader*, edited by Linda Glenn and Rudolf Müller-Schwefe. Albuquerque: Radix Institute, 1999.

Dispenza, Joe. *Evolve Your Brain: The Science of Changing Your Mind.* Deerfield Beach, FL: Health Communications, 2007.

Egger, Joseph, "Möglichkeiten von Diätbehandlungen bei hyperkinetischen Störungen." In *Hyperkinetische Störungen bei Kindern, Jugendlichen und Erwachsenen,* 2nd edition, edited by Hans-Christoph Steinhausen. Stuttgart, Germany: W. Kohlhammer, 2000.

Egger, Joseph, C. M. Carter, P. J. Graham, D. Gumley, and John F. Soothill. "A Controlled Trial Oligoantigenic Diet Treatment in the Hyperkinetic Syndrome." *The Lancet* 1:8428 (1985), 940–45.

Egger, Joseph, Adelheid Stolla, and Leonard M. McEwen. "Controlled Trial of Hyposensitisation in Children with Food-induced Hyperkinetic Syndrome." *The Lancet* 339:8802 (1992), 1150–53.

Egger, Joseph, C. M. Carter, J. Wilson, M. W. Turner, and John F. Soothill. "Is Migraine Food Allergy? A Double-blind Controlled Trial of Oligoantigenic Diet Treatment." *The Lancet* 2:8355 (1983), 865–69.

Emerson, William. "Birth and Life: The Hazy Mirrors." *European Journal of Humanistic Psychology* 6 (1978): 17–23.

———. *Infant and Child Birth Refacilitation.* Guildford, UK: University of Surrey Press, 1984.

Enkin, Murray, Marc J. N. C. Keirse, James Neilson, Caroline Crowther, Leila Duley, Ellen Hodnett, and Justus Hofmeyr. *A Guide to Effective Care in Pregnancy and Childbirth.* 3rd ed. Oxford, UK: Oxford University Press, 2000.

Frei, Heiner, Regula Everts, Klaus von Ammon, Franz Kaufmann, Daniel Walther, Shu-fang Hsu-Schmitz, Marco Collenberg, et al. "Homeopathic Treatment of Children with Attention Deficit Hyperactivity Disorder: A Randomised, Double Blind, Placebo Controlled Crossover Trial." *European Journal of Pediatrics* 164:12 (December 2005), 758–67.

Frei, Heiner, Regula Everts, Klaus von Ammon, Franz Kaufmann, Daniel Walther, Shu-fang Hsu-Schmitz, Marco Collenberg, et al. "Randomised Controlled Trials of Homeopathy in Hyperactive Children: Treatment Procedure Leads to an Unconventional Study Design. Experience with Open-label Homeopathic Treatment Preceding the Swiss ADHD Placebo Controlled, Randomised, Double-Blind, Cross-Over Trial." *Homeopathy* 96:1 (2007), 35–41.

Frei, Heiner, Klaus von Ammon, and André Thurneysen. "Treatment of Hyper-
    active Children: Increased Efficiency Through Modifications of Homeo-
    pathic Diagnostic Procedure." *Homeopathy* 95:3 (2006), 163–70.

Gershon, Michael D. *The Second Brain: A Groundbreaking New Understand-
    ing of Nervous Disorders of the Stomach and Intestine*. New York: Harp-
    erCollins, 1998.

Grey, Alex. *Sacred Mirrors: The Visionary Art of Alex Grey*. Rochester, VT:
    Inner Traditions, 1990.

Grof, Stanislav. *Beyond the Brain: Birth, Death and Transcendence in Psycho-
    therapy*. Albany, NY: State University of New York Press, 1985.

———.*The Cosmic Game: Explorations of the Frontiers of Human Conscious-
    ness*. Albany, NY: State University of New York Press, 1998.

Grossinger, Richard. *Embryos, Galaxies, and Sentient Beings: How the Uni-
    verse Makes Life*. Berkeley, CA: North Atlantic Books, 2003.

Handoll, Nicholas. *Anatomy of Potency*. Portland, OR: Stillness Press, 2000.

Heller, Laurence, and Aline Lapierre. *Healing Developmental Trauma: How
    Early Trauma Affects Self-Regulation, Self-Image, and the Capacity for
    Relationship*. Berkeley, CA: North Atlantic Books, 2012.

Hüther, Gerald, and Helmuth Bonney. *Neues vom Zappelphilipp: ADS ver-
    stehen, vorbeugen und behandeln*. Mannheim, Germany: Patmos, 2010.

Jealous, James. *The Biodynamics of Osteopathy: An Introductory Overview*.
    Compact disc. Apollo Beach, FL: Marnee Jealous Long, 2001.

Jung, Carl G. *Synchronicity: An Acausal Connecting Principle*. Translated by
    R. F. C. Hull. Princeton, NJ: Princeton University Press, 1973.

Kafkalides, Athanassios. *The Knowledge of the Womb: Autopsychognosia with
    Psychedelic Drugs*. Bloomington, IN: AuthorHouse, 2005.

Kern, Michael. *Wisdom in the Body: The Craniosacral Approach to Essential
    Health*. Berkeley, CA: North Atlantic Books, 2005.

King, Hollis H., ed. *The Collected Papers of Viola M. Frymann, DO: Legacy of
    Osteopathy to Children*. Indianapolis: American Academy of Osteopathy,
    1998.

Laing, Ronald D. *The Divided Self: A Study of Sanity and Madness*. London:
    Tavistock, 1960.

Lake, Frank. *Mutual Caring: A Manual of Depth Pastoral Care*. Lexington,
    KY: Emeth Press, 2009.

La Mettrie, Julien Offray de. *Machine Man and Other Writings*. Edited by
    Anne Thomson. New York: Cambridge University Press, 1996.

———. *Man a Machine; and Man a Plant*. Translated by Richard A. Watson and Maya Rybalka. Indianapolis: Hackett, 1994.

Leboyer, Frédérick. *Birth without Violence*. Rev. ed. Rochester, VT: Healing Arts Press, 2002.

Leo, Pam. *Connection Parenting: Parenting through Connection Instead of Coercion, through Love Instead of Fear*. Deadwood, OR: Wyatt-MacKenzie, 2007.

Levine, Peter A. *In an Unspoken Voice: How the Body Releases Trauma and Restores Goodness*. Berkeley, CA: North Atlantic Books, 2010.

Levine, Peter A., and Maggie Kline. *Trauma through a Child's Eyes: Awakening the Ordinary Miracle of Healing*. Berkeley, CA: North Atlantic Books, 2006.

Liem, Torsten. *Cranial Osteopathy: A Practical Textbook*. Seattle: Eastland Press, 2009.

———. *Cranial Osteopathy: Principles and Practice*. Edinburgh: Churchill Livingstone, 2004.

Lippincott, Rebecca Conrow. *A Manual of Cranial Technique*. Ann Arbor, MI: Edwards, 1948.

Lipton, Bruce H. *The Biology of Belief: Unleashing the Power of Consciousness, Matter and Miracles*. Santa Rosa, CA: Mountain of Love, 2005.

———. *An Introduction to Spontaneous Evolution*. DVD. Carlsbad, CA: Hay House, 2012.

Lipton, Bruce H., and Steve Bhaerman. *Spontaneous Evolution: Our Positive Future (and a Way to Get There from Here)*. Carlsbad, CA: Hay House, 2009.

Magoun, Harold Ives, ed. *Osteopathy in the Cranial Field*. Kirksville, MO: Journal Printing Company, 1976.

McCann, Donna, Angelina Barrett, Alison Cooper, Debbie Crumpler, Lindy Dalen, Kate Grimshaw, Elizabeth Kitchin, et al. "Food Additives and Hyperactive Behaviour in 3-year-old and 8/9-year-old Children in the Community: A Randomised, Double-Blinded, Placebo-controlled Trial." *The Lancet* 370:9598 (November 2007), 1560–67.

Meaney, Michael J. "Nature, Nurture, and the Disunity of Knowledge." *Annals of the New York Academy of Sciences* 935 (May 2001): 50–61.

Milne, Hugh. *The Heart of Listening: A Visionary Approach to Craniosacral Work*. Vols. 1 and 2. Berkeley, CA: North Atlantic Books, 1998.

Mindell, Arnold. *The Quantum Mind and Healing: How to Listen and*

Respond to Your Body's Symptoms. Charlottesville, VA: Hampton Roads, 2004.

Odent, Michel. *The Scientification of Love.* Rev. ed. London: Free Association Books, 1999.

Oschman, James L. *Energy Medicine: The Scientific Basis.* Edinburgh: Churchill Livingstone, 2000.

———. *Energy Medicine in Therapeutics and Human Performance.* London: Butterworth-Heinemann, 2003.

Pert, Candace. *Molecules of Emotion: The Science behind Mind-Body Medicine.* New York: Simon & Schuster, 1999.

Pienta, Kenneth J., and Donald S. Coffey. "Cellular Harmonic Information Transfer through a Tissue Tensegrity-Matrix System." *Medical Hypotheses* 34:1 (January 1991), 88–95.

Pischinger, Alfred. *The Extracellular Matrix and Ground Regulation: Basis for a Holistic Biological Medicine.* Berkeley, CA: North Atlantic Books, 2007.

Pointelli, Alessandra. *Twins: From Fetus to Child.* London and New York: Routledge, 2002.

Porges, Stephen W. *The Polyvagal Theory: Neurophysiological Foundations of Emotions, Attachment, Communication, and Self-Regulation.* New York: W. W. Norton, 2011.

Rank, Otto. *The Trauma of Birth.* Eastford, CT: Martino Fine Books, 2010.

Reich, Wilhelm. *Character Analysis.* 3rd ed. New York: Farrar, Straus & Giroux, 1980.

———. *Children of the Future: On the Prevention of Sexual Pathology.* New York: Farrar, Straus and Giroux, 1983.

Ridley, Charles. *Stillness: Biodynamic Cranial Practice and the Evolution of Consciousness.* Berkeley, CA: North Atlantic Books, 2006.

Rizzolatti, Giacomo, and Corrado Sinigaglia. *Mirrors in the Brain: How Our Minds Share Actions and Emotions.* Oxford, UK: Oxford University Press, 2008.

Rohen, Johannes W. *Functional Morphology: The Dynamic Wholeness of the Human Organism.* Hillsdale, NY: Adonis Press, 2007.

Rothschild, Babette. *The Body Remembers: The Psychophysiology of Trauma and Trauma Treatment.* New York: W. W. Norton, 2000.

Shea, Michael J. *Biodynamic Craniosacral Therapy.* Vol. 1. Berkeley, CA: North Atlantic Books, 2007.

———. *Biodynamic Craniosacral Therapy.* Vol. 2. Berkeley, CA: North Atlantic Books, 2008.

Sheldrake, Rupert. *A New Science of Life: The Hypothesis of Formative Causation.* Los Angeles: Jeffrey P. Tarcher, 1981.

Sills, Franklyn. *Foundations in Craniosacral Biodynamics: The Breath of Life and Fundamental Skills.* Vol. 1. Berkeley, CA: North Atlantic Books, 2011.

Still, Andrew Taylor. *Autobiography of Andrew T. Still, with a History of the Discovery and Development of the Science of Osteopathy.* 1897. Reprinted New York: Arno Press, 1972.

———. *The Philosophy and Mechanical Principles of Osteopathy.* Kansas City, MO: Hudson-Kimberly, 1902.

Stone, Hal, and Sidra Winkelman. *Embracing Our Selves: Voice Dialogue Manual.* Los Angeles: De Vorss, 1985.

Sutherland, William Garner. *Teachings in the Science of Osteopathy.* Fort Worth, TX: Sutherland Teaching Foundation, 1991.

Sutherland, William Garner. *Contributions of Thought: The Collected Writings of W. G. Sutherland.* Portland, OR: Rudra Press, 1998.

Terry, Karlton. "Observations in Treatment of Children Conceived by In Vitro Fertilization." In *Pränatale Psychologie und Psychotherapie,* edited by Ludwig Janus. Heidelberg, Germany: Mattes, 2004.

Upledger, John. E. *A Brain Is Born: Exploring the Birth and Development of the Central Nervous System.* Berkeley, CA: North Atlantic Books, 2010.

———. *Cell Talk: Transmitting Mind into DNA.* Berkeley, CA: North Atlantic Books, 2010.

———. *Craniosacral Therapy II: Beyond the Dura.* Seattle: Eastland Press, 1987.

———. *SomatoEmotional Release: Deciphering the Language of Life.* Berkeley, CA: North Atlantic Books, 2002.

Upledger, John. E., and Jon D. Vredevoogd. *Craniosacral Therapy.* Seattle: Eastland Press, 1983.

Uvnäs Moberg, Kerstin. *The Oxytocin Factor: Tapping the Hormone of Calm, Love, and Healing.* Cambridge, MA: Da Capo Press, 2003.

Van der Wal, Jaap. *The Embryo in Us: A Phenomenological Search for Soul and Consciousness in the Prenatal Body.* 2012. www.portlandbranch.org/march-2012-newsletter.

Verny, Thomas. *The Secret Life of the Unborn Child: How You Can Prepare Your Unborn Baby for a Happy, Healthy Life.* New York: Dell, 1982.

Werner, Emmy E., and Ruth S. Smith. *Journeys from Childhood to Midlife: Risk, Resilience, and Recovery.* Ithaca, NY: Cornell University Press, 2001.

———. *Kauai's Children Come of Age.* Honolulu: University of Hawaii Press, 1977.

———. *Overcoming the Odds: High Risk Children from Birth to Adulthood.* Ithaca, NY: Cornell University Press, 1992.

Whitfield, Geoffrey Victor. *The Prenatal Psychology of Frank Lake and the Origins of Sin and Human Dysfunction.* Lexington, KY: Emeth Press, 2007.

INDEX

ABOUT THE AUTHOR

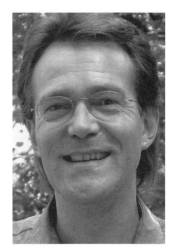

The founder and director of the Sphinx Craniosacral Institute in Basel, Switzerland, DANIEL AGUSTONI has been practicing Craniosacral Therapy for over twenty years. In addition to Craniosacral Therapy, Agustoni has trained in classical and biodynamic massage, Myofacial Release, conscious breathing, systemic family constellation, Gestalt therapy, Somatic Experiencing®, and treatment methods in the field of alternative medicine. With his extensive experience and education, Agustoni has developed his own approach, called Craniosacral_Flow®, which has been designed to balance the different systems of the body and stimulate self-healing. He is the author of *Harmonizing Your Craniosacral System: Self-Treatments for Improving Your Health; Craniosacral Rhythm: A Practical Guide to a Gentle Form of Bodywork Therapy;* and the audio CD *Harmonizing Your Craniosacral System: 17 Exercises for Relaxation and Self-Treatment.* His books have been published in six languages.

You can contact Daniel Agustoni at:

SPHINX CRANIOSACRAL INSTITUTE
P.O. Box/Postfach 629
CH-4003 Basel
Switzerland
email: sphinx@craniosacral.ch
website: www.craniosacral.ch